KU-825-728

ROYAL GLAMORGAN HOSPITAL
LIBRARY

DISPOSED OF FROM
CWM TAF LIBRARY
SERVICES 2024
NEWER INFORMATION
MAYBE AVAILABLE

E13880

ESSENTIALS IN OPHTHALMOLOGY: **Glaucoma.** F. Grehn · R. Stamper (Eds.)

ESSENTIALS IN OPHTHALMOLOGY

G. K. Krieglstein · R. N. Weinreb
Series Editors

Glaucoma

Cataract and Refractive Surgery

Uveitis and Immunological Disorders

Vitreo-retinal Surgery

Medical Retina

Oculoplastics and Orbit

Paediatric Ophthalmology,
Neuro-ophthalmology, Genetics

Cornea and External Eye Disease

Springer

Berlin
Heidelberg
New York
Hong Kong
London
Milan
Paris
Tokyo

Editors   Franz Grehn
Robert Stamper

Glaucoma

With 74 Figures, Mostly in Colour,
and 19 Tables

DISPOSED OF FROM
CWM TAF LIBRARY
SERVICES 2024
NEWER INFORMATION
MAYBE AVAILABLE

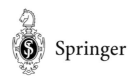

Springer

Series Editors

GÜNTHER K. KRIEGLSTEIN, MD
Professor and Chairman
Department of Ophthalmology
University of Cologne
Joseph-Stelzmann-Straße 9
D-50931 Cologne
Germany

ROBERT N. WEINREB, MD
Professor and Director
Hamilton Glaucoma Center
Department of Ophthalmology – 0946
University of California at San Diego
9500 Gilman Drive
La Jolla, CA 92093-0946
USA

Volume Editors

FRANZ GREHN, MD
Professor and Chairman
Department of Ophthalmology
University of Wuerzburg
Josef-Schneider-Straße 11
D-97080 Würzburg
Germany

ROBERT STAMPER, MD
Director of Glaucoma Service
Department of Ophthalmology
UCSF
10 Kirkham Street, Rm K301
San Francisco, CA 94143
USA

ISBN 3-540-40608-5
Springer Verlag Berlin Heidelberg New York

ISSN 1612-3212

Library of Congress Cataloging-in-Publication Data
Glaucoma / Franz Grehn, Robert Stamper (eds).
p. ; cm. – (Essentials in ophthalmology,
ISSN 1612-3212)
Includes bibliographical references and index.
ISBN 3-540-40608-5 (alk. paper)
1. Glaucoma. I. Grehn, Franz. II. Stamper, Robert L.,
1939- III. Series.
[DNLM: 1. Glaucoma. WW 290 G54928 2004]
RE871.G5432 2004   617.7'41–dc22   2004042952

This work is subject to copyright. All rights are
reserved, whether the whole or part of the material is
concerned, specifically the rights of translation,
reprinting, reuse of illustrations, recitation, broad-
casting, reproduction on microfilm or in any other
way, and storage in data banks. Duplication of this
publication or parts thereof is permitted only under
the provisions of the German Copyright Law of Sep-
tember 9, 1965, in its current version, and permission
for use must always be obtained from Springer-Verlag. Violations are liable for prosecution under the
German Copyright Law.

Springer-Verlag is a part of
Springer Science + Business Media

springeronline.com

© Springer-Verlag Berlin Heidelberg 2004
Printed in Germany

Cover picture "Cataract and Refractive Surgery" from
Kampik A, Grehn F (eds) Augenärztliche Therapie.
Georg Thieme Verlag Stuttgart, with permission.

The use of general descriptive names, registered
names, trademarks, etc. in this publication does not
imply, even in the absence of a specific statement, that
such names are exempt from the relevant protective
laws and regulations and therefore free for general use.

Product liability: The publishers cannot guarantee
the accuracy of any information about dosage and
application contained in this book. In every individual case the user must check such information by
consulting the relevant literature.

Editor: Marion Philipp, Heidelberg
Desk editor: Martina Himberger, Heidelberg
Production editor: Ute Pfaff, Heidelberg
Cover design: Erich Kirchner, Heidelberg
Typesetting and reproduction of the figures:
AM-productions GmbH, Wiesloch
Printing and binding: Mercedes-Druck, Berlin

Printed on acid-free paper
24/3150PF   5 4 3 2 1 0

Foreword

Essentials in Ophthalmology is a new review series covering all of ophthalmology categorized in eight subspecialties. It will be published quarterly; thus each subspecialty will be reviewed biannually.

Given the multiplicity of medical publications already available, why is a new series needed? Consider that the half-life of medical knowledge is estimated to be around 5 years. Moreover, it can be as long as 8 years between the description of a medical innovation in a peer-reviewed scientific journal and publication in a medical textbook. A series that narrows this time span between journal and textbook would provide a more rapid and efficient transfer of medical knowledge into clinical practice, and enhance care of our patients.

For the series, each subspecialty volume comprises 10 chapters selected by two distinguished editors and written by internationally renowned specialists. The selection of these contributions is based more on recent and note-worthy advances in the subspecialty than on systematic completeness. Each article is structured in a standardized format and length, with citations for additional reading and an appropriate number of illustrations to enhance important points. Since every subspecialty volume is issued in a recurring sequence during the 2-year cycle, the reader has the opportunity to focus on the progress in a particular subspecialty or to be updated on the whole field. The clinical relevance of all material presented will be well established, so application to clinical practice can be made with confidence.

This new series will earn space on the bookshelves of those ophthalmologists who seek to maintain the timeliness and relevance of their clinical practice.

G. K. Krieglstein
R. N. Weinreb
Series Editors

Preface

This first volume in the series *Essentials in Ophthalmology* seeks to bring the ophthalmic practitioner up to date on the important new advances or changes in glaucoma diagnosis and management occurring in the last 10 years. The last decade has seen significant changes in our understanding of the pathophysiology of some glaucomas, in our diagnostic approaches and in our management. Toward the goal of providing the most up-to-date information in a readable fashion, we have asked some of the world's experts to discuss areas to which they have contributed in a way that will be useful for the practicing doctor. For example, we have begun to chip away at the genetic secrets of glaucoma; Professor Tamm discusses this complicated and exciting field. Our comprehension of angle closure glaucoma has also changed markedly. Ten years ago, angle closure was simple with only a few mechanisms identified. The ultrasound biomicroscope has radically changed our understanding of this disease and added several previously unknown mechanisms to this common and often frustrating condition. Tello et al. give us the latest information on angle closure with beautifully illustrated ultrasound images that clearly show the mechanisms involved. Schlötzer-Schrehardt describes the latest findings in exfoliative glaucoma. Ritch updates our understanding of pigmentary glaucoma. New diagnostic devices that image the optic nerve and help detect change have appeared; Zangwill and coworkers help us to understand what works and what doesn't in this rapidly evolving field. It wasn't too long ago that the treatment basis of glaucoma was questioned. Brandt and Wilson review the several large studies that have outlined the modern treatment of open angle glaucoma. Discussions of the pathophysiology of some of the secondary glaucomas are also included. New surgical approaches are dissected and evaluated. Many of the mechanisms discussed and illustrated in this volume have not appeared in textbook format before. We hope that the topics and authors that we have selected are helpful in improving the understanding of the many faces of glaucoma and, ultimately, will contribute to reduced visual loss and better care for our patients.

FRANZ GREHN
ROBERT L. STAMPER

Contents

Chapter 7
Childhood Glaucoma and Amblyopia
Karim F. Tomey

Chapter 8
What Have We Learned
from the Major Glaucoma Clinical Trials?
J.D. Brandt, M.R. Wilson

Chapter 9
The Concept of Target IOP at Various Stages
of Glaucoma
C. Migdal

Chapter 10
A Practical Approach to the Management
of Normal Tension Glaucoma
R. A. Hitchings

Chapter 11
Pseudoexfoliation Glaucoma
Ursula Schlötzer-Schrehardt,
Gottfried O.H. Naumann

CHAPTER 13

Wound Modulation in Glaucoma Surgery
HOLGER MIETZ

CHAPTER 12

Pigment Dispersion Syndrome – Update 2003
ROBERT RITCH

CHAPTER 14

**Non-penetrating vs Penetrating Surgery
of Primary Open-Angle Glaucoma**
STEFANO A. GANDOLFI, LUCA CIMINO

Contributors

Bowd, Christopher, PhD
Assistant Research Scientist
Hamilton Glaucoma Center
Department of Ophthalmology – 0946
University of California at San Diego
9500 Gilman Drive
La Jolla, CA 92093-0946, USA

Brandt, James D., MD
Professor of Ophthalmology & Director
Glaucoma Service
University of California at Davis
4860 Y Street, Suite 2400
Sacramento, CA 95817-2307, USA

Cimino, Luca
Sezione di Oftalmologia
Dipartimento di Scienze
Otorino Odonto Oftalmologiche
e Cervico Facciali
Università di Parma
Via Gramsci, 14
43100 Parma, Italy

Gandolfi, Stefano A., Professor Dr.
Sezione di Oftalmologia
Dipartimento di Scienze
Otorino Odonto Oftalmologiche
e Cervico Facciali
Università di Parma
Via Gramsci, 14,
43100 Parma, Italy

Higginbotham, Eve J., MD
Professor and Chair
Department of Ophthalmology
University of Maryland
School of Medicine
419 Redwood Street, Suite 580
Baltimore, MD 21201-1595, USA

Hitchings, R.A., Professor Dr.
Moorfields Eye Hospital
City Road,
London EC1V 2PD, UK

Levin, Leonard A., MD, PhD
Department of Ophthalmology
and Visual Sciences
University of Wisconsin Medical School
K6/456 Clinical Science Center
600 Highland Avenue
Madison, WI 53792-4673, USA

Liebmann, Jeffrey M., MD
Clinical Professor of Ophthalmology
Director, Glaucoma Services
Manhattan Eye, Ear & Throat Hospital
and New York University Medical Center
121 East 60th Street
New York, NY 10022, USA

Medeiros, Felipe A., MD
Assistant Clinical Professor
Hamilton Glaucoma Center
Department of Ophthalmology – 0946
University of California at San Diego
9500 Gilman Drive
La Jolla, CA 92093-0946, USA

Mietz, Holger, Prof. Dr.
Universitäts-Augenklinik
Josef-Stelzmann-Straße 9
50931 Köln, Germany

Migdal, Clive, MD, FRCS, FRCOphth
Consultant Ophthalmologist
Western Eye Hospital
Marylebone Road
London, NW1 5YE, UK

Naumann, Gottfried O.H.
Prof. emer. Dr. Dr. h.c. mult.
Augenklinik der Universität
Erlangen-Nürnberg
Schwabachanlage 6
91054 Erlangen, Germany

Nowomiejska, Katarzyna
Tadeusz Krwawicz Chair of Ophthalmology
and 1st Eye Clinic, Medical Academy in Lublin
ul. Chmielna 1
20-079 Lublin, Poland

Paetzold, Jens, Dr. rer. nat.
University Eye Hospital Tübingen
Department of Pathophysiology
of Vision and Neuro-Ophthalmology
Schleichstr. 12-16
72076 Tübingen, Germany

Ritch, Robert, MD
Professor and Chief, Glaucoma Service
The New York Eye and Ear Infirmary
310 East 14 St.
New York, NY 10003, USA

Schiefer, Ulrich, Prof. Dr. med.
University Eye Hospital Tübingen
Department of Pathophysiology of Vision
and Neuro-Ophthalmology
Schleichstr. 12-16
72076 Tübingen, Germany

Schlötzer-Schrehardt, Ursula, PD Dr.
Augenklinik der Universität
Erlangen-Nürnberg
Schwabachanlage 6
91054 Erlangen, Germany

Tamm, Ernst R., Prof. Dr. med.
Friedrich-Alexander-Universität
Erlangen-Nürnberg
Anatomisches Institut, Lehrstuhl II
Molekulare Anatomie und Embryologie
Universitätsstraße 19
91054 Erlangen, Germany

Tello, Celso, MD
Assistant Professor
of Clinical Ophthalmology
Associate Director, Glaucoma Service
The New York Eye and Ear Infirmary
310 East 14 St.
New York, NY 10003, USA

Tomey, Karim F., MD, FACS, FRCOphth
Beirut Eye Specialist Center
Rizk Hospital
P.O. Box 11-3288, Beirut, Lebanon

Weinreb, Robert N., MD
Professor and Director
Hamilton Glaucoma Center
Department of Ophthalmology – 0946
University of California at San Diego
9500 Gilman Drive
La Jolla, CA 92093-0946, USA

Wilson, M. Roy, MD, MS
President
Texas Tech University
Health Sciences Center
Lubbock, TX, USA

Zangwill, Linda M., PhD
Associate Professor
Director, Diagnostic Imaging Laboratory
Hamilton Glaucoma Center
Department of Ophthalmology – 0946
University of California at San Diego
9500 Gilman Drive
La Jolla, CA 92093-0946, USA

Genetic Changes and Their Influence on Structure and Function of the Eye in Glaucoma

ERNST R. TAMM

Core Messages

- Developmental glaucoma is associated with *Axenfeld-Rieger's syndrome, Peters' anomaly, aniridia,* or other variants of anterior segment dysgenesis, which are all caused by mutations in a variety of different transcription factors
- Primary congenital glaucoma is caused by mutations in the gene *CYP1B1* which codes for the enzyme cytochrome P4501B1
- The ocular substrate for cytochrome P4501B1 is very likely part of an important developmental signaling pathway that has not yet been identified
- Linkage analysis of larger families with autosomal-dominant inherited POAG have led to the discovery of six POAG loci (GLC1A-GLC1F) on different chromosomes
- For two of these loci, the mutated gene has been identified

- Mutations in myocilin are responsible for GLC1A-linked glaucoma, mutations in optineurin cause GLC1E-linked glaucoma
- Myocilin is a secreted glycoprotein that is expressed in very high amounts in the trabecular meshwork
- So far, a specific function of myocilin has not been identified, but some experiments indicate that it might play a role in the modulation of aqueous humor outflow resistance
- Depending on the site of mutation, patients with mutated myocilin may suffer from very high intraocular pressure
- A considerable number of patients with mutations in optineurin suffer from normal pressure glaucoma
- The specific ocular function(s) of optineurin has/have not been identified

1.1
Introduction

Over the past decade, substantial promise for a future understanding of glaucoma has been seen due to the dramatic progress in medical and molecular genetics. While the research on glaucoma genetics was entirely descriptive for more than a century, recent advances in molecular genetics have transformed this field completely. In recent years, a considerable number of specific mutations have been identified in the genetic code of patients that segregate with specific glaucomatous disease phenotypes. As the human genome has been sequenced and the methods that are used to identify disease-related genes are rapidly improving, more genes that are causatively involved in the pathogenesis of glaucoma will be discovered. This will finally lead to a new and better concept to classify different forms of glaucoma, but will also enable scientists and clinicians to better understand the pathogenesis of glaucoma at the level of cell and molecular biology. For many of those genes that have already been identified, transgenic animal models were developed, which have considerably improved our understanding of the biological function of glaucoma-related genes and their gene products. The development of animal models based on the molecular changes in the genome of glaucoma patients will continue and provide controlled biological systems to study the biological role of the respective genes and their interaction with genetic and environmental factors. Subsequently, new concepts and targets for a rational and ultimately causative therapy of glaucoma will emerge. This chapter summarizes our current knowledge on the role of genes in glaucoma, and discusses some novel and older (but still relevant) ideas on how genetic alterations may lead to changes in structure and function of the eye in glaucoma.

take place during anterior eye development. Further studies may lead to a full and complete understanding of one of the most fascinating problems in ocular biology, namely how the development of the anterior eye is organized and successfully completed. Finally, research is needed to solve the question, why glaucoma develops in some but not all of the patients with comparable developmental abnormalities of the anterior eye. Such studies will result in novel therapeutic approaches that will prevent or ameliorate the manifestation of glaucoma in affected patients.

1.2
Glaucoma in Developmental Disorders

Glaucoma in developmental disorders is caused by a dysfunction of the aqueous outflow system, which is associated with structural defects in the anterior eye that occur during embryonic and fetal development. As a result, the resistance to aqueous humor outflow may become abnormally high causing an increase in intraocular pressure at birth or any time thereafter. Traditionally, developmental glaucomas are classified according to the nature of the structural abnormalities in the anterior eye that are associated with glaucoma. In recent years, a number of genes, which are causative for developmental glaucomas have been identified. All of these genes encode for transcription factors, which are DNA-binding proteins controlling the transcription of the large array of genes that is needed to organize anterior eye development. Our understanding of how this process is regulated at the molecular level is still in its infancy. It has become clear though that there is no strict correlation between the type of the genetic change and the resulting structural phenotype. Mutations in different genes may cause the same anatomical changes, whereas the same mutations in an individual gene may cause different anatomical phenotypes in different patients. Knockout mouse models have been developed that are deficient in those genes that cause glaucoma in humans. The analysis of these mouse models has already provided important insight into the complex regulatory mechanisms that

1.2.1
Development of the Ocular Mesenchyme in the Anterior Eye

The structural defects in the anterior eye that are associated with developmental glaucomas take place during the morphogenesis of the anterior eye segment in embryonic and fetal life. Involved in this group of disorders are primarily those tissues of the anterior eye that derive from the ocular mesenchyme. Ocular mesenchyme is first seen around the sixth week of human development, shortly after the lens stalk has become separated from the surface epithelium and the lens vesicle has invaginated into the optic cup. Fate mapping studies of avian eye development using quail-chick chimeras showed that most of the ocular mesenchyme derives from cells of the cranial neural crest [52]. More recent cell grafting and cell labelling experiments of craniofacial morphogenesis in the mouse confirmed a neural crest contribution during mammalian eye development, but also provided evidence for the presence of additional cranial paraxial mesoderm-derived cells in the ocular mesenchyme [127]. Mesenchymal cells migrate into the space between surface epithelium and lens epithelium to form several layers of loosely aggregated, star-shaped cells [24, 60, 145]. In a next step, most of these cells condense to a dense layer that will give rise to the future corneal endothelium [24, 25, 60]. Some cells remain in the stromal space between surface ectoderm and future corneal endothelium, which thickens again while mesenchyme

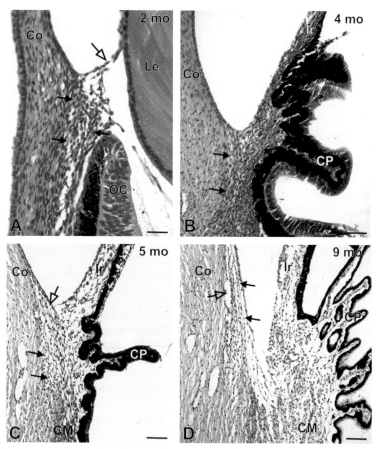

Fig. 1.1 A–D. Development of the chamber angle and trabecular meshwork in human embryonic and fetal eyes at 2 (**A**), 4 (**B**), 5 (**C**), and 9 (**D**) months of development. **A** At 2 months, mesenchymal cells (*solid arrows*) are seen between the anterior edge of the optic cup (*OC*) and the future cornea (*Co*). Cells of the anterior pupillary membrane (*open arrow*) extend from the peripheral cornea to the anterior surface of the lens. **B** At 4 months, mesenchymal cells (*arrows*) form a dense mass at the chamber angle, which extends on to the anterior surface of the developing iris (*Ir*). *CP*, ciliary process.

C In 5-month-old fetal eyes, the cells of the future trabecular meshwork (*solid arrows*) are separated from each other by small open spaces. Uveal tissue (*open arrow*) covers the anterior surface of the trabecular meshwork. *CM*, ciliary muscle. **D** At term, most of the trabecular meshwork (*solid arrows*) is exposed to the anterior chamber. Schlemm's canal (*open arrow*) is seen at the outer side of the trabecular meshwork. Sections kindly provided by Dr. Christian Vorwerk, Department of Ophthalmology, University of Magdeburg, Germany. Magnification bars: **A** 20 μm; **B** 30 μm; **C**, 40 μm; **D**, 60 μm

cells proliferate and/or continue to migrate to the future cornea. Finally, the mesenchyme cells between surface ectoderm and corneal endothelium differentiate into corneal stroma fibroblasts or keratocytes, the only cell type which is capable of synthesizing the distinct extracellular matrix compounds that are needed for transparency of the cornea. The surface ec-

toderm that covers the anterior side of the mesenchyme will become the corneal epithelium.

During differentiation of the corneal endothelium, the lens detaches from the future cornea and a fluid-filled chamber is generated between both structures. A new group of mesenchyme cells migrates now to the anterior eye and arrives at the chamber angle (Fig. 1.1 A). The peripheral edge of the optic cup grows into the cavity between lens and cornea, along the anterior lens surface to give rise to the iris and ciliary body. The formation of the iris separates the cavity between lens and cornea into the anterior and posterior chamber. When the optic cup enlarges to form the iris and ciliary body, the mesenchyme cells in the chamber angle continue to migrate along the epithelial layers of both structures and finally differentiate into the stroma of the iris and ciliary body (Fig. 1.1 B).

The last structures that become differentiated during anterior eye development are the trabecular meshwork and Schlemm's canal [5, 90, 144]. Shortly after the beginning of iris elongation around the 15th to 17th week, the chamber angle is occupied by a dense mass of mesenchymal cells (Fig. 1.1 B). These cells become separated from each other by small open spaces that are partially filled with extracellular fibers, while vessels appear in the immediate adjacent sclera (Fig. 1.1 C). At that time, the chamber angle is level with the anterior border of the future trabecular meshwork, which is covered by uveal tissue that is continuous with the root of the iris. Subsequently, the extracellular fibers in the chamber angle organize themselves into trabecular beams that become covered by trabecular meshwork cells, while the scleral vessels next to the chamber angle coalesce to Schlemm's canal. In parallel, the peripheral margin of the anterior chamber moves posteriorly and the inner surface of the trabecular meshwork becomes exposed to the anterior chamber. Around birth, the major morphogenesis of the trabecular meshwork is complete (Fig. 1.1 D), but some minor modeling and maturation of the inner aspects of the trabecular meshwork continues throughout the first years of life. Between the trabecular meshwork lamellae and the endothelial lining of Schlemm's canal, some cells with a stellate phenotype remain to form the juxtacanalicular or cribriform layer of the trabecular meshwork, a region of 5–10 μm in thickness, in which most of the resistance to aqueous humor outflow is located [50].

Summary for the Clinician

Critical steps during development of the anterior eye in sequential order:

- Separation of the lens from the surface epithelium
- Migration of mesenchymal cells into the space between surface epithelium and lens
- Differentiation of mesenchymal cells into keratocytes and corneal endothelium
- Formation of the anterior chamber
- Migration of mesenchymal cells to the chamber angle
- Formation of iris and ciliary body
- Differentiation of chamber angle mesenchyme into trabecular meshwork, formation of Schlemm's canal

1.2.2
Axenfeld-Rieger's Syndrome, Peters' Anomaly and Anterior Segment Dysgenesis

1.2.2.1
Structural Characteristics – Phenotype

Failure of correct mesenchyme differentiation during anterior eye development may result in a broad spectrum of clinical disorders, which are part of Axenfeld-Rieger's syndrome (for reviews see [2, 71]). In general, patients with Axenfeld-Rieger's syndrome develop glaucoma in about 50% of cases. Subtypes of Axenfeld-Rieger's syndrome include Rieger's anomaly or syndrome, Axenfeld's anomaly, and iridogoniodysgenesis, all of which are commonly inherited in an autosomal-dominant fashion [44, 104]. In Rieger's anomaly, midperipheral adhesions from the iris to cornea are seen (Fig. 1.2 B). In addition, there is a marked iris hypoplasia and structural defects such as polycoria and corectopia. When the ocular findings of Rieger's anomaly are associated with characteristic systemic developmental defects such as dental or facial abnormalities, the term Rieger's syndrome is used. Axenfeld's anomaly is characterized by iris strands that attach to a structure called posterior embryotoxon, which is a ring of collagenous fibers at the peripheral end of De-

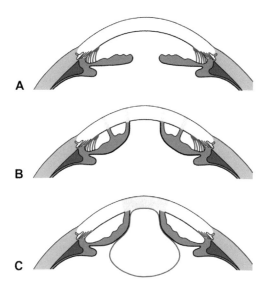

Fig. 1.2 A–C. Typical phenotypes seen in the spectrum of anterior segment dysgenesis. **A** In Axenfeld's anomaly, iris strands traverse the chamber angle and insert into a prominent Schwalbe's line (posterior embryotoxon). **B** In Rieger's anomaly, midperipheral adhesions from the iris to cornea are seen in addition to Axenfeld's anomaly. **C** The phenotype of Peters' anomaly consists of a central corneal opacity (leukoma), with local absence of the corneal endothelium. The lens may adhere to the back of the corneal opacity. Peters' anomaly is usually associated with iridocorneal adhesions that arise from the pupillary region. (Modified from [44])

scemet's membrane forming a prominent Schwalbe's line (Fig. 1.2 A). It is clinically recognized as a ring-shaped opacity in the peripheral cornea. Patients with iridogoniodysgenesis have an iris with hypoplastic stroma, abnormal chamber angle tissue, and glaucoma.

1.2.2.2
Genetic Changes

It has been shown that the broad spectrum of abnormalities with different specific clinical phenotypes, which characterize Axenfeld-Rieger's syndrome, results from mutations in the bicoid-like homeobox gene, *PITX2*, or the forkhead/winged-helix transcription factor gene, *FOXC1* [81, 98]. Both genes code for transcription factors that have a critical role for the

control of anterior eye morphogenesis. In the mouse eye, *Pitx2* is expressed in periocular mesenchyme, presumptive cornea, eyelids and extraocular muscle [70,72], and *Foxc1* in periocular mesenchyme, presumptive cornea and trabecular meshwork [57]. In addition to an important role during morphogenesis of the anterior eye, *PITX2* might also have a critical role for controlling gene expression in the chamber angle tissues of the adult anterior eye. In the course of the NEIBank project of the National Eye Institute in Bethesda, MD, an un-normalized cDNA library was generated from RNA, which had been extracted from dissected trabecular meshwork pooled from 28 healthy adult human donors [124]. A total of 3459 independent cDNA clones were obtained, and transcripts for *PITX2* were found among those most highly expressed. This strongly indicates that *PITX2* is part of the control mechanisms which regulate the expression of those distinct genes that are needed for proper function of the aqueous humor outflow pathways.

1.2.2.3
Spectrum of Phenotypes

Some patients with mutations in *PITX2* or *FOXC1* have been reported that express the phenotype of Peters' anomaly [22, 45, 84]. Peter's anomaly is characterized by central corneal opacities (leukoma) with abnormalities of the deepest corneal stromal layers and local absence of the corneal endothelium (Fig. 1.2 C) [97]. The lens may adhere to the back of the corneal opacity and show signs of an anterior polar cataract. Peters' anomaly is usually associated with iridocorneal adhesions that arise from the pupillary region, and with iris hypoplasia and corectopia. Most cases of Peters' anomaly are sporadic; 50 %–70 % of cases have abnormally high intraocular pressure and develop glaucoma, very likely due to dysgenesis and/or malfunction of the aqueous humor outflow tissues in the iridocorneal angle. The reasons for the wide spectrum of phenotypes caused by mutations in *PITX2* or *FOXC1* are not clear and have been discussed recently [40]. Mutant proteins may retain partial functions resulting in milder phenotypes. However, individuals with the same mutation may have different phenotypes, even within the same family [45, 84]. There is the distinct possibility that different phenotypes result from the action of modifying genes that interact with the mutant genes. Indeed, *Foxc1*$^{+/-}$ mice express a phenotype comparable to that of human patients with mutations in *FOXC1* depending on strain, and therefore genetic background (for review see [40]). Still, even within mice from the same inbred strain (with essentially the same background), the severity of the phenotype varies between animals, and right and left eye within the same animal. It has been suggested that stochastic developmental events and/or the local environment during development influence the outcome for each individual eye [40]. Such events may lead to the presence of a more or less active gene product at a given critical point during development. Indeed, the data from mouse mutants strongly suggest that dosage is an important factor. Heterozygous *Foxc1*$^{-/+}$ mutant mice show phenotypes that resemble those of humans with Axenfeld-Rieger's syndrome, whereas homozygous mutant mice show persistent corneolenticular adhesions and failure of anterior chamber development similar to the phenotype of Peters' anomaly [57]. Comparable defects are seen in homozygous *Pitx2*$^{-/-}$ deficient mice, which show a persistence of both corneolenticular adhesions and lens stalk [34].

1.2.2.4
Lens Genes
and Anterior Segment Dysgenesis

In some patients with anterior segment dysgenesis and Peters' anomaly, mutations have been found in the genes *MAF*, *FOXE3* and *PITX3* which encode for transcription factors that are primarily expressed during lens development where they are involved in closure of the lens vesicle and fiber cell elongation. *MAF* encodes for a basic region leucine zipper (bZIP) transcription factor and human patients with mutations in *MAF* suffer from developmental abnormalities in both lens, iris and cornea such as congenital cataracts, iris coloboma, opaque corneas and Peters' anomaly [47]. *FOXE3* encodes a forkhead transcription factor and muta-

tions in *FOXE3* cause Peters' anomaly, a prominent Schwalbe's line (posterior embryotoxon) and cataracts in humans [83, 101]. *PITX3* is a homeobox-containing gene expressed in the lens [100]. Mutations in *PITX3* are associated with autosomal-dominant congenital cataracts, central opacity of the cornea and adhesions between iris and cornea [99]. A common theme of all these disorders appears to be the fact that problems during early lens development such as delayed or incomplete separation of the lens vesicle from the surface ectoderm or incomplete closure of the lens vesicle by failure of lens fiber elongation almost invariably interferes with signals that are required for early differentiation of the corneal mesenchyme. Inductive signals from the lens are known to be important for corneal development and differentiation of anterior eye mesenchyme [9], and those genes that organize the structural changes of the developing lens may also be involved, directly or indirectly, in the formation of such signals.

Summary for the Clinician

- Developmental glaucoma is associated with Axenfeld-Rieger's syndrome, Peters' anomaly or other variants of anterior segment dysgenesis
- Mutations in a variety of different transcription factors have been identified as causative for anterior segment dysgenesis
- Transcription factors are DNA-binding proteins that control or coordinate the transcription of their specific set of target genes
- No clear genotype–phenotype correlation has been shown and, for as yet unidentified reasons, the same mutation may cause different clinical forms of anterior segment dysgenesis in different patients

1.2.2.5
The Role of Signaling Molecules

It appears reasonable to assume that the various transcription factors which are involved in the control of the morphogenesis of the anterior eye coordinate their signals by modulating the expression of secreted signaling molecules. There is considerable evidence from studies on mutant mouse models that the signaling molecules bone morphogenetic protein 4 (BMP4) and/or transforming growth factor-β2 (TGF-β2) are directly involved in the developing processes that occur during mesenchyme morphogenesis in the anterior eye. Both proteins are members of the TGF-β superfamily and are involved in many developmental processes including cell proliferation, differentiation, apoptosis, and intercellular interactions. BMP4 is expressed in the iris, ciliary body, and retinal pigment epithelium of embryonic and adult mouse eyes [16]. Mice heterozygous for a null allele of *Bmp4* (*Bmp4^{tm1BLh}*) show a variety of ocular segment abnormalities involving the iris (irregular shaped pupils, anterior synechiae), cornea (opacity at the periphery, diffuse haze), and chamber angle (displaced Schwalbe's line, small or absent Schlemm's canal, hypoplastic or absent trabecular meshwork) [16]. The extent of structural changes in the chamber angle varies along the circumference of individual eyes, and animals with severe structural abnormalities show an increase in intraocular pressure. Similar to the structural changes in *Foxc1* heterozygote mice, the severity of the changes depends on the genetic background, and there is phenotypic variability between eyes of genetically uniform mice. It seems reasonable to assume that BMP4 is not only required for the proper formation of the anterior segment of the mouse eye, but also for that of humans. In addition, it might be an important signaling molecule for regulatory processes in the adult chamber angle, as BMP4 has been found to be secreted in the adult human trabecular meshwork [143].

Similar to BMP4, TGF-β2 is expressed during ocular development and in the adult anterior eye. High levels of TGF-β2 are found in the normal aqueous humor, which are elevated in some patients with primary open-angle glaucoma (POAG) [85, 129]. Homozygous TGF-β2 knock-out mice, which die at birth because of cardiac defects, show the phenotype of Peters' anomaly. The cornea is markedly thinner than normal and an anterior chamber is not present. The lens and iris are in contact with the corneal stoma and the corneal endothelium is completely absent [94]. Transgenic overexpression of TGF-β1 (which is closely related to TGF-β2 and utilizes the same receptors) in the anterior eye causes the formation of a thick and opaque cornea, and prevents the formation of the anterior chamber and that of the tissues in the chamber angle [30]. In addition, the corneal endothelium, iris and ciliary body are absent, underlying that the dose of TGF-βs must be critically maintained during development to avoid severe malformations in anterior eye development. The availability of TGF-βs at the right dose might also be very important for the proper function of the trabecular meshwork in the adult eye. It is interesting to note that an interaction between TGF-β signaling and *FOXC1* expression has been observed in cell culture studies. Treatment with TGF-β1 up-regulates the expression of *FOXC1* in several human cancer cell lines [148]. Mesenchyme cells from mouse embryos show a characteristic response to added TGF-β, which is not observed in cells from *Foxc1* null mouse embryos [64].

1.2.2.6
Causal Factors for Glaucoma

About 50% of patients with Axenfeld-Rieger's syndrome develop glaucoma, which commonly develops in childhood or young adulthood. The extent of iris defects such as the tissue strands that bridge the chamber angle from the peripheral iris to the prominent Schwalbe's line, or the insertion of the iris into the posterior trabecular meshwork appear not to correlate precisely with the presence or severity of glaucoma [104]. This observation is in line with the current concept of the localization of outflow resistance in the trabecular meshwork, which implies that there is no significant resistance to aqueous humor outflow in the inner parts of the TM [50]. In contrast, most of the resistance to aqueous outflow is localized in the juxtacanalicular or cribriform layer of the trabecular meshwork, a region of 5–10 μm in thickness immediately adjacent to the inner wall endothelium of Schlemm's canal. Ultrastructural analyses of the juxtacanalicular layer in specimens from patients with Axenfeld-Rieger's anomaly described the presence of considerable amounts of amorphous extracellular material in the extracellular spaces of this region [103]. In addition, the connective tissue core of the trabecular lamellae was markedly thickened and surrounded by a thick layer of extracellular

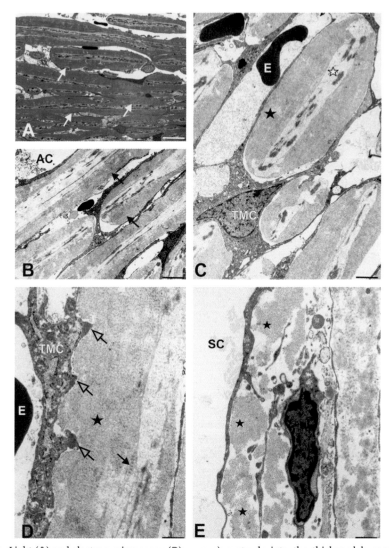

Fig. 1.3 A–E. Light (**A**) and electron microscopy (**B**) of the trabecular meshwork (TM) in a 24-year-old patient with Axenfeld's syndrome and glaucoma.

A, B The intertrabecular spaces are markedly narrowed because of an abnormally thickened basement membrane in the TM lamellae (*arrows*). **C** The basement membrane (*black asterisk*) surrounds the central core of TM lamellae (*white asterisk*), which is of normal thickness. **D** Processes of TM cells (*open arrows*) protrude into the thickened basement membrane (*asterisk*), which appears granular and contains aggregates of broad-banded material (*solid arrow*). **E** The extracellular spaces of the juxtacanalicular meshwork contain numerous aggregates of sheath-derived plaque material (*asterisks*). *AC*, anterior chamber; *TMC,*: trabecular meshwork cell; *SC*, Schlemm's canal; *E*, erythrocyte. Magnification bars: **A** 4 μm; **B** 1.7 μm; **C, E** 1 μm; **D** 0.7 μm

material, which frequently contained large amounts of broad-banded collagen of 128 nm periodicity. This increase appeared to cause a marked narrowing of the intertrabecular spaces. We observed essentially similar ultrastructural changes in two trabeculectomy specimen from both eyes of a 24-year-old patient with Axenfeld's syndrome and glaucoma (E.R. Tamm, F. Hoffmann, E. Lütjen-Drecoll, unpublished observations). The trabecular lamellae of the corneoscleral and uveal trabecular meshwork were markedly thickened due to an increase in electron dense material in the basement membrane of trabecular meshwork cells (Fig. 1.3 A–C). This material was homogenous or fine granular and contained broad-banded aggregates (Fig. 1.3 D). The extracellular spaces of the juxtacanalicular meshwork were filled with large aggregates of sheath-derived plaque material (Fig. 1.3 E). This material derives from the sheath of the elastic fibers in the cribriform or juxtacanalicular region and has been shown to be significantly increased in the eyes of patients with adult-onset POAG [73]. The amount of sheath-derived plaque material in the eyes of patients with POAG correlates with the extent of axonal damage in the optic nerve [39]. Overall these findings suggest that haploinsufficieny in factors like *FOXC1* or *PITX2* may lead to an abnormal turnover of the extracellular matrix in the juxtacanalicular trabecular meshwork during development, which continues during childhood and adolescence. An abnormal quantity and/or quality of the extracellular matrix in the trabecular meshwork may finally lead to an increase in aqueous humor outflow resistance and cause glaucoma in Axenfeld-Rieger's syndrome.

Summary for the Clinician

- About 50% of patients with Axenfeld-Rieger's syndrome develop glaucoma, which commonly becomes manifest in childhood or young adulthood
- The extent of iris defects appears not to correlate precisely with the presence or severity of glaucoma
- Available data indicate that glaucoma in Axenfeld-Rieger's syndrome is associated with an increase of extracellular matrix in the trabecular meshwork

1.2.3
Aniridia

1.2.3.1
Structural Abnormalities

Another gene that is critically required for the morphogenesis of mesenchyme-derived tissues in the anterior eye is *PAX6*, which codes for a paired domain and paired-like homeodomain transcription factor. Pax6 is a key regulator of eye development that is both essential for eye formation in different organisms as well as capable of inducing ectopic eyes in flies and frogs upon misexpression [7, 18, 35]. Humans with heterozygote mutations in *PAX6* express the phenotype *aniridia*, a panocular disease that is associated with iris hypoplasia, corneal opacification, cataract, and foveal dysplasia [37,53,125]. In addition, mutations in *PAX6* have also been found in patients with Peters' anomaly, autosomal dominant keratitis, and isolated foveal hypoplasia [88]. About 50%–75% of patients with aniridia develop glaucoma, which is thought to be due to developmental abnormalities in the chamber angle that obstruct aqueous humor outflow to the trabecular meshwork and Schlemm's canal. The exact nature of the developmental defects that cause glaucoma in aniridia are unclear. It has been discussed that the stump of the hypoplastic iris progressively obstructs those parts of the trabecular meshwork which are important for the outflow of aqueous humor [41]. In contrast, histopathological analyses of several case reports have provided evidence of abnormal trabecular meshwork differentiation and/or complete absence of Schlemm's canal in patients with aniridia [75]. Still, for most of these case reports, the genetic type of aniridia is not clear, and in most cases later stages of glaucoma have been examined in which secondary changes may have been present. More insight into the pathological changes of the chamber angle that are caused by mutations in Pax6 have come again from studies of genetically engineered mouse models. Heterozygous *Pax6*[lacZ/+] mutant mice have a null allele of *Pax6* and show a reduction in eye size and cataracts [8]. The trabecular meshwork of

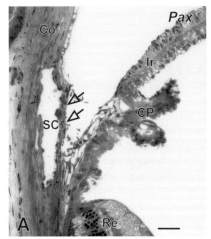 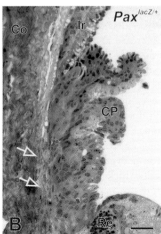

Fig. 1.4 A,B. Chamber angle mesenchyme of a normal (A) and a heterozygous Pax6-deficient *Pax6^{lacZ/+}* mouse eye at P21.
A In wild-type mice, a well differentiated trabecular meshwork (*open arrows*) is in contact with Schlemm's canal (*SC*).

B In *Pax6^{lacZ/+}* animals, a differentiated trabecular meshwork or Schlemm's canal are not present. Instead, a compact strand of closely aggregated cells is observed in the narrowed chamber angle (*open arrows*). *CB*, ciliary body; *Co*, cornea; *Ir*, iris; *Re*, retina. Magnification bars: 30 μm

Pax6^{lacZ/+} mutant mice remains undifferentiated, Schlemm's canal is absent, and the chamber angle is very narrow [8] (Fig. 1.4). The iris of the animals remains hypoplastic and corneal abnormalities are present. In a third of *Pax6^{lacZ/+}* mutant mice, the separation of the cornea from the lens is incomplete, the epithelial layers of lens and cornea are continuous and iridocorneal adhesions are present, all hallmarks of Peters' anomaly [8]. Persistence of the lens stalk, and an irregular lamellar alignment of the corneal stroma together with cellular infiltrates and vascularization has also been observed in *Small eye* (*Sey*) mice, another mouse strain with a null allele of *Pax6* [89].

1.2.3.2
The Role of Pax6

Overall, the phenotypes of Pax6 haploinsufficiency in mice and humans indicate that Pax6 is critically required for the differentiation of those tissues of the anterior eye segment that are of mesenchymal origin. Pax6 could indirectly act on the morphogenesis of ocular mesenchyme as strong Pax6 expression has been described in cells that derive from the neuroectoderm of the optic cup or from the anterior surface ectoderm [21, 42, 62, 137]. This strong expression is seen during ocular development and is maintained in adulthood. More recent data indicate, however, that Pax6 also acts directly on mesenchymal differentiation in the developing eye, as Pax6 was also shown to be expressed in ocular cells of mesenchymal origin. The intensity of the expression is weaker than in cells of surface ectodermal or neuroepithelial origin and only observed in mid-fetal stages, but not in adult animals [8, 20]. In addition, studies on gene expression and distribution of *Pax6^{-/-}* cells in *Pax6^{+/+}* ⟺ *Pax6^{-/-}* mouse chimeras confirmed that *Pax6* is autonomously required for cells to contribute to corneal stroma and corneal endothelium [20]. The high and continuous expression of Pax6 in cells that derive from surface ectoderm and optic cup (lens, corneal epithelium, iris, and ciliary epithelium) appears to be required for the expression of transcription factors, structural genes, and signaling molecules, which are critical for the morphogenesis of those tissues, and probably also for the migration of neural crest cells into the eye

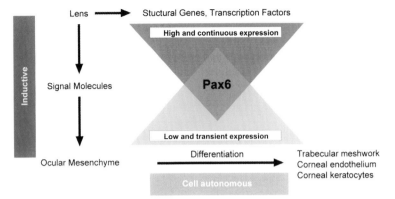

Fig. 1.5. The proposed role of *PAX6* for anterior eye development. A high and continuous expression of *PAX6* in cells of ectodermal origin (lens, corneal epithelium, iris, and ciliary epithelium) is important for the expression of regulatory and structural genes in these tissues, as well as for the expression of signaling molecules that act on cells of mesenchymal origin in the anterior eye (trabecular meshwork, stroma of iris, ciliary body, and cornea). In addition, a low and transient expression of Pax6 is observed in cells of mesenchymal origin during development of the trabecular meshwork, chamber angle, iris, and ciliary body. This expression is important for proper differentiation of trabecular meshwork and chamber angle

by inductive processes (Fig. 1.5) [8]. In addition, a low and transient expression of Pax6 plays cell-autonomous roles in the subsequent differentiation of the trabecular meshwork, and in the formation of corneal endothelium, keratocytes, and cells of the iris stroma [8, 20] (Fig. 1.5). It is tempting to speculate that Pax6, which is active in both epithelial and mesenchymal cells during ocular development, is a key element to synchronize the complex interaction of cells types of different origin that is needed for proper morphogenesis of the anterior eye.

| Summary for the Clinician |

- *Aniridia* is caused by mutations in Pax6
- Data from mouse models with mutations in pax6 indicate that glaucoma in aniridia is due to a malformation of trabecular meshwork and Schlemm's canal

1.2.4
Primary Congenital Glaucoma

1.2.4.1
Structural Defects

Primary congenital glaucoma (primary infantile glaucoma, trabeculodysgenesis) is a specific, inherited developmental defect in the trabecular meshwork and chamber angle that manifests itself in the neonatal or infantile period with increased intraocular pressure, corneal enlargement, and optic nerve cupping. There has been some debate as to the exact nature of the structural changes in the chamber angle that are associated with primary congenital glaucoma (PCG). Early authors have described the presence of an imperforate mesodermal membrane covering the outflow tissue. In later studies, such a membrane could not be verified. Several histopathological studies observed that the iris insertion and anterior ciliary body overlap the posterior portion of the trabecular meshwork, but leave the angle open. It was concluded that during chamber angle development, the iris and ciliary body failed to recede posteriorly (see Sect. 1.2.1) [5]. Tawara and Inomata

[119], who studied trabeculectomy specimens from the eyes of six patients with PCG, observed that the juxtacanalicular area was markedly thickened and consisted of many layers of spindle-shaped cells with surrounding extracellular matrix. In contrast, the corneoscleral and uveal trabecular meshwork was smaller in size and had fewer lamellae than normal. The extracellular spaces of the juxtacanalicular region contained large amounts of amorphous and fibrillar extracellular matrix, and whorls of basal lamina-like material. An increase in extracellular material in the juxtacanalicular areas was also described by other researchers [5, 77]. In addition, the trabecular beams were found to be thicker than normal. In general, structural studies agree that the developmental defects in the trabecular meshwork affect all regions of the trabecular meshwork. Nevertheless, the success rate of goniotomy, where presumably only the superficial layers of the trabecular meshwork are incised, appears to indicate that these layers are more critical for impaired outflow resistance in patients with PCG.

1.2.4.2
Genetic Defects

Most cases of PCG are sporadic in occurrence. In familial cases of PCG, an autosomal recessive mode of inheritance is commonly observed. PCG has a higher incidence in Gypsies (1:2500) and in the Middle East (1:2500) as compared with that of Western Societies (1:5,000–1:22,000) [32, 36]. For the hereditary forms, two loci were identified and mapped to chromosomal regions 2p21 (GLC3A) [95] and 1p36.2-p36.1 (GLC3B) [1], respectively. According to the Humane Genome Organization (HUGO) Nomenclature Committee, loci for congenital glaucoma are designated by *GLC3*, and letters are added to distinguish specific loci in order of their discovery. For GLC3A-linked families, mutations in the gene *CYP1B1* coding for the enzyme cytochrome P4501B1 were found to be causative for PCG [107]. In the meantime, a series of various mutations in *CYP1B1* have been identified in patients with PCG from distinct populations [10, 54, 78, 106, 109, 134]. Mutant *CYP1B1* can associate with ocular phenotypes other than PCG, as it

has been found in patients with Peters' anomaly [106, 133], with glaucoma of later onset than typical PCG [10, 11], and is suggested to be a factor altering the presentation of adult-onset glaucoma [134]. In a Saudi Arabian population a variable expression of the phenotype was observed, as apparently unaffected individuals had haplotypes identical to their affected siblings [10, 11]. These data might be explained by the presence of a dominant modifier locus that is not genetically linked to *CYP1B1*.

The ocular substrate for the enzyme cytochrome P4501B1 is not known. In general, enzymes of the cytochrome P450 multigene family mediate detoxification reactions including that of drugs or toxic foreign compounds. In the case of cytochrome P4501B, it is obvious that the substrate is very likely endogenous and part of an important developmental signaling pathway. Possible candidates are steroids, all-trans retinol, fatty acids, or arachidonic acid [108]. In the mouse anterior eye, expression of cytochrome P4501B1 mRNA is confined to the pigmented ciliary epithelium and is not observed before the ciliary body develops from the optic cup [12]. If cytochrome P4501B1 is involved in the metabolization or production of signaling molecules, they need to be secreted from the ciliary epithelium to reach the trabecular meshwork.

Summary for the Clinician

- Primary congenital glaucoma is caused by mutations in the gene *CYP1B1* which codes for the enzyme cytochrome P4501B1
- The ocular substrate for cytochrome P4501B1 is very likely part of an important developmental signaling pathway that has not yet been identified

1.2.4.3
Mouse Models
for Primary Congential Glaucoma

In a recent study, Libby and coworkers [68] showed that mutant $Cyp1b1^{-/-}$ mice, which are deficient in cytochrome P4501B1 showed focal defects in chamber angle development including an increase in basal lamina material in the trabecular meshwork, and a small or absent

Schlemm's canal. When *Cyp1b1*$^{-/-}$ mice were crossed in mouse strains with different genetic background, pigmented mice of the B6 background had mild abnormalities, while albino (tyrosinase-deficient) mice of the 129X1/SvJ background had more severe and extensive angle abnormalities. These observations suggested that the presence of tyrosinase protects *Cyp1b1*$^{-/-}$ mice against developmental abnormalities. Similar findings were observed for the structural changes of *Foxc1*$^{+/-}$ mice (see Sect. 1.2.2.3) leading to the hypothesis that tyrosinase might affect chamber angle development through modulation of L-dihydroxyphenylalanine (L-dopa) levels, as tyrosinase converts tyrosine to L-dopa. In support of this, treatment of mothers with L-dopa prevented the severe chamber angle dysgenesis in their offspring that was present in untreated mice lacking cytochrome P4501B1 and tyrosinase. L-dopa has been shown to play a role in development in other systems and might well play a role during the development of the anterior eye. Interestingly, anterior segment dysgenesis and congenital glaucoma have been reported in a few humans with albinism [15, 132].

1.2.5
Nail-Patella Syndrome

Nail-patella syndrome is inherited in an autosomal dominant fashion and is typically characterized by skeletal anomalies including hypoplastic or absent patellae, absent, hypoplastic, or dystrophic nails, elbow abnormalities and the presence of iliac horns. Glaucoma has been recognized as a feature of nail-patella syndrome only relatively recently [69]. In a recent study involving 123 affected patients, the prevalence of glaucoma and ocular hypertension was reported at 9.6% and 7.5%, respectively [113]. When participants under the age of 40 were excluded, the numbers rose to 16.7%. In many patients, glaucoma seems to be phenotypically identical to primary open-angle glaucoma (POAG) and no discernible structural anomalies are found that accompany the elevated intraocular pressure. In a small number of affected patients with glaucoma, anterior segment anomalies have been reported such as iris processes, mild iris stromal thinning, and "cloudy" corneas. No published reports describing the structural changes in the trabecular meshwork of patients with nail-patella syndrome are available.

The gene defect that is responsible for nail-patella syndrome involves haploinsufficiency of the LIM-homeodomain transcription factor *LMX1B* and was identified subsequent to the findings of anatomical abnormalities in *lmx1b* null mice [23], and independently by positional cloning [136]. In the mouse eye, *lmx1b* is expressed in periocular mesenchyme during development, and in corneal and iris stroma, and trabecular meshwork in the adult eye [87]. Mice that are homozygous for a targeted mutation of *lmx1b* display iris and ciliary body hypoplasia, a reduction in anterior chamber depth and defects in the corneal stroma [87]. The abnormalities in the corneal stroma seem to be related to the fact that collagen fibrillogenesis is disturbed in mutant corneas and that specific components of the corneal extracellular matrix such as the keratin sulfate proteoglycan keratocan are not expressed. It is tempting to speculate that haploinsufficiency of *LMX1b* may similarly affect the synthesis of some specific trabecular meshwork genes in affected patients and cause POAG.

1.3
Genes and Primary Open-Angle Glaucoma (POAG)

While there has been significant progress in our understanding of the inheritance pattern and genetic contributions for developmental forms of glaucoma and PCG, the underlying causes for most cases of POAG remain unknown. There is considerable evidence though that genetic factors do also contribute to POAG. It has long been recognized that POAG is more likely to occur in people who have relatives with POAG and recent epidemiological studies have confirmed that a family history of POAG is a major risk factor for this disease [17, 66, 123]. Between monozygotic twins, concordance of glaucoma is higher than between dizygotic twins supporting the concept of a genetic predisposition [120]. Finally, the prevalence of glaucoma differs in particular racial or ethnic groups. POAG is more prevalent in black than in white populations. In a population-based prevalence survey, age-adjusted prevalence rates for POAG were four to five times higher in blacks as compared with whites. Rates among blacks ranged from 1.23% in those aged 40 through 49 years to 11.26% in those 80 years or older, whereas rates for whites ranged from 0.92% to 2.16%, respectively [122]. POAG is particularly frequent among Afro-Caribbeans, with prevalences of 7% in Barbados [65] and 8.8% in St. Lucia [76].

1.3.1
Loci for POAG

Because of the relatively late onset of POAG in affected individuals, there are usually only a few affected family members alive at the same time, which makes it difficult to determine an exact modus of inheritance and to collect sufficient material for genetic analyses. Therefore, the search for genes that cause POAG has first focused on several selected large families worldwide, in which the disease was mostly shown to be inherited in an autosomal dominant mendelian fashion. In the course of these studies, genetic loci contributing to POAG susceptibility have been identified on chromosome 1q23–24 (GLC1A) [102], 2cen–q13 (GLC1B) [110], 3q21–q24 (GLC1C) [141]), 8q23 (GLC1D) [128], 10p15–10p14 (GLC1E) [96], and 7q35–q36 (GLC1F) [142]. According to the Human Genome Organization (HUGO) Nomenclature Committee, loci for open-angle glaucoma are designated by GLC1, and letters are added to distinguish specific loci in order of their discovery.

To date, the genes that underlie two of the six named POAG loci have been identified. MYOC is the gene for GLC1A and OPTN is the gene for GLC1E. MYOC and OPTN encode for the proteins myocilin or optineurin, respectively (see Sect. 1.3.2). The GLC1B locus was identified in patients with low to moderate intraocular pressures, an onset of the disease in the fifth decade and a good response to medical treatment. In an independent study, in which a genome-wide scan of sibling pairs (sibpairs) with POAG was

performed, significant results were also observed with markers located near the GLC1B locus [140]. GLC1C was identified in a family from Oregon with 12 affected family members with autosomal-dominant POAG. Linkage on the same chromosomal region was subsequently also observed in a Greek family with autosomal-dominant POAG, which showed clinical characteristics similar to the Oregon family [59]. As a candidate gene that maps to this region, the PCOLCE2 gene was identified, which codes for a type I procollagen C-proteinase enhancer protein-like gene [146]. However, no coding sequence mutations were detected in PCOLCE2 in a POAG patient from the GLC1C family and the nature of the specific gene defect at this locus is still unclear. GLC1D and GLC1F were found in families with adult-onset POAG, again the nature of the mutated genes is unknown. More recently, some researchers focused on approaches which do not require the assumption of a specific mode of inheritance, such as an autosomal dominant mendelian inheritance. In a genome-wide scan for adult-onset POAG based on a sib-pair multipoint analysis, additional linkages to loci in regions of chromosomes 14, 17p, 17q, and 19 were reported [140]. Nemesure and colleagues performed a genome-wide scan on 1327 individuals of Afro-Caribbean origin from 146 families in Barbados, West Indies, and concluded that POAG in this black population is with high probability linked to regions on the chromosome arms 2q and 10p [79]. Mutations in myocilin or optineurin were excluded as causative for POAG in this population. Overall, it has become very clear that POAG is genetically very complex and that within the general population affected with POAG, many different genes may be causatively involved.

Summary for the Clinician

- Linkage analysis of larger families with autosomal-dominant inherited POAG have led to the discovery of six POAG loci (GLC1A-GLC1F) on different chromosomes
- For two of these loci, the mutated gene has been identified
- Mutations in myocilin are responsible for GLC1A-linked glaucoma, mutations in optineurin cause GLC1E-linked glaucoma

1.3.2
Myocilin

In 1997, Stone and coworkers identified mutations in the myocilin gene as causative for *GLC1A*-linked inherited juvenile open-angle glaucoma [111]. In the meantime, these results have been confirmed by numerous other investigators (for review see [114]). Primary juvenile open-angle glaucoma refers to a subgroup of POAG with autosomal dominant heredity, which is usually accompanied by high intraocular pressure that often requires early surgical treatment [3]. In addition to patients with inherited juvenile open-angle glaucoma, mutations in *MYOC* were observed in 3 % of patients living in the middle west of the USA, which suffered from adult-onset POAG [111]. In a broader study that analyzed the worldwide distribution of mutations in myocilin, 1703 patients from four continents were investigated and mutations in myocilin were found in 2 %–4 % of patients [29].

The product of *MYOC*, the protein myocilin, had originally been identified in studies that were undertaken to analyze proteins, which were inducible by long-term treatment of trabecular meshwork cells with dexamethasone [80, 86]. In this cell culture model for steroid-induced glaucoma, an induction of a specific protein (originally named TIGR, for trabecular meshwork inducible glucocorticoid response protein) was shown at a time course similar to that observed during the manifestation of steroid-induced glaucoma. In parallel and independent studies, Kubota and colleagues identified the same protein in porcine retina and termed it myocilin [63]. This is also the name that was assigned to gene and gene product by the nomenclature committee of HUGO.

The finding that mutations in myocilin cause some subgroups of POAG attracted substantial attention, as for the first time, a specific gene product had been identified that is responsible for the development of at least some forms of POAG. As patients with mutated myocilin can suffer from very high IOP, it appeared to be obvious that more knowledge about the function of myocilin could provide the clue for a better understanding of the molecular mechanisms that cause elevated intraocular pressure in POAG. After all, despite decades of research, the molecular mechanisms involved in the formation of aqueous humor outflow resistance and its increase in POAG are still almost completely unclear.

1.3.2.1
The Structure of Myocilin

Myocilin consists of 504 amino acids and has an approximate molecular weight of 55–57 kDa [80]. At the N-terminus, myocilin contains a signaling sequence as well as motive characteristic for a leucine zipper or a coiled-coil domain (Fig. 1.6). Leucine zippers can form protein dimers by using hydrophobic residues on the amino acid leucine. In addition, two major domains could be identified by sequence alignment: a myosin-like domain at the N-terminus and an olfactomedin-like domain at the C-terminus (Fig. 1.6). The homology of the myosin-like domain is low when compared to myosin, whereas the homology to olfactomedin is substantial (for review see [114]). Olfactomedin is a main component of the mucus layer of the olfactory epithelium in the frog. The homologous protein in mammals, olfactomedin-related glycoprotein was identified in nerve cells of the brain, but also in the kidney and lung, as well as in the ciliary body, cornea, and iris (for review see [114]). The olfactomedin domain of myocilin is highly conserved across mammalian species. Furthermore, most clinically significant mutations occur in this region. Secreted myocilin can form dimers or multimers with a molecular weight of 120–200 kDa [80]. These myocilin-myocilin interactions are probably arranged by the leucine zipper as well as by intermolecular disulfide bonds [26]. In addition, studies of myocilin interactions with optimedin, an olfactomedin-like protein with an olfactomedin domain homologous to that of myocilin, show that these interactions seem to involve the olfactomedin domains of both proteins [126].

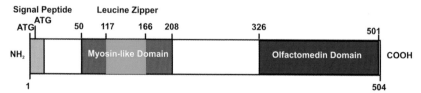

Fig. 1.6. Human myocilin. Colored areas mark the position of the signaling sequence with its two ATG initiation sites, the leucine zipper, and the myosin-like and olfactomedin domains

1.3.2.2
The Localization of Myocilin

In human eyes, mRNA of myocilin has been found in the trabecular meshwork, the retina, the ciliary body, the choroid, and the iris (for review see [114]). The amount of myocilin mRNA in the tissues of the anterior eye is high, whereas only smaller amounts can be isolated from that of the posterior eye segment. Extremely high amounts are observed in the trabecular meshwork [114]. In an un-normalized trabecular meshwork cDNA library generated through the NEIBank project, transcripts for myocilin formed the third most abundant cluster among 3459 independent clones [124]. By immunohistochemistry, myocilin was detected between the collagen fibers of sclera and cornea, as well as in keratocytes and cells of the corneal endothelium [56]. In the trabecular meshwork, staining for myocilin was observed in cells of the uveoscleral and corneoscleral region. In addition, the cells and the extracellular matrix within the cribriform or juxtacanalicular region, were intensely labeled (Fig. 1.7). Electron microscopy showed myocilin to be associated with the sheath-derived plaque material [131], which forms the largest part of the extracellular matrix in this region [73]. Myocilin was also seen in the ciliary epithelium, in the stromal cells of the iris and in the smooth muscle cells of the iris and the ciliary body [56]. Considerable amounts of secreted myocilin were also detected in the aqueous humor of the eye [93].

In the posterior eye segment, an immunostaining for myocilin was seen within the vitreous. In the retina, myocilin was observed at the inner and outer nuclear layer, as well as in axons of the ganglion cells. Staining for myocilin was also detected in axons of the optic nerve in the prelaminar and postlaminar region, as well as in the lamina cribrosa. In addition, myocilin was observed in astrocytes of the glia columns and the cribriform plates of the lamina cribrosa (for review see [114]).

Outside the eye, low amounts of myocilin mRNA were detected in the skeletal muscle, heart, mammary gland, thymus, prostate, testis, small intestine, colon, thyroid, trachea, and bone marrow (for review see [114]). Only little is known about the exact localization of myocilin in these organs. Recent data of our laboratory indicate that the broad distribution of myocilin throughout the body may be partly caused by a strong expression of myocilin in Schwann cells of peripheral nerves. Immunohistochemistry showed immunoreactivity for myocilin in paranodal terminal loops of the nodes of Ranvier, and outer mesaxons and basal/abaxonal regions of the myelin sheath [82]. Double-labeling experiments with antibodies against myelin basic protein showed no overlapping, while overlapping immunoreactivity was observed with antibodies against myelin-associated glycoprotein. By northern blotting, the mRNA levels for myocilin in peripheral nerves and the eye were comparable.

It is remarkable that myocilin has such a broad distribution in the body and in different tissues of the eye, while patients with a mutation in myocilin have only an elevated risk for glaucoma and apparently not for any other diseases. Outside the eye, mutations in myocilin are obviously compensated for by other mechanisms. This assumption is supported by investigations of homozygous mice with a targeted null-mutation for myocilin (myocilin knock-out). These animals are fertile and viable, and do not show a pathological phenotype [58].

Fig. 1.7. Immunohistochemistry for myocilin in the trabecular meshwork of a 64-year-old human donor. Positive labeling is seen in trabecular meshwork cells covering the corneoscleral lamellae (CS, *open arrows*), and in cells and extracellular matrix of the cribriform or juxta-canalicular region (JCT, *solid arrows*) directly adjacent to Schlemm's canal (SC, original magnification, ×600). (Reproduced from [115], with permission)

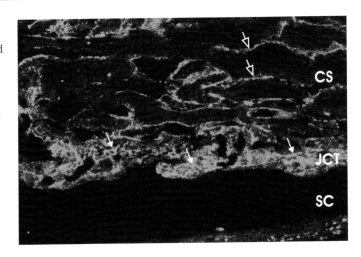

1.3.2.3
Myocilin and Aqueous Humor Outflow

Depending on the respective localization of a disease-causing mutation in the myocilin gene, most of the patients suffer from higher IOP and a more severe course of the disease than patients with other types of glaucoma. This phenotype of the affected patients indicates that mutated myocilin influences directly or indirectly the normal outflow of aqueous humor through the trabecular meshwork. It is unclear though, if normal myocilin is important for aqueous humor outflow under physiological conditions. The data from *Myoc*-deficient mice with a targeted null-mutation for myocilin (myocilin knock-out) indicate that myocilin is not essential to generate a normal outflow resistance for aqueous humor, as the mice do not show structural abnormalities at the chamber angle and have normal intraocular pressures [58]. Still, it needs to be considered that there are similarities, but also marked differences in the anatomical structures of the chamber angle between mice and humans, which have been reviewed recently [114]. The most pronounced differences relate to the fact that the ciliary muscle is relatively large in size in humans, but only vestigial in mice. Consequently, there is no comparable influence of ciliary muscle tone on trabecular meshwork structure and function in the mouse eye, as it is in humans and primates with

a highly developed accommodative system. During accommodation, the human trabecular meshwork is continuously stretched and structurally remodeled, which correlates with the observation that there are much more extracellular fibrillar matrix components relative to the size of the meshwork in the human than in the mouse eye. In addition, there is experimental evidence that stretch of trabecular meshwork cells in vitro and in situ causes significant changes in its gene expression [130]. Moreover, the expression of myocilin is upregulated in human trabecular meshwork cells after mechanical stretch in vitro and in situ after stretch due to increased perfusion pressure in perfused anterior eye segment organ culture [13, 117]. In the living eye, similarly increased amounts of myocilin could well influence the outflow resistance of the trabecular meshwork and be more relevant in the human than in the mouse eye.

1.3.2.4
Myocilin and Steroid-Induced Elevated IOP

The strong induction of myocilin after treatment of human trabecular meshwork cells with dexamethasone, clearly indicates that there is a direct association between the induction of myocilin and the onset of steroid-induced glaucoma. In vitro, an approximately 90-fold induction of myocilin mRNA was observed in trabecular meshwork cells after treatment with dexamethasone for 3 days [117]. An association between myocilin and steroid-induced glaucoma is also supported by electron microscopy of surgical samples from glaucoma patients. These studies demonstrated morphological changes in the trabecular meshwork of patients with steroid-induced glaucoma that were highly similar to those of patients with juvenile glaucoma [33, 49]. Both forms of glaucoma showed a characteristic increase of the extracellular matrix in the trabecular meshwork. Comparable ultrastructural changes were also seen in the trabecular meshwork of monkeys that were treated with cortisol acetate for one year [19]. Still, up until now, a direct association of myocilin with the newly formed extracellular matrix has not been shown and, so far, there is no evidence that myocilin is directly involved in the structural and functional changes of steroid-induced glaucoma. In theory, an increased synthesis of myocilin could directly cause the glaucomatous changes, but it might well occur parallel to and independently from the real disease-causing mechanisms.

1.3.2.5
Myocilin in Late-Onset POAG

Immunohistochemical investigations concerning the localization of myocilin in the trabecular meshwork of patients with late-onset POAG, normal tension glaucoma, and pseudoexfoliation glaucoma showed an increase in immunoreactivity for myocilin in the trabecular meshwork in combination with an increased staining for αB-crystallin [74]. αB-crystallin is a molecular chaperon that is inducible by heat-shock, oxidative stress, and treatment with transforming growth factor-β1 (TGF-β) [116, 138]. Such an expression is also observed for myocilin after treatment with TGF-β1 and H_2O_2 [86, 117]. Myocilin is also induced in trabecular meshwork cells by mechanical stress [117]. It is tempting to speculate that some of these factors are involved in the increased expression of myocilin in eyes of patients with POAG. In support of this, the levels of TGF-β1 in the aqueous humor of patients with POAG are elevated when compared to normals [129] and an elevated IOP

should cause an increased mechanical tension and stretch of the trabecular meshwork. Still, as long as we do not know if and why the resistance in the trabecular meshwork is influenced by myocilin, it will remain unclear, if the increased staining for myocilin in the trabecular meshwork of patients with POAG is cause or symptom of this disease.

1.3.2.6
Myocilin and the Resistance to Flow in the Trabecular Meshwork

To investigate the influence of myocilin on the resistance of aqueous humor outflow, recombinant myocilin was produced in a bacterial expression system and isolated by Fautsch and Johnson [27]. The addition of 25 µg recombinant myocilin to culture medium of perfused anterior eye segments caused a significant increase in aqueous humor outflow resistance. However, the mechanism of protein biosynthesis in prokaryotic, bacterial expression systems differs from that in eucaryotic cells. Bacteria do not have an endoplasmatic reticulum and do not undertake certain post-translational protein modifications, i.e. glycosylation. To clarify, if eucaryotic myocilin also shows a comparable influence on outflow resistance, Goldwich and coworkers tested the influence of a C-terminal fragment of myocilin, purified from an eucaryotic expression system, on trabecular meshwork outflow facility [38]. The myocilin fragment contained the entire olfactomedin domain, which appears to be important for the function of myocilin. Perfusion with the recombinant myocilin fragment containing this domain did not change outflow facility. It is possible that post-translational modifications of myocilin may have a major impact on protein function. Alternatively, both the olfactomedin and N-terminal domains (including the leucine zipper), which has been shown to be important in dimer and multimer formation, must be present for myocilin to have full function. Multimer formation would be expected to be efficient at influencing aqueous outflow dynamics, particularly if it were to occur within the narrow flow regions of the juxtacanalicular tissue. Additionally, the N-terminal region of the protein may contain binding sequences for extracellular matrix proteins, and the interaction of myocilin with extracellular proteins could be important in determining outflow facility. For example, myocilin is known to bind to the HepII domain of fibronectin, although a specific binding sequence on myocilin has not yet been identified [28].

A different experimental approach was chosen by Russell and coworkers to gain a better understanding of the influence of myocilin on aqueous humor outflow [93]. Their studies were based on earlier investigations in which unknown proteins within the aqueous humor blocked the flow through polycarbon filters with a pore diameter of 0.2 µm (analogous to the pore diameter within the trabecular meshwork) [51]. In a retrial of these experiments, it was observed that myocilin was bound to the filters that were blocked by aqueous humor. Myocilin in the aqueous humor is obviously involved in the blocking of polycarbon filters when perfused with aqueous humor. This indicates that myocilin has the tendency to decrease aqueous humor flow rather than to increase it; however, the mechanisms for this decrease are completely unclear. Myocilin might interact with other proteins and block the pores of the filters by forming larger aggregates.

1.3.2.7
Characteristics of Mutated Myocilin

In many diseases that are caused by point mutations, the synthesis of the affected polypeptide is not disturbed but rather the three-dimensional folding of the protein or its stability. Most secreted proteins are folded in the endoplasmatic reticulum (ER) where special proteins are localized to support correct folding. If protein folding in the ER is perturbed, incorrectly folded proteins are detected by the control mechanisms in the ER and subsequently eliminated. A well studied example for such a process is cystic fibrosis [61]. In these patients, the incorrect gene product remains within the ER and is not transported to the cellular surface. Experimental data suggest a similar scenario for myocilin. In cultured trabecular meshwork cells, myocilin containing typical glaucoma-associated muta-

tions is not secreted but withhold within the cytoplasm [46]. Under normal conditions, incorrectly folded proteins are degraded via proteasomes. In certain cases, however, this mechanism does not function. Mutated or incorrectly folded proteins accumulate in the ER, block the physiological secretion pathway and cause dysfunction of the ER that can result in cell death [139]. A similar scenario that finally leads to a loss of trabecular meshwork function might happen in patients with mutated myocilin, but so far, direct experimental support of this is lacking.

Summary for the Clinician

- Mutations in myocilin are responsible for GLC1A-linked autosomal dominant inherited juvenile POAG, and 2%–4% of cases with adult-onset POAG
- Myocilin is a secreted glycoprotein that is expressed in very high amounts in the trabecular meshwork
- So far, a specific function of myocilin has not been identified, but some experiments indicate that it might play a role in the modulation of aqueous humor outflow resistance
- Depending on the site of mutation, patients with mutations in myocilin may suffer from very high intraocular pressure
- In cultured trabecular meshwork cells, mutated myocilin is not secreted but withheld within the cell. In glaucoma patients with mutated myocilin, a similar scenario might lead to a loss of trabecular meshwork function

1.3.3
Optineurin

1.3.3.1
Genetic Findings

A missense mutation in the *OPTN* gene was identified in affected members of the family, in which glaucoma had been shown to segregate as an autosomal dominant trait with the *GLC1E* locus on chromosome 10p14-p15 [91]. This mutation resulted in a Glu^{50}Lys (E50 K) amino acid change in the protein optineurin. In a subsequent broader search of 54 additional families with autosomal dominant POAG, the E50 K mutation was again found in some of the families. Two additional mutations were identified in two other families. The majority of the families that were investigated presented with normal intraocular pressures (IOP) (<22 mm Hg), whereas others had mixed clinical pictures of both normal and moderately raised IOP (23–26 mm Hg). So far, no other report has been published, which shows mutations in optineurin in POAG patients different from that investigated by Rezaie and coworkers. Tang and colleagues investigated 148 unrelated Japanese patients with normal pressure glaucoma, 165 patients with POAG, and 196 unrelated controls, and did not find glaucoma-specific mutations in the *OPTN* gene [118]. Forsman et al. investigated eight Finnish families with open-angle glaucoma, in which glaucoma was diagnosed in 53 subjects, and did not find evidence for disease causing mutations in *OPTN* [31].

1.3.3.2
Localization and Functional Roles of Optineurin

OPTN contains three noncoding exons in the 5'-untranslated region and 13 exons that code for a 577-amino acid protein. Alternative splicing generates different isoforms, but all have the same reading frame. The E50 K mutation is located within a putative basic region leucine zipper (bZIP) motif, which is typically involved in DNA binding or protein dimerization. The bZIP motif is conserved in sequences from mouse, cow, and monkey. The expression of mRNA for optineurin has been shown in heart, brain, placenta, liver, skeletal muscle, and pancreas. In the eye, optineurin transcripts were detected by RT-PCR in the trabecular meshwork, nonpigmented ciliary epithelium and retina. Rezaie and coworkers generated antibodies against optineurin and detected its presence in the aqueous humor, which would suggest that optineurin is a secreted protein [91]. Cultured cells showed staining in vesicular structures and the Golgi apparatus, consistent with the idea of a secreted protein. An association of optineurin with the Golgi apparatus was also found by other authors [112].

Optineurin had originally been identified as FIP-2. FIP-2 was shown to block the anti-apoptotic activity of adenovirus E3–14.7 K on tumor necrosis factor-α (TNF-α)-mediated cell death [67]. In addition, the expression of FIP-2 was induced by TNF-α treatment in a time-dependent manner [67]. TNF-α secreted by glial cells was shown to facilitate the apoptotic death of retinal ganglion cells, while retinal ganglion cell apoptosis was attenuated approximately 66% by a neutralizing antibody against TNF-α [121]. In the optic nerve heads of patients with POAG, the expression of both TNF-α and its receptor TNF-R1 were found to be upregulated, and appeared to parallel the progression of optic nerve degeneration [147]. Because of the induction of FIP-2 by TNF-α, the links between TNF-α and retinal ganglion cell death, and the fact that mutations in *OPTN* were identified in a considerable number of patients with normal pressure glaucoma, Rezaie and collaborators speculated that optineurin may play a neuroprotective role in the eye, but when defective contributes to the glaucomatous optic neuropathy [91].

Other functions for optineurin are suggested by the observation that FIP-2 was reported to link Huntingtin (a Huntington's disease protein) to the Rab8 protein to form a complex that is supposed to regulate membrane trafficking and cellular morphogenesis [43].

Vittitow and Borrás investigated the effects of TNF-α, dexamethasone, and elevated perfusion pressure on optineurin mRNA expression in the trabecular meshwork of anterior segment perfused organ cultures [135]. Using normalized RT-PCR, the authors found that treatment with TNF-α and dexamethasone moderately induced the expression of optineurin. In addition, after raising the perfusion pressure at relatively high levels (ΔP of 35 mmHg) for 2, 4 and 7 days, a substantial increase in optineurin mRNA was observed at longer perfusion times. These results were not confirmed in parallel studies by Kamphuis and Schneemann, who used a similar perfusion system and quantitative real-time PCR [55]. In their experiments, raising the perfusion pressure from 10 to 30 mmHg for periods ranging between 1 and 24 h did not cause significant changes in the amount of optineurin mRNA. So far, any functional roles of optineurin in the trabecular meshwork are unclear.

Summary for the Clinician

- Mutations in optineurin are causative for GLC1E-linked autosomal-dominant inherited POAG
- A considerable number of patients with mutations in optineurin suffer from normal pressure glaucoma
- The specific ocular function(s) of optineurin has/have not been identified

1.4
Genes and Pigmentary Glaucoma

Pigmentary glaucoma is a condition that characteristically develops in young myopic patients suffering from pigment dispersion syndrome [14]. Melanin granules are liberated from the iris pigment epithelium and carried by aqueous humor into the anterior chamber, where they become deposited in the trabecular meshwork. The accumulation of pigment in the trabecular meshwork leads to an increase in outflow resistance that may result in the development of glaucoma. Andersen and coworkers studied 54 members of four families in which pigment dispersion syndrome and pigmentary glaucoma was inherited as an autosomal dominant trait [4]. The gene, which is responsible for pigment dispersion syndrome in these four families was mapped to the telomeric end of the long arm of chromosome 7 (i.e., 7q35-q36). So far, the nature of this gene is unknown. John and colleagues identified a mouse strain (DBA/2 J mice) with iris stroma atrophy and pigment dispersion quite similar to the situation in humans [48]. Intraocular pressure increases with age in DBA/2 J mice, which finally develop glaucoma. Iris pigment dispersion in DBA/2 J mice was subsequently found to result from mutations in the *Gpnmb* gene, while the iris stroma atrophy in these animals is caused by the recessive *Tyrp1*[b] mutant allele [6]. The predicted full-length GP-NMB and TYRP1 proteins contain several motifs common to melanosomal proteins. It has been hypothesized that mutations in the *Gpnmb*

and *Tyrp1* genes alter melanosomes, allowing pigment production to occur while cytotoxic intermediates of pigment production escape, inducing iris disease, changes in the chamber angle and subsequently glaucoma. The structural anomalies in the chamber angle of DBA/2 J mice appear to be induced by marked anterior synechiae, which completely occlude trabecular meshwork and Schlemm's canal. Marked structural changes in the trabecular meshwork have also been observed in specimens from patients with pigmentary glaucoma, which appeared relatively acellular with collapse of the trabecular sheets. Cells covering the trabecular sheets were filled with pigment and showed various stages of degeneration, while the intertrabecular spaces contained free pigment granules as well as cell debris [92, 105]. While a comparable mechanism may be responsible for the development of pigmentary glaucoma in humans and DBA/2 J mice, different genes are likely to be affected. The *GPNMD* coding region from the affected individuals of an autosomal dominant form of pigment dispersion syndrome was sequenced and no mutations were detected. Known human *TRRP1* mutations cause OCA3, a form of oculocutaneous albinism with no reported increased risk of pigmentary glaucoma.

References

1. Akarsu AN, Turacli ME, Aktan SG, Barsoum-Homsy M, Chevrette L, Sayli BS, Sarfarazi M (1996) A second locus (GLC3B) for primary congenital glaucoma (Buphthalmos) maps to the 1p36 region. Hum Mol Genet 5:1199–1203
2. Alward WL (2000) Axenfeld-Rieger syndrome in the age of molecular genetics. Am J Ophthalmol 130:107–115
3. Alward WL, Fingert JH, Coote MA, Johnson AT, Lerner SF, Junqua D, Durcan FJ, McCartney PJ, Mackey DA, Sheffield VC, Stone EM (1998) Clinical features associated with mutations in the chromosome 1 open-angle glaucoma gene (GLC1A). N Engl J Med 338:1022–1027
4. Andersen JS, Pralea AM, DelBono EA, Haines JL, Gorin MB, Schuman JS, Mattox CG, Wiggs JL (1997) A gene responsible for the pigment dispersion syndrome maps to chromosome 7q35-q36. Arch Ophthalmol 115:384–388

5. Anderson DR (1981) The development of the tra-becular meshwork and its abnormality in primary infantile glaucoma. Trans Am Ophthalmol Soc 79:458–485

6. Anderson MG, Smith RS, Hawes NL, Zabaleta A, Chang B, Wiggs JL, John SW (2002) Mutations in genes encoding melanosomal proteins cause pigmentary glaucoma in DBA/2J mice. Nat Genet 30:81–85

7. Ashery-Padan R, Gruss P (2001) Pax6 lights-up the way for eye development. Curr Opin Cell Biol 13:706–714

8. Baulmann DC, Ohlmann A, Flügel-Koch C, Goswami S, Cvekl A, Tamm ER (2002) Pax6 heterozygous eyes show defects in chamber angle differentiation that are associated with a wide spectrum of other anterior eye segment abnormalities. Mech Dev 118:3–17

9. Beebe DC, Coats JM (2000) The lens organizes the anterior segment: specification of neural crest cell differentiation in the avian eye. Dev Biol 220:424–431

10. Bejjani BA, Lewis RA, Tomey KF, Anderson KL, Dueker DK, Jabak M, Astle WF, Otterud B, Leppert M, Lupski JR (1998) Mutations in CYP1B1, the gene for cytochrome P4501B1, are the predominant cause of primary congenital glaucoma in Saudi Arabia. Am J Hum Genet 62:325–333

11. Bejjani BA, Stockton DW, Lewis RA, Tomey KF, Dueker DK, Jabak M, Astle WF, Lupski JR (2000) Multiple CYP1B1 mutations and incomplete penetrance in an inbred population segregating primary congenital glaucoma suggest frequent de novo events and a dominant modifier locus. Hum Mol Genet 9:367–374

12. Bejjani BA, Xu L, Armstrong D, Lupski JR, Reneker LW (2002) Expression patterns of cytochrome P4501B1 (Cyp1b1) in FVB/N mouse eyes. Exp Eye Res 75:249–257

13. Borrás T, Rowlette LL, Tamm ER, Gottanka J, Epstein DL (2002) Effects of elevated intraocular pressure on outflow facility and TIGR/MYOC expression in perfused human anterior segments. Invest Ophthalmol Vis Sci 43:33–40

14. Campbell DG, Schertzer RM (1996) Pigmentary glaucoma. In:Ritch R, Shields MB, Krupin T (eds) The glaucomas. Clinical Science. Mosby, St. Louis, p2

15. Catalano RA, Nelson LB, Schaffer DB (1988) Oculocutaneous albinism associated with congenital glaucoma. Ophthalmic Paediatr Genet 9:5–6

16. Chang B, Smith RS, Peters M, Savinova OV, Hawes NL, Zabaleta A, Nusinowitz S, Martin JE, Davisson ML, Cepko CL, Hogan BL, John SW (2001) Haploinsufficient Bmp4 ocular phenotypes include anterior segment dysgenesis with elevated intraocular pressure. BMC Genet 2:18

17. Charliat G, Jolly D, Blanchard F (1994) Genetic risk factor in primary open-angle glaucoma: a case-control study. Ophthalmic Epidemiol 1:131–138

18. Chow RL, Lang RA (2001) Early eye development in vertebrates. Annu Rev Cell Dev Biol 17:255–296

19. Clark AF, Steely HT, Dickerson JE, English-Wright S, Stropki K, McCartney MD, Jacobson N, Shepard AR, Clark JI, Matsushima H, Peskind ER, Leverenz JB, Wilkinson CW, Swiderski RE, Fingert JH, Sheffield VC, Stone EM (2001) Glucocorticoid induction of the glaucoma gene MYOC in human and monkey trabecular meshwork cells and tissues. Invest Ophthalmol Vis Sci 42:1769–1780

20. Collinson JM, Quinn JC, Hill RE, West JD (2003) The roles of Pax6 in the cornea, retina, and olfactory epithelium of the developing mouse embryo. Dev Biol 255:303–312

21. Davis JA, Reed RR (1996) Role of Olf-1 and Pax-6 transcription factors in neurodevelopment. J Neurosci 16:5082–5094

22. Doward W, Perveen R, Lloyd IC, Ridgway AE, Wilson L, Black GC (1999) A mutation in the RIEG1 gene associated with Peters' anomaly. J Med Genet 36:152–155

23. Dreyer SD, Zhou G, Baldini A, Winterpacht A, Zabel B, Cole W, Johnson RL, Lee B (1998) Mutations in LMX1B cause abnormal skeletal patterning and renal dysplasia in nail patella syndrome. Nat Genet 19:47–50

24. Duke-Elder S, Cook C (1963) Normal and Abnormal Development. Part 1. Embryology. Henry Kimpton, London, pp164–170

25. Düblin I (1970) Comparative embryologic studies of the early development of the cornea and the pupillary membrane in reptiles, birds and mammals. Acta Anat (Basel) 76:381–408

26. Fautsch MP, Johnson DH (2001) Characterization of myocilin-myocilin interactions. Invest Ophthalmol Vis Sci 42:2324–2331

27. Fautsch MP, Bahler CK, Jewison DJ, Johnson DH (2000) Recombinant TIGR/MYOC increases outflow resistance in the human anterior segment. Invest Ophthalmol Vis Sci 41:4163–4168

28. Filla MS, Liu X, Nguyen TD, Polansky JR, Brandt CR, Kaufman PL, Peters DM (2002) In vitro localization of TIGR/MYOC in trabecular meshwork extracellular matrix and binding to fibronectin. Invest Ophthalmol Vis Sci 43:151–161

29. Fingert JH, Héon E, Liebmann JM, Yamamoto T, Craig JE, Rait J, Kawase K, Hoh ST, Buys YM, Dickinson J, Hockey RR, Williams-Lyn D, Trope G, Kitazawa Y, Ritch R, Mackey DA, Alward WL, Sheffield VC, Stone EM (1999) Analysis of myocilin mutations in 1703 glaucoma patients from five different populations. Hum Mol Genet 8:899–905

30. Flügel-Koch C, Ohlmann A, Piatigorsky J, Tamm ER (2002) Overexpression of TGF-β1 alters early development of cornea and lens in transgenic mice. Dev Dyn 225:111–125

31. Forsman E, Lemmelä S, Varilo T, Kristo P, Forsius H, Sankila EM, Järvelä I (2003) The role of TIGR and OPTN in Finnish glaucoma families: a clinical and molecular genetic study. Mol Vis 9:217–222

32. Francois J (1980) Congenital glaucoma and its inheritance. Ophthalmologica 181:61–73

33. Furuyoshi N, Furuyoshi M, Futa R, Gottanka J, Lütjen-Drecoll E (1997) Ultrastructural changes in the trabecular meshwork of juvenile glaucoma. Ophthalmologica 211:140–146

34. Gage PJ, Suh H, Camper SA (1999) Dosage requirement of Pitx2 for development of multiple organs. Development 126:4643–4651

35. Gehring WJ, Ikeo K (1999) Pax 6: mastering eye morphogenesis and eye evolution. Trends Genet 15:371–377

36. Gencik A (1989) Epidemiology and genetics of primary congenital glaucoma in Slovakia. Description of a form of primary congenital glaucoma in gypsies with autosomal-recessive inheritance and complete penetrance. Dev Ophthalmol 16:76–115

37. Glaser T, Walton DS, Maas RL (1992) Genomic structure, evolutionary conservation and aniridia mutations in the human PAX6 gene. Nat Genet 2:232–239

38. Goldwich A, Ethier CR, Chan DW, Tamm ER (2003) Perfusion with the olfactomedin domain of myocilin does not affect outflow facility. Invest Ophthalmol Vis Sci 44:1953–1961

39. Gottanka J, Johnson DH, Martus P, Lütjen-Drecoll E (1997) Severity of optic nerve damage in eyes with POAG is correlated with changes in the trabecular meshwork. J Glaucoma 6:123–132

40. Gould DB, John SW (2002) Anterior segment dysgenesis and the developmental glaucomas are complex traits. Hum Mol Genet 11:1185–1193

41. Grant WM, Walton DS (1974) Progressive changes in the angle in congenital aniridia, with development of glaucoma. Am J Ophthalmol 78:842–847

42. Grindley JC, Davidson DR, Hill RE (1995) The role of Pax-6 in eye and nasal development. Development 121:1433–1442

43. Hattula K, Peranen J (2000) FIP-2, a coiled-coil protein, links Huntingtin to Rab8 and modulates cellular morphogenesis. Curr Biol 10:1603–1606

44. Hohlbach LM, Hinzpeter EN, Naumann GOH (1997) Kornea und Sklera. In:Naumann GOH (ed) Pathologie des Auges. Springer, Berlin, Heidelberg, pp507–692

45. Honkanen RA, Nishimura DY, Swiderski RE, Bennett SR, Hong S, Kwon YH, Stone EM, Sheffield VC, Alward WL (2003) A family with Axenfeld-Rieger syndrome and Peters Anomaly caused by a point mutation (Phe112Ser) in the FOXC1 gene. Am J Ophthalmol 135:368–375

46. Jacobson N, Andrews M, Shepard AR, Nishimura D, Searby C, Fingert JH, Hageman G, Mullins R, Davidson BL, Kwon YH, Alward WL, Stone EM, Clark AF, Sheffield VC (2001) Non-secretion of mutant proteins of the glaucoma gene myocilin in cultured trabecular meshwork cells and in aqueous humor. Hum Mol Genet 10:117–125

47. Jamieson RV, Perveen R, Kerr B, Carette M, Yardley J, Heon E, Wirth MG, van Heyningen V, Donnai D, Munier F, Black GC (2002) Domain disruption and mutation of the bZIP transcription factor, MAF, associated with cataract, ocular anterior segment dysgenesis and coloboma. Hum Mol Genet 11:33–42

48. John SW, Smith RS, Savinova OV, Hawes NL, Chang B, Turnbull D, Davisson M, Roderick TH, Heckenlively JR (1998) Essential iris atrophy, pigment dispersion, and glaucoma in DBA/2J mice. Invest Ophthalmol Vis Sci 39:951–962

49. Johnson D, Gottanka J, Flügel C, Hoffmann F, Futa R, Lütjen-Drecoll E (1997) Ultrastructural changes in the trabecular meshwork of human eyes treated with corticosteroids. Arch Ophthalmol 115:375–383

50. Johnson M, Erickson K (2000) Mechanisms and routes of aqueous humor drainage. In:Albert DM, Jakobiec FA (eds) Principles and practice of ophthalmology. W.B. Saunders, Philadelphia, pp 2577–2595

51. Johnson M, Ethier CR, Kamm RD, Grant WM, Epstein DL, Gaasterland D (1986) The flow of aqueous humor through micro-porous filters. Invest Ophthalmol Vis Sci 27:92–97

52. Johnston MC, Noden DM, Hazelton RD, Coulombre JL, Coulombre AJ (1979) Origins of avian ocular and periocular tissues. Exp Eye Res 29:27–43

53. Jordan T, Hanson I, Zaletayev D, Hodgson S, Prosser J, Seawright A, Hastie N, van Heyningen V (1992) The human PAX6 gene is mutated in two patients with aniridia. Nat Genet 1:328–332

54. Kakiuchi-Matsumoto T, Isashiki Y, Ohba N, Kimura K, Sonoda S, Unoki K (2001) Cytochrome P450 1B1 gene mutations in Japanese patients with primary congenital glaucoma(1). Am J Ophthalmol 131:345–350

55. Kamphuis W, Schneemann A (2003) Optineurin gene expression level in human trabecular meshwork does not change in response to pressure elevation. Ophthalmic Res 35:93–96

56. Karali A, Russell P, Stefani FH, Tamm ER (2000) Localization of myocilin/trabecular meshwork-inducible glucocorticoid response protein in the human eye. Invest Ophthalmol Vis Sci 41:729–740

57. Kidson SH, Kume T, Deng K, Winfrey V, Hogan BL (1999) The forkhead/winged-helix gene, Mf1, is necessary for the normal development of the cornea and formation of the anterior chamber in the mouse eye. Dev Biol 211:306–322

58. Kim BS, Savinova OV, Reedy MV, Martin J, Lun Y, Gan L, Smith RS, Tomarev SI, John SW, Johnson RL (2001) Targeted disruption of the myocilin gene (Myoc) suggests that human glaucoma-causing mutations are gain of function. Mol Cell Biol 21:7707–7713

59. Kitsos G, Eiberg H, Economou-Petersen E, Wirtz MK, Kramer PL, Aspiotis M, Tommerup N, Petersen MB, Psilas K (2001) Genetic linkage of autosomal dominant primary open angle glaucoma to chromosome 3q in a Greek pedigree. Eur J Hum Genet 9:452–457

60. Kolmer W (1936) Entwicklung des Auges. In: Kolmer W, Lauber H (eds) Handbuch der mikroskopischen Anatomie des Menschen, Haut und Siinesorgane. Part 2:Auge. Verlag von Julius Springer, Berlin, pp 623–676

61. Kopito RR (1999) Biosynthesis and degradation of CFTR. Physiol Rev 79:S167–173

62. Koroma BM, Yang JM, Sundin OH (1997) The Pax-6 homeobox gene is expressed throughout the corneal and conjunctival epithelia. Invest Ophthalmol Vis Sci 38:108–120

63. Kubota R, Noda S, Wang Y, Minoshima S, Asakawa S, Kudoh J, Mashima Y, Oguchi Y, Shimizu N (1997) A novel myosin-like protein (myocilin) expressed in the connecting cilium of the photoreceptor: molecular cloning, tissue expression, and chromosomal mapping. Genomics 41:360–369

64. Kume T, Deng KY, Winfrey V, Gould DB, Walter MA, Hogan BL (1998) The forkhead/winged helix gene Mf1 is disrupted in the pleiotropic mouse mutation congenital hydrocephalus. Cell 93:985–996

65. Leske MC, Connell AM, Schachat AP, Hyman L (1994) The Barbados Eye Study. Prevalence of open angle glaucoma. Arch Ophthalmol 112:821–829

66. Leske MC, Connell AM, Wu SY, Hyman LG, Schachat AP (1995) Risk factors for open-angle glaucoma. The Barbados Eye Study. Arch Ophthalmol 113:918–924

67. Li Y, Kang J, Horwitz MS (1998) Interaction of an adenovirus E3 14.7-kilodalton protein with a novel tumor necrosis factor alpha-inducible cellular protein containing leucine zipper domains. Mol Cell Biol 18:1601–1610

68. Libby RT, Smith RS, Savinova OV, Zabaleta A, Martin JE, Gonzalez FJ, John SW (2003) Modification of ocular defects in mouse developmental glaucoma models by tyrosinase. Science 299:1578–1581

69. Lichter PR, Richards JE, Downs CA, Stringham HM, Boehnke M, Farley FA (1997) Cosegregation of open-angle glaucoma and the nail-patella syndrome. Am J Ophthalmol 124:506–515

70. Lin CR, Kioussi C, O'Connell S, Briata P, Szeto D, Liu F, Izpisúa-Belmonte JC, Rosenfeld MG (1999) Pitx2 regulates lung asymmetry, cardiac positioning and pituitary and tooth morphogenesis. Nature 401:279–282

71. Lines MA, Kozlowski K, Walter MA (2002) Molecular genetics of Axenfeld-Rieger malformations. Hum Mol Genet 11:1177–1184

72. Lu MF, Pressman C, Dyer R, Johnson RL, Martin JF (1999) Function of Rieger syndrome gene in left-right asymmetry and craniofacial development. Nature 401:276–278

73. Lütjen-Drecoll E, Shimizu T, Rohrbach M, Rohen JW (1986) Quantitative analysis of 'plaque material' in the inner- and outer wall of Schlemm's canal in normal- and glaucomatous eyes. Exp Eye Res 42:443–455

74. Lütjen-Drecoll E, May CA, Polansky JR, Johnson DH, Bloemendal H, Nguyen TD (1998) Localization of the stress proteins alpha B-crystallin and trabecular meshwork inducible glucocorticoid response protein in normal and glaucomatous trabecular meshwork. Invest Ophthalmol Vis Sci 39:517–525

75. Margo CE (1983) Congenital aniridia: a histopathologic study of the anterior segment in children. J Pediatr Ophthalmol Strabismus 20:192–198

76. Mason RP, Kosoko O, Wilson MR, Martone JF, Cowan CL, Gear JC, Ross-Degnan D (1989) National survey of the prevalence and risk factors of glaucoma in St. Lucia, West Indies. Part I. Prevalence findings. Ophthalmology 96:1363–1368

77. Maul E, Strozzi L, Muñoz C, Reyes C (1980) The outflow pathway in congenital glaucoma. Am J Ophthalmol 89:667–673

78. Michels-Rautenstrauss KG, Mardin CY, Zenker M, Jordan N, Gusek-Schneider GC, Rautenstrauss BW (2001) Primary congenital glaucoma: three case reports on novel mutations and combinations of mutations in the GLC3A (CYP1B1) gene. J Glaucoma 10:354–357

79. Nemesure B, Jiao X, He Q, Leske MC, Wu SY, Hennis A, Mendell N, Redman J, Garchon HJ, Agarwala R, Schaffer AA, Hejtmancik F (2003) A genome-wide scan for primary open-angle glaucoma (POAG): the Barbados family study of open-angle glaucoma. Hum Genet 112:600–609

80. Nguyen TD, Chen P, Huang WD, Chen H, Johnson D, Polansky JR (1998) Gene structure and properties of TIGR, an olfactomedin-related glycoprotein cloned from glucocorticoid-induced trabecular meshwork cells. J Biol Chem 273:6341–6350

81. Nishimura DY, Swiderski RE, Alward WL, Searby CC, Patil SR, Bennet SR, Kanis AB, Gastier JM, Stone EM, Sheffield VC (1998) The forkhead transcription factor gene FKHL7 is responsible for glaucoma phenotypes which map to 6p25. Nat Genet 19:140–147

82. Ohlmann A, Goldwich A, Flügel-Koch C, Fuchs AV, Schwager K, Tamm ER (2003) Secreted glycoprotein myocilin is a component of the myelin sheath in peripheral nerves. Glia 43:128–140

83. Ormestad M, Blixt A, Churchill A, Martinsson T, Enerbäck S, Carlsson P (2002) Foxe3 haploinsufficiency in mice: a model for Peters' anomaly. Invest Ophthalmol Vis Sci 43:1350–1357

84. Perveen R, Lloyd IC, Clayton-Smith J, Churchill A, van Heyningen V, Hanson I, Taylor D, McKeown C, Super M, Kerr B, Winter R, Black GC (2000) Phenotypic variability and asymmetry of Rieger syndrome associated with PITX2 mutations. Invest Ophthalmol Vis Sci 41:2456–2460

85. Picht G, Welge-Luessen U, Grehn F, Lütjen-Drecoll E (2001) Transforming growth factor beta 2 levels in the aqueous humor in different types of glaucoma and the relation to filtering bleb development. Graefes Arch Clin Exp Ophthalmol 239:199–207

86. Polansky JR, Fauss DJ, Chen P, Chen H, Lütjen-Drecoll E, Johnson D, Kurtz RM, Ma ZD, Bloom E, Nguyen TD (1997) Cellular pharmacology and molecular biology of the trabecular meshwork inducible glucocorticoid response gene product. Ophthalmologica 211:126–139

87. Pressman CL, Chen H, Johnson RL (2000) LMX1B, a LIM homeodomain class transcription factor, is necessary for normal development of multiple tissues in the anterior segment of the murine eye. Genesis 26:15–25

88. Prosser J, van Heyningen V (1998) PAX6 mutations reviewed. Hum Mutat 11:93–108

89. Ramaesh T, Collinson JM, Ramaesh K, Kaufman MH, West JD, Dhillon B (2003) Corneal abnormalities in Pax6+/- small eye mice mimic human aniridia-related keratopathy. Invest Ophthalmol Vis Sci 44:1871–1878

90. Remé C, d'Epinay SL (1981) Periods of development of the normal human chamber angle. Doc Ophthalmol 51:241–268

91. Rezaie T, Child A, Hitchings R, Brice G, Miller L, Coca-Prados M, Heon E, Krupin T, Ritch R, Kreutzer D, Crick RP, Sarfarazi M (2002) Adult-onset primary open-angle glaucoma caused by mutations in optineurin. Science 295:1077–1079

92. Richardson TM, Hutchinson BT, Grant WM (1977) The outflow tract in pigmentary glaucoma: a light and electron microscopic study. Arch Ophthalmol 95:1015–1025

93. Russell P, Tamm ER, Grehn FJ, Picht G, Johnson M (2001) The presence and properties of myocilin in the aqueous humor. Invest Ophthalmol Vis Sci 42:983–986

94. Saika S, Liu CY, Azhar M, Sanford LP, Doetschman T, Gendron RL, Kao CW, Kao WW (2001) TGFbeta2 in corneal morphogenesis during mouse embryonic development. Dev Biol 240:419–432

95. Sarfarazi M, Akarsu AN, Hossain A, Turacli ME, Aktan SG, Barsoum-Homsy M, Chevrette L, Sayli BS (1995) Assignment of a locus (GLC3A) for primary congenital glaucoma (Buphthalmos) to 2p21 and evidence for genetic heterogeneity. Genomics 30:171–177

96. Sarfarazi M, Child A, Stoilova D, Brice G, Desai T, Trifan OC, Poinoosawmy D, Crick RP (1998) Localization of the fourth locus (GLC1E) for adult-onset primary open-angle glaucoma to the 10p15-p14 region. Am J Hum Genet 62:641–652

97. Schottenstein EM (1996) Peters' anomaly. In:Ritch R, Shields MB, Krupin T (eds) The glaucomas. Mosby, St. Louis, pp 887–897

98. Semina EV, Reiter R, Leysens NJ, Alward WL, Small KW, Datson NA, Siegel-Bartelt J, Bierke-Nelson D, Bitoun P, Zabel BU, Carey JC, Murray JC (1996) Cloning and characterization of a novel bicoid-related homeobox transcription factor gene, RIEG, involved in Rieger syndrome. Nat Genet 14:392–399

99. Semina EV, Ferrell RE, Mintz-Hittner HA, Bitoun P, Alward WL, Reiter RS, Funkhauser C, Daack-Hirsch S, Murray JC (1998) A novel homeobox gene PITX3 is mutated in families with autosomal-dominant cataracts and ASMD. Nat Genet 19:167–170

100. Semina EV, Murray JC, Reiter R, Hrstka RF, Graw J (2000) Deletion in the promoter region and altered expression of Pitx3 homeobox gene in aphakia mice. Hum Mol Genet 9:1575–1585

101. Semina EV, Brownell I, Mintz-Hittner HA, Murray JC, Jamrich M (2001) Mutations in the human forkhead transcription factor FOXE3 associated with anterior segment ocular dysgenesis and cataracts. Hum Mol Genet 10:231–236

102. Sheffield VC, Stone EM, Alward WL, Drack AV, Johnson AT, Streb LM, Nichols BE (1993) Genetic linkage of familial open angle glaucoma to chromosome 1q21-q31. Nat Genet 4:47–50

103. Shields MB (1983) Axenfeld-Rieger syndrome: a theory of mechanism and distinctions from the iridocorneal endothelial syndrome. Trans Am Ophthalmol Soc 81:736–784

104. Shields MB (1996) Axenfeld-Rieger Syndrome. In:Ritch R, Shields MB, Krupin T (eds) The glaucomas. Clinical Science. Mosby, St. Louis, pp 875–885

105. Shimizu T, Hara K, Futa R (1981) Fine structure of trabecular meshwork and iris in pigmentary glaucoma. Albrecht Von Graefes Arch Klin Exp Ophthalmol 215:171–180

106. Sitorus R, Ardjo SM, Lorenz B, Preising M (2003) CYP1B1 gene analysis in primary congenital glaucoma in Indonesian and European patients. J Med Genet 40:E9

107. Stoilov I, Akarsu AN, Sarfarazi M (1997) Identification of three different truncating mutations in cytochrome P4501B1 (CYP1B1) as the principal cause of primary congenital glaucoma (Buphthalmos) in families linked to the GLC3A locus on chromosome 2p21. Hum Mol Genet 6:641–647

108. Stoilov I, Jansson I, Sarfarazi M, Schenkman JB (2001) Roles of cytochrome p450 in development. Drug Metabol Drug Interact 18:33–55

109. Stoilov IR, Costa VP, Vasconcellos JP, Melo MB, Betinjane AJ, Carani JC, Oltrogge EV, Sarfarazi M (2002) Molecular genetics of primary congenital glaucoma in Brazil. Invest Ophthalmol Vis Sci 43:1820–1827

110. Stoilova D, Child A, Trifan OC, Crick RP, Coakes RL, Sarfarazi M (1996) Localization of a locus (GLC1B) for adult-onset primary open angle glaucoma to the 2cen-q13 region. Genomics 36:142–150

111. Stone EM, Fingert JH, Alward WL, Nguyen TD, Polansky JR, Sunden SL, Nishimura D, Clark AF, Nystuen A, Nichols BE, Mackey DA, Ritch R, Kalenak JW, Craven ER, Sheffield VC (1997) Identification of a gene that causes primary open angle glaucoma. Science 275:668–670

112. Stroissnigg H, Repitz M, Miloloza A, Linhartova I, Beug H, Wiche G, Propst F (2002) FIP-2, an IkappaB-kinase-gamma-related protein, is associated with the Golgi apparatus and translocates to the marginal band during chicken erythroblast differentiation. Exp Cell Res 278:133–145

113. Sweeney E, Fryer A, Mountford R, Green A, McIntosh I (2003) Nail patella syndrome: a review of the phenotype aided by developmental biology. J Med Genet 40:153–162

114. Tamm ER (2002) Myocilin and glaucoma: facts and ideas. Prog Retin Eye Res 21:395–428

115. Tamm ER, Polansky J (2001) The TIGR/MYOC gene and glaucoma: opportunities for new understandings. J. Glaucoma 10[Suppl 1]:9–12

116. Tamm ER, Russell P, Johnson DH, Piatigorsky J (1996) Human and monkey trabecular meshwork accumulate alpha B-crystallin in response to heat shock and oxidative stress. Invest Ophthalmol Vis Sci 37:2402–2413

117. Tamm ER, Russell P, Epstein DL, Johnson DH, Piatigorsky J (1999) Modulation of myocilin/TIGR expression in human trabecular meshwork. Invest Ophthalmol Vis Sci 40:2577–2582

118. Tang S, Toda Y, Kashiwagi K, Mabuchi F, Iijima H, Tsukahara S, Yamagata Z (2003) The association between Japanese primary open-angle glaucoma and normal tension glaucoma patients and the optineurin gene. Hum Genet 113:276–279

119. Tawara A, Inomata H (1981) Developmental immaturity of the trabecular meshwork in congenital glaucoma. Am J Ophthalmol 92:508–525

120. Teikari JM (1987) Genetic factors in open-angle (simple and capsular) glaucoma. A population-based twin study. Acta Ophthalmol (Copenh) 65:715–720

121. Tezel G, Wax MB (2000) Increased production of tumor necrosis factor-alpha by glial cells exposed to simulated ischemia or elevated hydrostatic pressure induces apoptosis in cocultured retinal ganglion cells. J Neurosci 20:8693–8700

122. Tielsch JM, Sommer A, Katz J, Royall RM, Quigley HA, Javitt J (1991) Racial variations in the prevalence of primary open-angle glaucoma. The Baltimore Eye Survey. JAMA 266:369–374

123. Tielsch JM, Katz J, Sommer A, Quigley HA, Javitt JC (1994) Family history and risk of primary open angle glaucoma. The Baltimore Eye Survey. Arch Ophthalmol 112:69–73

124. Tomarev SI, Wistow G, Raymond V, Dubois S, Malyukova I (2003) Gene expression profile of the human trabecular meshwork: NEIBank sequence tag analysis. Invest Ophthalmol Vis Sci 44:2588–2596

125. Ton CC, Hirvonen H, Miwa H, Weil MM, Monaghan P, Jordan T, van Heyningen V, Hastie ND, Meijers-Heijboer H, Drechsler M et al (1991) Positional cloning and characterization of a paired box- and homeobox-containing gene from the aniridia region. Cell 67:1059–1074

126. Torrado M, Trivedi R, Zinovieva R, Karavanova I, Tomarev SI (2002) Optimedin: a novel olfactomedin-related protein that interacts with myocilin. Hum Mol Genet 11:1291–1301

127. Trainor PA, Tam PP (1995) Cranial paraxial mesoderm and neural crest cells of the mouse embryo: co-distribution in the craniofacial mesenchyme but distinct segregation in branchial arches. Development 121:2569–2582

128. Trifan OC, Traboulsi EI, Stoilova D, Alozie I, Nguyen R, Raja S, Sarfarazi M (1998) A third locus (GLC1D) for adult-onset primary open-angle glaucoma maps to the 8q23 region. Am J Ophthalmol 126:17–28

129. Tripathi RC, Li J, Chan WF, Tripathi BJ (1994) Aqueous humor in glaucomatous eyes contains an increased level of TGF-beta 2. Exp Eye Res 59:723–727

130. Tumminia SJ, Mitton KP, Arora J, Zelenka P, Epstein DL, Russell P (1998) Mechanical stretch alters the actin cytoskeletal network and signal transduction in human trabecular meshwork cells. Invest Ophthalmol Vis Sci 39:1361–1371

131. Ueda J, Wentz-Hunter K, Yue BY (2002) Distribution of myocilin and extracellular matrix components in the juxtacanalicular tissue of human eyes. Invest Ophthalmol Vis Sci 43:1068–1076

132. van Dorp DB, Delleman JW, Loewer-Sieger DH (1984) Oculocutaneous albinism and anterior chamber cleavage malformations. Not a coincidence. Clin Genet 26:440–444

133. Vincent A, Billingsley G, Priston M, Williams-Lyn D, Sutherland J, Glaser T, Oliver E, Walter MA, Heathcote G, Levin A, Héon E (2001) Phenotypic heterogeneity of CYP1B1: mutations in a patient with Peters' anomaly. J Med Genet 38:324–326

134. Vincent AL, Billingsley G, Buys Y, Levin AV, Priston M, Trope G, Williams-Lyn D, Héon E (2002) Digenic inheritance of early-onset glaucoma: CYP1B1, a potential modifier gene. Am J Hum Genet 70:448–460

135. Vittitow J, Borrás T (2002) Expression of optineurin, a glaucoma-linked gene, is influenced by elevated intraocular pressure. Biochem Biophys Res Commun 298:67–74

136. Vollrath D, Jaramillo-Babb VL, Clough MV, McIntosh I, Scott KM, Lichter PR, Richards JE (1998) Loss-of-function mutations in the LIM-homeodomain gene, LMX1B, in nail- patella syndrome [published erratum appears in Hum Mol Genet 1998 Aug;7(8):1333]. Hum Mol Genet 7:1091–1098

137. Walther C, Gruss P (1991) Pax-6, a murine paired box gene, is expressed in the developing CNS. Development 113:1435–1449

138. Welge-Lussen U, May CA, Eichhorn M, Bloemendal H, Lutjen-Drecoll E (1999) AlphaB-crystallin in the trabecular meshwork is inducible by transforming growth factor-beta. Invest Ophthalmol Vis Sci 40:2235–2241

139. Welihinda AA, Tirasophon W, Kaufman RJ (1999) The cellular response to protein misfolding in the endoplasmic reticulum. Gene Expr 7:293–300

140. Wiggs JL, Allingham RR, Hossain A, Kern J, Auguste J, DelBono EA, Broomer B, Graham FL, Hauser M, Pericak-Vance M, Haines JL (2000) Genome-wide scan for adult onset primary open angle glaucoma. Hum Mol Genet 9:1109–1117

141. Wirtz MK, Samples JR, Kramer PL, Rust K, Topinka JR, Yount J, Koler RD, Acott TS (1997) Mapping a gene for adult-onset primary open-angle glaucoma to chromosome 3q. Am J Hum Genet 60:296–304

142. Wirtz MK, Samples JR, Rust K, Lie J, Nordling L, Schilling K, Acott TS, Kramer PL (1999) GLC1F, a new primary open-angle glaucoma locus, maps to 7q35-q36. Arch Ophthalmol 117:237–241

143. Wordinger RJ, Agarwal R, Talati M, Fuller J, Lambert W, Clark AF (2002) Expression of bone morphogenetic proteins (BMP), BMP receptors, and BMP associated proteins in human trabecular meshwork and optic nerve head cells and tissues. Mol Vis 8:241–250@ref.reference:144.
    Wulle KG (1972) The development of the productive and draining system of the aqueous humor in the human eye. Adv Ophthalmol 26:269–355

145. Wulle KG, Lerche W (1969) Electron microscopic observations of the early development of the human corneal endothelium and Descemet's membrane. Ophthalmologica 157:451–461

146. Xu H, Acott TS, Wirtz MK (2000) Identification and expression of a novel type I procollagen C-proteinase enhancer protein gene from the glaucoma candidate region on 3q21-q24. Genomics 66:264–273

147. Yuan L, Neufeld AH (2000) Tumor necrosis factor-alpha: a potentially neurodestructive cytokine produced by glia in the human glaucomatous optic nerve head. Glia 32:42–50

148. Zhou Y, Kato H, Asanoma K, Kondo H, Arima T, Kato K, Matsuda T, Wake N (2002) Identification of FOXC1 as a TGF-beta1 responsive gene and its involvement in negative regulation of cell growth. Genomics 80:465–472

Leonard A. Levin

Core Messages

- Retinal ganglion cells are central nervous system neurons and thus do not have the protective mechanisms of peripheral nerves
- Neuroprotection consists of prevention of injury, maintenance of the cellular connections and preservation of the internal and external cellular requirements
- Current studies of neuroprotection are directed at interfering with mechanisms of retinal ganglion cell death
- Agents inhibiting retinal ganglion cell death that have been successfully utilized in the laboratory include NMDA inhibitors, nitric oxide synthase inhibitors, α-adrenergic agonists, β-adrenergic antagonists reactive species inhibitors, immune vaccination and neurotrophic factors
- None of the agents shown to be effective in cell culture or animal models have been proven effective yet in clinical glaucoma settings. Intraocular pressure lowering is at present the only clinically proven neuroprotective strategy
- Memantine is an NMDA inhibitor that has been FDA-approved for the treatment of Alzheimer's disease and might be considered as an off-label adjunct when progression is occurring despite maximum practical pressure lowering

2.1
Introduction

2.1.1
Basics

Neuroprotection refers to a set of therapies for preventing neurons from dying as the result of a disease process. It is thus applicable to many ophthalmic disorders of varied etiology. Examples include diseases due to ischemia (as in central retinal artery occlusion or anterior ischemic optic neuropathy), inflammation (as might be seen with a posterior uveitis or cystoid macular edema), hereditary disorders (such as inherited macular and peripheral retinal degenerations, or Leber's hereditary optic neuropathy). Neuroprotection may be particularly valuable for glaucoma, a disorder of complex etiology which results in loss of retinal ganglion cells.

Retinal ganglion cells are inner retinal neurons, receiving inputs from bipolar and amacrine cells, and projecting their axons via the optic nerve to target areas in the brain. Retinal ganglion cells thus subserve transmission of visual information. The main target in humans is the lateral geniculate nucleus, which connects to the visual cortex and is responsible for visual processing. Other targets include the pretectal nuclei (for the pupillary response), the suprachiasmatic nucleus of the hypothalamus (for maintenance of diurnal rhythm), and the superior colliculus (for orienting responses). Retinal ganglion cells will die if their axon is injured; we and others have shown that their death in optic nerve transection, ischemia, or as a result of glaucoma occurs by apoptosis [2, 22, 38], a type of programmed cell death. The mechanisms by

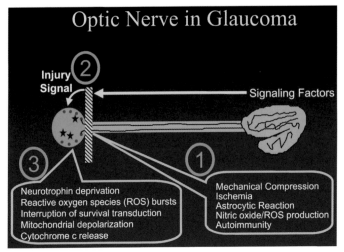

Fig. 2.1. Optic nerve in glaucoma. Retinal ganglion cells carry visual information from the retina to target areas in the brain. At the same time, one or more of the target areas release neuronal signaling factors (including neurotrophins) that support neuronal survival. These are transported back to the retina via retrograde axonal transport along the retinal ganglion cell axon. Glaucomatous optic neuropathy probably starts with pathophysiology at the optic nerve head which both interferes with the transport of signaling factors and induces an injury signal within the retina. The nature of the axonal injury is unclear, and may be multifactorial. This is followed by retinal ganglion cell death (via apoptosis), which can occur through the several mechanisms listed

which retinal ganglion cells die in glaucoma is controversial; some of the possible pathways are depicted in Fig. 1.1.

2.1.2
Rationale for Neuroprotection in Glaucoma

Since glaucomatous optic neuropathy eventually results in loss of retinal ganglion cells, it is reasonable to expect that protecting them from death might serve as one component of any treatment. With rare exception, neurons within higher vertebrates are unable to divide after birth. This implies that the supply of neurons that is available at birth must last the life of the organism. At the present state of biomedical research it is not yet possible to replace dead retinal ganglion cells with functional new ones using stem cells. The ramification of this chain of reasoning is that protecting the retinal ganglion cell from death is necessary to prevent its irreversible loss of functional capacity, as replacement or substitution is not yet possible.

Furthermore, while most organs and extracranial tissues are innervated by nerves of the peripheral nervous system, the eye is unusual in that it contains central nervous system type neurons. The difference is significant: peripheral nerve axons are usually capable of regeneration after injury, while central nervous system axons are not. The human neural retina contains approximately 1,000,000 retinal ganglion cells. Significant loss of these neurons from glaucoma can result in visual disability. Because these neurons cannot be replaced, this inescapably implies permanent loss of function. In some cases, the functional loss is not as dramatic as the quantitative loss of neurons, simply because there is enough plasticity within the rest of the central nervous system to compensate for some loss of neurons. In addition, there is built-in redundancy within the visual system, so that there are usually more than enough neurons for specific visual tasks under most clinical setting. Therefore, loss of even a sizable proportion of neurons will not necessarily become manifest on standard tests of visual function.

This is most commonly observed in early glaucomatous optic neuropathy, where the visual field may be relatively normal by automated visual field analysis, yet there is anatomical evidence (optic nerve head cupping, thinning of the nerve fiber layer) for axonal loss from retinal ganglion cells.

2.1.3
Necessary Steps for Neuroprotection

To maintain sufficient neuronal function for useful vision in the face of damage to retinal neurons or their axons, several steps are required. First, the death of the neuron must be prevented. Second, either the integrity of its connections (dendrites and axons) must be maintained, or some mechanism for dendritic sprouting and axonal regeneration must be introduced. Third, the electrical, biochemical, and energetic requirements needed for transmission of the impulses that code for vision must be preserved. Fourth, and most importantly, the disease process that necessitated the first three steps must be arrested. If this is not done, then the neuroprotective strategy may eventually fail in the face of overwhelming attack.

For the most part, standard therapies for glaucoma focus on the fourth step, i.e., arresting progression of the disease process by lowering the intraocular pressure. However, in many cases there is progressive structural and functional loss despite excellent pressure lowering, and in these cases neuroprotection may be the only viable therapy. In other cases pressure lowering requires use of pharmacological or surgical therapies with the potential for substantial side effects, and the use of neuroprotection can be adjunctive to ocular hypotensive treatment. In some patients there is pressure-independent progression, for which no glaucoma therapy may be useful. A major advantage of a neuroprotective therapy is that it may be effective when there is no known therapy.

The majority of research on neuroprotection has focused on preventing death of neurons, while maintenance of neuronal connections and their functional capacity has usually been considered subordinate to this. In part, this reflects the fact that if a neuron cannot be saved, then a therapy addressed to its function becomes moot. However, since methods for maintaining neuronal survival in the face of disease have increasingly been validated in a variety of *in vitro* and animal models, the ensuing prospects for clinical therapy will demand attention to these issues.

2.2
Preclinical Evidence
for Neuroprotection in Glaucoma

Retinal ganglion cells and their axons die in glaucoma, and the mechanisms by which they are damaged and undergo apoptosis represent targets for neuroprotection. This section will discuss each of the major class of therapies for which neuroprotection has been used in preclinical models of glaucoma. Although many drugs and approaches have been used to protect against retinal ganglion cell death in various paradigms, the therapies listed in Table 2.1 have all shown efficacy in *experimental models of ocular hypertension*.

2.2.1
NMDA Receptor Antagonists

Neurotoxicity by the excitatory amino acid glutamate occurs via binding of glutamate to the NMDA receptor, as well as AMPA/kainate receptors. In vitro animal models of excitotoxicity use intravitreal NMDA or glutamate to induce retinal ganglion cell death. One neuroprotective strategy is to interrupt the excitotoxic cascade, e.g., by blockade of the receptors that cause cell death when retinal ganglion cells are exposed to glutamate. The classic pharmacological approach for this is to block the NMDA subtype glutamate receptor with specific antagonists, and several such compounds have been used in tissue culture and animal models. MK801, a non-competitive NMDA antagonist, demonstrated neuroprotective properties in pressure-induced and reperfusion-injury animal models of retinal ganglion cell toxicity [6, 20], but is unsuitable for clinical use because of its psy-

Table 2.1. Therapies showing efficacy in experimental models of ocular hypertension

Drug	Mechanism
2-Aminoguanidine	iNOS inhibitor
L-N(6)-(1-iminoethyl)lysine 5-tetrazole amide	Prodrug for iNOS inhibitor
Brimonidine	α_2-Agonist
Cop-1 vaccine	T-cell activator
Heat stress	Heat shock protein activator
BDNF/S-PBN	Neurotrophin and reactive oxygen species scavenger
Memantine	NMDA antagonist
MK-801	NMDA antagonist

chotropic side effects. Memantine is a clinically well tolerated NMDA receptor antagonist [23]. Experimental evidence in animal models [11, 19], including rat and monkey ocular hypertension, suggests its utility in glutamate-mediated excitatory retinal ganglion cell death in glaucoma.

Human trials with NMDA antagonists have been performed for stroke and similar disorders; however, with disappointing results. More recently, memantine has been shown to be effective in Alzheimer's disease in randomized clinical trials [39]. It remains to be seen whether this drug will be effective for glaucomatous optic neuropathy, which differs greatly in pathophysiology from stroke, and in some ways is more similar to a chronic neurodegenerative disorder. Memantine's role in neuroprotection is currently being evaluated [36].

2.2.2
α_2-Adrenergic Receptor Agonists

Agonists of α_2-adrenergic receptors, e.g., clonidine, have been shown to induce production of basic fibroblast growth factor (bFGF) and brain-derived neurotrophic factor (BDNF; see below), which are known neuroprotective agents [5, 9, 46]. α_2-Adrenergic receptor agonists have been demonstrated to enhance retinal ganglion cell survival in multiple models, including ischemic injury, optic nerve crush, and rat intraocular hypertension [45, 48, 51]. Mechanisms of action include induction of growth factors, inhibition of glutamate excitotoxicity, increase in phosphorylated Akt, increase in Bcl-x_L levels, and reduction of calcium influx [44, 47].

2.2.3
β_1-Adrenergic Receptor Antagonists

There is excellent experimental evidence that β_1-adrenergic antagonists are neuroprotective in animal models of optic nerve injury [7, 35, 49, 50], although experimental glaucoma has not yet been reported. The neuroprotective effects of β_1-adrenergic antagonists probably occur by different mechanisms from α_2-adrenergic agonists, as they do not cause a similar change in bFGF expression, although the closely related agonist levobetaxolol increases bFGF and CNTF expression [1]. In neurons, betaxolol, a β_1-adrenoceptor antagonist, has been shown to decrease sodium and calcium influx [52] predominantly through L-type calcium channels [28]. In an experimental model of ischemia and reperfusion, produced by temporary elevation of IOP, ganglion cell damage is indicated by both electrophysiology with loss of the ERG b-wave and by decreased choline acetyltransferase (ChAT) immunoreactivity [5, 7, 29]. Topical administration of betaxolol, prior to induced ischemia and reperfusion, significantly preserved the ERG b-wave and preserved ChAT immunoreactivity [49].

2.2.4
Nitric Oxide Synthase Antagonists

Inducible nitric oxide synthase (iNOS) is present in the optic nerve head of glaucoma patients and, in vitro, optic nerve astrocytes are capable of up-regulating the production of iNOS under conditions of increased hydrostatic pressure [24, 25, 42]. Inhibition of iNOS using 2-aminoguanidine in a rat ocular hypertension model reduced retinal ganglion cell loss by about 70% [34]. Similar results were seen with a prodrug of an iNOS inhibitor, L-N(6)-(1-iminoethyl)lysine 5-tetrazole amide [33]. NOS is postulated to play a role in retinal ganglion cell axonal toxicity, and strategies to reduce NOS are potential therapeutic targets in glaucoma and other optic neuropathies.

Interestingly, nipradilol, a β- and α_1-antagonist which increases nitric oxide release, is neuroprotective for cultured retinal ganglion cells [15] and retinal ganglion cells after optic nerve transection [32].

2.2.5
Reactive Oxygen Species Scavengers and Lipid Peroxidation Inhibitors

The role for reactive oxygen species scavenger and lipid peroxidation inhibitors in the prevention of retinal ganglion cell death is being studied. The lipid peroxidation inhibitor tirilazad mesylate partially blocked the death of retinal ganglion cells in mixed culture, where the processes of axotomy, dissociation, and absence of neurotrophins normally result in the gradual loss of these cells [21]. Cell death induced by chemical hypoxia (via inhibiting complex IV of the electron transport chain) and hypoglycemia was also decreased when lipid peroxidation was blocked. The blockage of retinal ganglion cell death by blocking lipid peroxidation could therefore result from inhibition of either a necrotic or apoptotic process. Specifically, reactive oxygen intermediates appear to have two separate roles, in that they can activate a neuronal cell death program [12, 14], as well as participate in the destruction of the cell [43].

There is a synergistic reduction of cell death through the use of both free-radical scavengers and neurotrophic factors [18]. Both glycolysis and oxidative phosphorylation are required for high levels of ATP production from glucose, and thus the inhibition of lipid peroxidation may be neuroprotective in conditions of decreased cellular metabolism, e.g., ischemia. Presumably, decreasing the ability of free radicals to damage membrane lipids directly protects cellular and subcellular integrity under conditions of substrate or hypoxic stress. Alternatively, inhibition of free radical-mediated lipid peroxidation may directly interfere with early steps in the apoptotic program, similar to the ability of superoxide dismutase to delay apoptosis of nerve growth factor-deprived sympathetic neurons [10].

2.2.6
Neurotrophic Factors

Neurotrophins increase retinal ganglion cell survival and are capable of being produced by retinal cells [4, 37]. Several groups have used BDNF and other neurotrophins to prolong retinal ganglion cell survival after axonal injury [3, 26, 27, 30], although this effect is not long-lasting [8]. Multiple strategies have been proposed to increase exogenous neurotrophin levels in order to prolong retinal ganglion cell survival. Addition of exogenous BDNF is able to block neuronal cell death in an excitotoxicity animal model, suggesting the potential usefulness of this agent in prolonging cell survival [17]. Other strategies involve delivery of a neurotrophin-producing viral vector to the retina and ganglion cells in order to have short-term in situ production of the agent [8]. Successful use of viral vector delivery of human BDNF was demonstrated in the rat optic neuropathy model, where retinal ganglion cell programmed cell death follows axotomy [13], and in a glaucoma model of retinal ganglion cell death [18].

Although the possibility of delivering neurotrophins to the retina is appealing, the mechanism of delivery is important to define. Repeated intravitreal injections may not be well tolerated. On the other hand, systemic therapy is difficult with neurotrophins, as they are large protein molecules, and therefore cannot readily cross the blood–retinal barrier. An alternative is a sustained-release intraocular implant or a transscleral delivery system, which would allow long-term delivery of a drug to the retina over the many years of chronic glaucoma. The validity of this approach has not yet been proven. Finally, the ability of neurotrophins alone to serve as neuroprotectants is unclear, as even in animal models, their administration incompletely blocks retinal ganglion cell loss after optic nerve injury.

Another neuroprotective strategy is to use small molecules that are able to substitute for the signaling cascade of neurotrophins or other survival agents, or blocks the signaling cascade for cell death. An example of this would be a drug that either mimics or activates a second or third messenger for one or more neurotrophins. Several such compounds may turn out to be useful for this approach, although as of yet the precise intracellular pathways by which retinal ganglion cells survive or die in glaucoma have not been completely mapped out.

2.2.7
Vaccination

Activated T cells are effective in the therapy of axonal injury as demonstrated in a rat optic nerve crush model [31, 41] and rat ocular hypertension [40]. The beneficial effect of immune T cells appears to be physiologic, antigen-specific, and possibly mediated by the local secretion of neurotrophins at the site of axonal injury [31, 41].

Summary for the Clinician

- Multiple therapies are neuroprotective in animal models of glaucoma

2.3
Clinical Experience
with the Described Substances

Although there is good to excellent evidence of efficacy for some of the approaches listed above in treating experimental models of glaucoma, there is scant clinical evidence proving effectiveness in human glaucoma. Proof of effectiveness is best obtained from properly conducted randomized controlled clinical trials. Although trials are ongoing and others are undoubtedly being planned, there are no published results of such trials to guide clinical use. The level of evidence for neuroprotection is depicted in Fig. 2.2.

On the other hand, there is clinical experience using drugs that happen to have neuroprotective properties, but approved for other paradigms. The drugs listed in Table 2.2 are approved by the United States Food and Drug Administration (FDA), and have been shown in preclinical research to be neuroprotective in animal models of ocular hypertension (see above). Both are the subject of clinical trials of neuroprotection in glaucoma and other optic neuropathies.

Brimonidine, an α_2-agonist, is neuroprotective in rats in experimental glaucoma [48]. Clonidine and apraclonidine should theoretically also be neuroprotective in these models, although they have relatively more α_1 activity. This means that there is more likelihood of an unwanted vasoconstrictive effect, and may be less preferable to a purer α_2 agonist. Brimonidine is dosed topically, and there is some human data to suggest that low nanomolar concentrations can be reached within the vitreous in phakic patients (aphakic and pseudophakic eyes reach much higher concentrations) [16]. Whether these concentrations will translate into clinical evidence of neuroprotection will depend on the results of clinical studies in which topically dosed brimonidine is compared with an ocular hypotensive agent (usually a β-antagonist) that does not have neuroprotective activity. These studies are ongoing.

Memantine is an NMDA antagonist, and therefore counteracts the excitotoxic effects of glutamate at the NMDA receptor. It is neuroprotective in monkeys and rats in experimental glaucoma, and was tested in monkeys at a concentration of 4 mg/kg per day [11] to reach the same plasma levels as that seen in human subjects treated for Parkinson's disease. Memantine has been shown to be effective in Alzheimer's disease in well-designed phase III randomized controlled clinical trials, and was approved in October 2003 by the USA FDA for that indication, at an oral dose of 20 mg daily [39]. The rate of adverse effects at that dose was not apprecia-

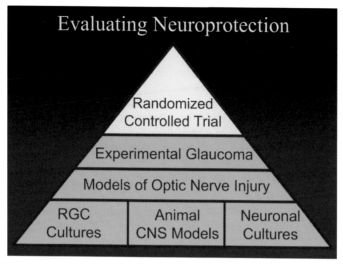

Fig. 2.2. Evaluating neuroprotection. Evidence for neuroprotection in glaucoma is manifold, and can be viewed as a hierarchy of support. The least direct evidence is from culture models or central nervous system models where there is no direct linkage to glaucoma. Better is evidence from animal models of optic nerve injury or disease. Better yet is evidence from animal models of experimental ocular hypertension or optic nerve head ischemia. The best evidence is from the results of randomized controlled clinical trials. The three lowest levels of the pyramid of evidence are highlighted to represent that there is adequate scientific support. The top level is in yellow, to indicate that clinical trials are ongoing, but have not yet provided proof of concept

Table 2.2. Therapies showing efficacy in experimental models of ocular hypertension which are also FDA-approved for other indications

Drug	Mechanism	Indication	References for neuroprotection in experimental glaucoma
Brimonidine	α_2-Agonist	Intraocular pressure lowering	[48]
Memantine	NMDA antagonist	Moderate to severe Alzheimer's disease	[11]

bly different from placebo [39]. Because the drug is systemically delivered, there is less concern about it reaching the retinal ganglion cell in sufficient concentrations.

Summary for the Clinician

- There are a small number of therapies available for the clinician which have been shown to be neuroprotective in animal models of glaucoma and which have been approved for other indications, making it possible to prescribe them
- Human clinical trial data is not yet available to guide clinical decision-making

2.4
Current Clinical Practice/Recommendations

The ophthalmologist taking care of patients with glaucoma does not yet have the results of clinical trials to guide the use of neuroprotective drugs, making decision-making very difficult. There are two groups of patients in which drugs with neuroprotective properties could be considered, as long as it is borne in mind that the evidence for their use is so far only from preclinical studies. First, patients who are unresponsive to pressure-lowering therapy and continue to progress, e.g., patients who have unequivocal glaucoma, have had filtering surgery with intraocular pressures below 10, and yet continue to progress theoretically could be candidates for off-label use of memantine. Obviously, a frank discussion with the patient of the unproven nature of the therapy, as well as excellent informed consent is necessary for this approach.

A second group that could be candidates for neuroprotective therapy are patients who are responsive to pressure lowering but for whom further pressure lowering is needed but difficult to achieve. In these patients, theoretically both ocular hypotensive agents and neuroprotection could be used. What is the best way to calculate the effects of neuroprotection with respect to pressure-lowering? One method is to normalize all therapies with respect to the effect on visual field progression. For example, the Ocular Hypertension Treatment Study (OHTS), Advanced Glaucoma Intervention Study (AGIS), Collaborative Initial Glaucoma Treatment Study (CIGTS), Collaborative Normal Tension Glaucoma Study (CNTGS), and Early Manifest Glaucoma Trial (EMGT) showed that there is roughly a 10% reduction in progression for each 1 mmHg lowering of intraocular pressure. Although we do not yet have data on how much (if at all) neuroprotective agents decrease field progression, we can envisage (as an example) that a drug decreasing progression by 30%–50% would therefore be equivalent to an additional lowering of intraocular pressure by 3–5 mmHg.

In summary, we do not yet have good clinical data to help the clinician in deciding the optimal use of neuroprotective drugs. These data will undoubtedly accrue over the next few years. At present, the best approach is to continue to maintain familiarity with the preclinical and clinical research going on in the field.

References

1. Agarwal N, Martin E, Krishnamoorthy RR, Landers R, Wen R, Krueger S, Kapin MA, Collier RJ (2002) Levobetaxolol-induced Up-regulation of retinal bFGF and CNTF mRNAs and preservation of retinal function against a photic-induced retinopathy. Exp Eye Res 74:445–453
2. Berkelaar M, Clarke DB, Wang YC, Bray GM, Aguayo AJ (1994) Axotomy results in delayed death and apoptosis of retinal ganglion cells in adult rats. J Neurosci 14:4368–4374
3. Castillo BJ, del CM, Breakefield XO, Frim DM, Barnstable CJ, Dean DO, Bohn MC (1994) Retinal ganglion cell survival is promoted by genetically modified astrocytes designed to secrete brain-derived neurotrophic factor (BDNF). Brain Res 647:30–36
4. Cellerino A, Kohler K (1997) Brain-derived neurotrophic factor/neurotrophin-4 receptor TrkB is localized on ganglion cells and dopaminergic amacrine cells in the vertebrate retina. J Comp Neurol 386:149–160
5. Chao HM, Chidlow G, Melena J, Wood JP, Osborne NN (2000) An investigation into the potential mechanisms underlying the neuroprotective effect of clonidine in the retina. Brain Res 877:47–57
6. Chaudhary P, Ahmed F, Sharma SC (1998) MK801-a neuroprotectant in rat hypertensive eyes. Brain Res 792:154–158
7. Chidlow G, Melena J, Osborne NN (2000) Betaxolol, a beta(1)-adrenoceptor antagonist, reduces Na(+) influx into cortical synaptosomes by direct interaction with Na(+) channels: comparison with other beta-adrenoceptor antagonists. Br J Pharmacol 130:759–766
8. DiPolo A, Aigner LJ, Dunn RJ, Bray GM, Aguayo AJ (1998) Prolonged delivery of brain-derived neurotrophic factor by adenovirus-infected Muller cells temporarily rescues injured retinal ganglion cells. Proc Natl Acad Sci USA 95:3978–3983
9. Gao H, Qiao X, Cantor LB, Wu Dunn D (2002) Up-regulation of brain-derived neurotrophic factor expression by brimonidine in rat retinal ganglion cells. Arch Ophthalmol 120:797–803
10. Greenlund LJ, Deckwerth TL, Johnson EM (1995) Superoxide dismutase delays neuronal apoptosis: a role for reactive oxygen species in programmed neuronal death. Neuron 14:303–315

11. Hare W, WoldeMussie E, Lai R, Ton H, Ruiz G, Feldmann B, Wijono M, Chun T, Wheeler L (2001) Efficacy and safety of memantine, an NMDA-type open-channel blocker, for reduction of retinal injury associated with experimental glaucoma in rat and monkey. Surv Ophthalmol 45[Suppl 3]: S284–289; discussion S295–286

12. Hockenbery DM, Oltvai ZN, Yin XM, Milliman CL, Korsmeyer SJ (1993) Bcl-2 functions in an antioxidant pathway to prevent apoptosis. Cell 75:241–251

13. Isenmann S, Klocker N, Gravel C, Bahr M (1998) Short communication: protection of axotomized retinal ganglion cells by adenovirally delivered BDNF in vivo. Eur J Neurosci 10:2751–2756

14. Kane DJ, Sarafian TA, Anton R, Hahn H, Gralla EB, Valentine JS, Ord T, Bredesen DE (1993) Bcl-2 inhibition of neural death: decreased generation of reactive oxygen species. Science 262:1274–1277

15. Kashiwagi K, Iizuka Y, Tsukahara S (2002) Neuroprotective effects of nipradilol on purified cultured retinal ganglion cells. J Glaucoma 11:231–238

16. Kent AR, Nussdorf JD, David R, Tyson F, Small D, Fellows D (2001) Vitreous concentration of topically applied brimonidine tartrate 0.2%. Ophthalmology 108:784–787

17. Kido N, Tanihara H, Honjo M, Inatani M, Tatsuno T, Nakayama C, Honda Y (2000) Neuroprotective effects of brain-derived neurotrophic factor in eyes with NMDA-induced neuronal death. Brain Res 884:59–67

18. Ko ML, Hu DN, Ritch R, Sharma SC (2000) The combined effect of brain-derived neurotrophic factor and a free radical scavenger in experimental glaucoma. Invest Ophthalmol Vis Sci 41:2967– 2971

19. Lagreze WA, Knorle R, Bach M, Feuerstein TJ (1998) Memantine is neuroprotective in a rat model of pressure-induced retinal ischemia. Invest Ophthalmol Vis Sci 39:1063–1066

20. Lam TT, Siew E, Chu R, Tso MO (1997) Ameliorative effect of MK-801 on retinal ischemia. J Ocul Pharmacol Ther 13:129–137

21. Levin LA, Clark JA, Johns LK (1996) Effect of lipid peroxidation inhibition on retinal ganglion cell death. Invest Ophthalmol Vis Sci 37:2744–2749

22. Levin LA, Louhab A (1996) Apoptosis of retinal ganglion cells in anterior ischemic optic neuropathy. Arch Ophthalmol 114:488–491

23. Lipton SA (2003) Possible role for memantine in protecting retinal ganglion cells from glaucomatous damage. Surv Ophthalmol 48[Suppl 11]:S38–46

24. Liu B, Neufeld AH (2000) Expression of nitric oxide synthase-2 (NOS-2) in reactive astrocytes of the human glaucomatous optic nerve head. Glia 30:178–186

25. Liu B, Neufeld AH (2001) Nitric oxide synthase-2 in human optic nerve head astrocytes induced by elevated pressure in vitro. Arch Ophthalmol 119: 240–245

26. Maffei L, Carmignoto G, Perry VH, Candeo P, Ferrari G (1990) Schwann cells promote the survival of rat retinal ganglion cells after optic nerve section. Proc Natl Acad Sci USA 87:1855–1859

27. Mansour-Robaey S, Clarke DB, Wang YC, Bray GM, Aguayo AJ (1994) Effects of ocular injury and administration of brain-derived neurotrophic factor on survival and regrowth of axotomized retinal ganglion cells. Proc Natl Acad Sci USA 91:1632–1636

28. Melena J, Stanton D, Osborne NN (2001) Comparative effects of antiglaucoma drugs on voltage-dependent calcium channels. Graefes Arch Clin Exp Ophthalmol 239:522–530

29. Melena J, Wood JP, Osborne NN (1999) Betaxolol, a beta1-adrenoceptor antagonist, has an affinity for L-type Ca2+ channels. Eur J Pharmacol 378: 317–322

30. Mey J, Thanos S (1993) Intravitreal injections of neurotrophic factors support the survival of axotomized retinal ganglion cells in adult rats in vivo. Brain Res 602:304–317

31. Moalem G, Gdalyahu A, Shani Y, Otten U, Lazarovici P, Cohen IR, Schwartz M (2000) Production of neurotrophins by activated T cells: implications for neuroprotective autoimmunity. J Autoimmun 15:331–345

32. Nakazawa T, Tomita H, Yamaguchi K, Sato Y, Shimura M, Kuwahara S, Tamai M (2002) Neuroprotective effect of nipradilol on axotomized rat retinal ganglion cells. Curr Eye Res 24:114–122

33. Neufeld AH, Das S, Vora S, Gachie E, Kawai S, Manning PT, Connor JR (2002) A prodrug of a selective inhibitor of inducible nitric oxide synthase is neuroprotective in the rat model of glaucoma. J Glaucoma 11:221–225

34. Neufeld AH, Sawada A, Becker B (1999) Inhibition of nitric-oxide synthase 2 by aminoguanidine provides neuroprotection of retinal ganglion cells in a rat model of chronic glaucoma. Proc Natl Acad Sci USA 96:9944–9948

35. Osborne NN, Cazevieille C, Carvalho AL, Larsen AK, DeSantis L (1997) In vivo and in vitro experiments show that betaxolol is a retinal neuroprotective agent. Brain Res 751:113–123

36. Parsons CG, Danysz W, Quack G (1999) Memantine is a clinically well tolerated N-methyl-D-aspartate (NMDA) receptor antagonist–a review of preclinical data. Neuropharmacology 38:735–767

37. Perez MT, Caminos E (1995) Expression of brain-derived neurotrophic factor and of its functional receptor in neonatal and adult rat retina. Neurosci Lett 183:96–99

38. Quigley HA, Nickells RW, Kerrigan LA, Pease ME, Thibault DJ, Zack DJ (1995) Retinal ganglion cell death in experimental glaucoma and after axotomy occurs by apoptosis. Invest Ophthalmol Vis Sci 36:774–786

39. Reisberg B, Doody R, Stoffler A, Schmitt F, Ferris S, Mobius HJ (2003) Memantine in moderate-to-severe Alzheimer's disease. N Engl J Med 348: 1333–1341

40. Schori H, Kipnis J, Yoles E, WoldeMussie E, Ruiz G, Wheeler LA, Schwartz M (2001) Vaccination for protection of retinal ganglion cells against death from glutamate cytotoxicity and ocular hypertension: implications for glaucoma. Proc Natl Acad Sci USA 98:3398–3403

41. Schwartz M (2001) Physiological approaches to neuroprotection. boosting of protective autoimmunity. Surv Ophthalmol 45[Suppl 3]:S256–260; discussion S273–256

42. Shareef S, Sawada A, Neufeld AH (1999) Isoforms of nitric oxide synthase in the optic nerves of rat eyes with chronic moderately elevated intraocular pressure. Invest Ophthalmol Vis Sci 40:2884–2891

43. Tappel AL (1973) Lipid peroxidation damage to cell components. Fed Proc. 32:1870–1874

44. Tatton WG, Chalmers-Redman RM, Tatton NA (2001) Apoptosis and anti-apoptosis signalling in glaucomatous retinopathy. Eur J Ophthalmol 11[Suppl 2]:S12–22

45. Vidal-Sanz M, Lafuente MP, Mayor S, de Imperial JM, Villegas-Perez MP (2001) Retinal ganglion cell death induced by retinal ischemia. neuroprotective effects of two alpha-2 agonists. Surv Ophthalmol 45:S261–267

46. Wen R, Cheng T, Li Y, Cao W, Steinberg RH (1996) Alpha 2-adrenergic agonists induce basic fibroblast growth factor expression in photoreceptors in vivo and ameliorate light damage. J Neurosci 16:5986–5992

47. Wheeler LA, Gil DW, WoldeMussie E (2001) Role of alpha-2 adrenergic receptors in neuroprotection and glaucoma. Surv Ophthalmol 45[Suppl 3]: S290–294; discussion S295–296

48. WoldeMussie E, Ruiz G, Wijono M, Wheeler LA (2001) Neuroprotection of retinal ganglion cells by brimonidine in rats with laser-induced chronic ocular hypertension. Invest Ophthalmol Vis Sci 42:2849–2855

49. Wood JP, DeSantis L, Chao HM, Osborne NN (2001) Topically applied betaxolol attenuates ischaemia-induced effects to the rat retina and stimulates BDNF mRNA. Exp Eye Res 72:79–86

50. Wood JP, Schmidt KG, Melena J, Chidlow G, Allmeier H, Osborne NN (2003) The beta-adrenoceptor antagonists metipranolol and timolol are retinal neuroprotectants: comparison with betaxolol. Exp Eye Res 76:505–516

51. Yoles E, Wheeler LA, Schwartz M (1999) Alpha2-adrenoreceptor agonists are neuroprotective in a rat model of optic nerve degeneration. Invest Ophthalmol Vis Sci 40:65–73

52. Zhang J, Wu SM, Gross RL (2003) Effects of beta-adrenergic blockers on glutamate-induced calcium signals in adult mouse retinal ganglion cells. Brain Res 959:111–119

Eve J. Higginbotham

Core Messages

- The value of screening for glaucoma has been debated
- High rates of visual impairment due to undiagnosed glaucoma support need for screening
- As many as 62% of patients with glaucoma are unaware of it
- Screening also educates the public
- Screening with tonometry alone has little value. Primary care physicians do not regularly screen appropriately for glaucoma
- Follow-up is a critical component of any screening program
- Risk factor questionnaire is helpful
- Frequency doubled perimetry has been shown to be an effective screening device. It may have to be repeated to be sure abnormality is real
- Scanning laser polarimetry has a large overlap between normal and glaucoma eyes. Perhaps new algorithms with corneal compensation will be more accurate
- While the cost of finding and managing early glaucoma may be relatively high, the benefit to the individual of preserving vision may be incalculable

3.1 Introduction

The value of screening for open angle glaucoma in the elderly has been a hotly debated topic for the last 20 years. When the Office of Technology Assessment (OTA) considered this question in a formal document in 1988, their conclusion essentially was that screening for glaucoma or those among the elderly at risk for glaucoma was expensive. Although the authors recognized that "the potential benefits of such a program (were) substantial, whether those benefits (could) actually be realized (was) still highly uncertain." The OTA document continued to note that value would be dependent upon "two unknown factors: first, on the true accuracy of the various screening tests in the settings in which they would be used; and second, on the effectiveness of treatment in preventing, halting, or delaying the progression of visual impairment due to OAG (open angle glaucoma)" [24].

Of course since the OTA document was completed there has been significant progress in clarifying both of these "unknown factors." Technology such as frequency doubling technology (FDT, Zeiss-Humphrey, San Leandro, CA) has significantly enhanced the ability of unskilled screeners to assess functional abnormalities in naive patients in public settings [31]. Moreover, nerve fiber imaging devices, such as scanning laser polarimetry (SLP) have improved our ability to assess early, structural signs of glaucoma [32]. Secondly, at least two randomized clinical trials directly address the "unknown" questions posed by the OTA, whether or not treatment of patients with ocular hypertension delays the onset of glaucoma and if treatment of patients with primary open angle glaucoma (POAG) is effective. This chapter will review current screening practices, specific screening methodologies, and the cost-effectiveness of screening. However, before embarking on these topics, it is important to review why we should be screening for glaucoma in the general population, particularly given the difficulties in rallying enthusiasm for screening among ophthalmologists over the last two decades. In order to attempt to abide by the guidelines set by the editors regarding the number of references, this chapter will focus on the most relevant and recent articles that address these four topics.

3.2
Why Screen for Glaucoma?

There are three primary reasons one should consider for supporting an argument for screening: (1) the burden of untreated disease; (2) the importance of early diagnosis; (3) the lack of knowledge regarding glaucoma in the lay community.

3.2.1
The Burden of Untreated Disease

There have been several studies that have documented the significant prevalence of glaucoma in the world population. Recent studies have examined populations that have been previously under-represented in the literature. Ramakrishnan and coworkers assessed the prevalence of glaucoma in a rural population of southern India. A cohort of 5150 individuals aged 40 years and older underwent a comprehensive eye examination including automated central 24–2 full threshold perimetric testing and dilated fundus examinations. The authors noted an overall prevalence of any glaucoma diagnosis that measured 2.6%, and when considering specifically POAG and primary angle closure glaucoma (PACG), the proportions were 1.7% and 0.5%, respectively. Of those patients who presented with POAG, 20.9% of the patients

were blind in either eye and 93% of patients with POAG had not been previously diagnosed [27]. In Thailand, Singalavanija and others reported a higher prevalence of glaucoma, 6.12% in a series of 2092 individuals. However, these individuals were 60 years of age and older. Visual fields were not performed in this survey; however, individuals underwent measurement of their visual acuity, tonometry, portable slit lamp biomicroscopy, and direct and indirect ophthalmoscopy. Approximately a third of these individuals evidenced low vision; however, cataract, age-related macular disease, corneal disease and nonglaucomatous optic nerve disease also contributed to the numbers of impaired individuals [29]. Both of these studies highlight the significant numbers of visually impaired individuals who are not being addressed by existing health care systems in these countries.

In the United States, there has been recent data on Mexican Americans and residents of Minnesota that reaffirm the position of glaucoma as a public health concern. In the Proyecto VER study that was conducted in Arizona, Hispanic individuals who were 40 years and older were screened. Participants underwent visual acuity testing, tonometry, gonioscopy, optic disc evaluation, and threshold perimetric testing. Among the 4774 individuals evaluated, an overall prevalence of 1.97% was noted; age-specific rates ranged from 0.50% among those 41–49 years of age to 12.63%, among those who were 80 years and older. A total of 62% of individuals were unaware of their diagnosis before the examination [26]. North of Arizona in Minnesota, the incidence rates were assessed among 60,666 residents of Olmstead County. This retrospective review used medical histories and information derived from the database of the Rochester Epidemiology Project to determine the new cases of either OAG, glaucoma suspect, or ocular hypertension between 1965 and 1980. These investigators noted an overall age- and gender-adjusted annual incidence rate of 14.5 per 100,000. These rates increased from 1.6 in the fourth decade to 94.3 in the eighth decade [28]. These two studies reaffirm the significant relationship between age and glaucoma in the general population.

The burden of the glaucoma will only increase if individuals remain undetected and then seek treatment at a time in their lives when other chronic illnesses that affect the aged will impact their compliance with therapy and appointments. Among treated patients, as Chen noted in his study, when patients present with blindness in at least one eye, poor optic nerve function, and noncompliance, the likelihood of developing severe visual impairment is greater [6]. Thus, in order to improve one's chances of preserving visual function, early detection is very important.

3.2.2
The Importance of Early Detection

The best evidence that treatment indeed is effective in reducing the progression of glaucoma is the Early Manifest Glaucoma Treatment Study (EMGT). This study randomized newly diagnosed patients with POAG to either no treatment or treatment with a combination of betaxolol and argon laser trabeculoplasty. This is a study that needed to be performed in order to definitively demonstrate that reducing intraocular pressure does indeed slow the progression of disease. Essentially, 255 patients were randomized; both groups were followed with perimetric testing every 3 months and optic nerve photography every 6 months. Among those individuals who were not treated, 62% (78/126) progressed versus 45% (58/129) among those patients who were treated. Benefits of treatment were noted among both young and older individuals and those patients with mild and advanced disease [14]. Thus, this study answers one of the "unknowns" posed by the OTA, treatment does indeed slow the progression of disease. Therefore, it is important that patients be identified prior to the stage of legal blindness to improve their chances of preserving their vision.

In addition, the benefits of identifying glaucoma suspects who have elevated intraocular pressure have been reaffirmed by the results of the Ocular Hypertension Treatment Study. This study randomized patients with elevated IOP, greater than 24 mmHg in at least one eye, normal optic nerves, and normal visual fields to either treatment or observation. The treatment goal was 20% below baseline and less than 24 mmHg. Patients who were not treated were more likely to progress over 5 years to glaucoma, 9.5% versus those who were treated, 4.4% [18]. Thus, identifying patients prior to the onset of functional loss will significantly delay the development of glaucoma.

3.2.3
The Lack of Knowledge Regarding Glaucoma in the Lay Community

One of the most under-appreciated features of screening is the indirect benefit of education. There are three studies that highlight the magnitude of the need for an educational initiative. In Germany, 2742 individuals were interviewed, 75% had either an active or passive knowledge of the term "glaucoma"; however, only 8.4% correctly identified the basic definition of glaucoma. Interestingly, a significant proportion felt either blurred vision (39%), pain (28%), or reading difficulty (22%) was associated with the onset of glaucoma. Information about glaucoma was more often learned from friends (44%) versus physicians (13%) [23].

Two other studies are even more disconcerting, considering that patients were surveyed who were already actively engaged in the health care system. In Australia, patients who presented to an urban emergency department were surveyed. Determinants of knowledge regarding glaucoma were assessed. Women, people over the age of 40, and those who had a family member with glaucoma were more likely to be aware of the disease rather than individuals who had a history of either systemic hypertension, diabetes, Raynaud's phenomenon, migraines, and myopia [20]. A study conducted at the Massachusetts Eye and Ear Infirmary found that patients who were either African American or Hispanic were more likely to be unfamiliar with glaucoma as an eye problem, as well as those who had less than a college education [10]. It is apparent that health care professionals can improve their own knowledge regarding glaucoma so that they can effectively communicate with their patients in a culturally sensitive fashion.

3.3
Current Screening Practices and Experience

It has been well established that screening for glaucoma by simply using tonometry has little value [8]. Certainly, when one considers that half of the newly diagnosed glaucoma patients enrolled in the EMGT [14] evidenced intraocular pressures less than 20.9 mmHg at baseline, the number of patients who may have been missed if only tonometry was used to identify them is a concern. Furthermore, in the Projector VER [26] study, if 22 mmHg had been set as a cut off for glaucoma patients, 80% of individuals would have been missed. So, if tonometry is not used as the primary screening tool, what is currently being done?

Since many individuals see only a primary care provider (PCP) as their only physician, it is important to know to what extent PCPs are looking for glaucoma in their patients. In a survey of family practitioners in Canada, only 53% claimed to routinely screen for glaucoma. Of those who stated they did not screen for glaucoma, the reasons cited were often lack of equipment and skills. Education seems to be an important issue. Of the 26 physicians who responded to the question regarding screening methods, 14 admitted to using ophthalmoscopy as a means to detect glaucoma, thirteen physicians queried their patients about their family history. One concern is the number of inappropriate methods that were revealed such as the assessment of pupillary reaction to light, ocular palpation, and eyelid abnormalities. Although the response rate in this study was only 30.4% out of a pool of 161 individuals, these data emphasize the importance of educating nonophthalmologists regarding glaucoma and appropriate methods to screen their patients [15].

Those screenings conducted by ophthalmic personnel use a combination of perimetric, tonometric, and ophthalmoscopic devices to assess large groups of individuals. The differences that exist between those individuals who are screened versus identified in a clinical practice was evaluated by Grodum and coworkers in Sweden. A total of 402 patients were identified through a mass screening process and another 354 individuals were identified via a retrospective chart review process in a clinical practice. Among the patients identified from the clinical practice, individuals were identified based on confirmed perimetric defects that were compatible with glaucoma; the diagnosis was determined independent of intraocular pressure. The community screening algorithm consisted of visual acuity, refraction, tonometry, and fundus photography. Individuals were considered positive for glaucoma if either their intraocular pressure was greater than 25 mmHg or if there were characteristic findings in the optic disc, specifically vertical cupping, a focal notch, or localized nerve fiber defects. The authors diagnosed 52.9% of newly identified patients as "normal tension" glaucoma patients. On the other hand patients who self-referred to a clinical practice evidenced a higher mean pressure of 32.5 mmHg versus the mean IOP of 22.9 mmHg in the screened group. Pseudoexfoliation was noted less frequently in the screened group, 16.4% versus 44% and the visual field was not as severely affected, median MD of –8.0 dB versus –16.2 dB. A remarkable finding was the relatively few numbers of individuals who had seen an ophthalmologist in the preceding 2 years, 17%, although as many as 62% of those identified following the screening attested to seeing an ophthalmologist at some point previously [13]. Others have noted that individuals who were screened at a health fair were more likely to have not visited an ophthalmologist versus those who were screened at a senior center, although individuals screened at a senior center had poorer visual acuity [9].

One of the biggest challenges facing any screening program is follow-up. As evidenced by Grodum and colleagues [13], a significant number of individuals fail to follow-up despite being diagnosed as a glaucoma suspect or having glaucoma. Quigley and coworkers reported that only 41% of individuals who were scheduled for an eye appointment successfully kept the appointment, despite the provision of transportation if necessary. Two of the primary reasons given for missing the appointment were that no appointment was given (26%) or failure to remember the appointment (20%) [25]. Thus, any effective screening program must include innovative ways to facilitate follow-up.

3.4
Specific Screening Tests

Most screening programs currently use a combination of risk factor questionnaire, visual acuity and perimetric testing. This combination can be performed by lay persons who are trained to perform these tests. If skilled personnel are available, then this combination of tests can be supplemented by tonometry, and either ophthalmoscopy or optic nerve or nerve fiber imaging technology. This portion of the chapter will focus on specific tests used in screening such as frequency-doubling technology (FDT) and SLP. Moreover, the promising technology involved in teleophthalmology will be briefly discussed. First of all, it is important to review the rationale for including a risk factor questionnaire in every screening event.

3.4.1
Rationale for a Risk Factor Questionnaire

Essential questions to include on any risk factor questionnaire are age, family history, history of either diabetes or hypertension, and the time since the last comprehensive eye examination. Age has been noted to be a significant risk factor for converting to glaucoma among patients with ocular hypertension [11]. As noted earlier, the incidence of glaucoma among the elderly is high [26, 28]. Family history is also very important, particularly given the findings of Nguyen and others. When the relatives of patients with POAG were screened using automated perimetry and optic nerve photography, it was noted siblings had the highest risk of evidencing disease at a rate of 64.7% versus the children, 13.2% and other blood relatives, 22.2% [22]. These rates, however, are all significantly higher than overall rates in the population. Although there is no consensus in the literature regarding diabetes and hypertension as risk factors for glaucoma, given the higher rates of these systemic diseases among the aged and the significant role they play in the health of the retina and optic nerve, it is important to identify the presence of these diseases when assessing the results of the

screening examination. Finally, if the patient is over 40 years of age and has at least one of these other risk factors and the time since the last comprehensive examination is more than 2 years, then a comprehensive examination should be recommended. Individuals should always be reminded that their screening experience is not a replacement for a dilated eye examination.

3.4.2
Frequency-Doubling Technology

FDT has been proven to be an effective method of detecting functional loss in a screening environment (see Fig. 3.1). This device is portable, does not require reduced ambient lighting, and the test can be performed by lay personnel. The test uses a low special frequency sinusoidal grating (<1 cyc/deg) which then undergoes a high temporal frequency counter-phase flicker at 15 Hz or above. The grating appears to be twice its original spatial grating; the perception of this illusion is mediated by the magnocellular pathway. This response presumably represents a subset of retinal ganglion cells that have minimal redundancy. Thus, the potential that this device can detect early functional damage is high [16].

Several recent studies have compared this device to other perimeters and high levels of sensitivity and specificity have been demonstrated. Yamada and coworkers compared FDT perimetry to Damato campimetry, a portable, inexpensive device that has also been used in mass screenings. Subjects in this study underwent both tests, as well as an ophthalmic examination, and Humphrey visual field testing using the 24–2 FASTPAC program. In all, 240 individuals underwent FDT testing and 175 participants underwent Damato campimetric testing. The sensitivity and specificity levels for the FDT were 92% and 93%, respectively; on the other hand, Damato campimetric testing yielded a sensitivity of 53% and specificity of 90% [31]. In another study, the C20–1 screening program on the FDT was compared to the HVF 24–2, standard full threshold test. A total of 36 experienced patients were tested. The investigators

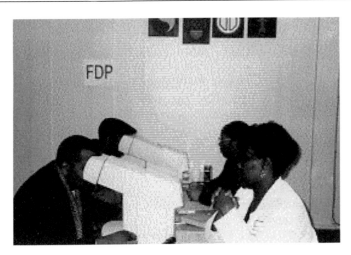

Fig. 3.1. Several FDT units can be used in large screening to detect early structural loss

devised a system to compare the output of the two devices and determined the kappa coefficient between FDT and threshold testing among those eyes with normal tension and high tension glaucoma. Agreement was greater among those patients with normal tension glaucoma versus high tension glaucoma, 0.520 and 0.288, respectively, when comparing thresholds. When comparing scotomata between the two devices, the agreement was similar, 0.439 for normal tension glaucoma and 0.480 for high tension glaucoma [19]. Of course, how one characterizes any given glaucoma patient will determine how well any functional device performs. Chandrasekhar and coworkers used disc findings as a determinant of disease and compared FDT to HVF 24–2 standard full threshold testing. Only patients with early glaucoma were included in this trial which involved 34 consecutive patients and 96 normal patients. The authors observed a sensitivity and specificity of 52.3 % and 57.3 %, respectively, for the HVF and 65.9 % and 61.5 %, respectively, for the FDT [5]. Thus, it appears that the FDT is comparable to HVF in most instances and as a screening device has an acceptable level of sensitivity and specificity.

As with another perimetric tests, some naive patients may need repeated testing to determine their true function. This phenomenon was evaluated in a series of normal patients using the C-20–5 screening mode of the FDT. The mean age of the patients in this cohort was 54.8 years. Of the 81 participants evaluated, 85.2 % of patients tested normal following one test and an additional 11.1 % required a second test. Only 2.5 % of the cohort of patients required three or more tests [17]. Thus, in a screening environment it is important to note that as many as 15 % of individuals may be false positives, just based on the effect of the learning curve. Combining this test with other modes of assessing individuals will improve the examiners ability to eliminate false positives.

3.4.3
Scanning Laser Polarimetry

Considering that patients may initially present with evidence of optic nerve deterioration rather that either functional loss or even elevated intraocular pressure, assessment of the optic nerve becomes an important feature of screening. SLP (Fig. 3.2) indirectly measures the peripapillary thickness of the nerve fiber and thus provides quantitative measures that can be compared to age-matched normals. Essentially, 780-nm laser light is projected onto to the retina; an ellipsometer detects the change in the polarization of the light once it returns to the device. The polarization or retardation of the light is proportional to the amount of tissue present. This device takes advantage of the birefringent properties of the retinal nerve layer. However,

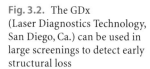

Fig. 3.2. The GDx
(Laser Diagnostics Technology,
San Diego, Ca.) can be used in
large screenings to detect early
structural loss

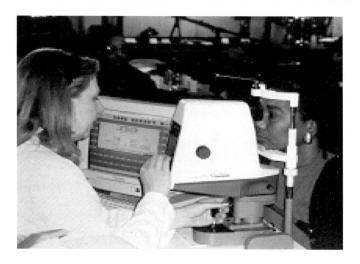

because other structures of the eye possess bire-fringent properties there may be artifact imposed on the output. A newer version of the SLP addresses the variability of the birefringence of the eye across patients by using a "variable corneal compensator" rather than a fixed compensator which was present in the older version of the polarimeter. SLP with variable corneal compensation has been shown to more closely correlate with optical coherence tomography when comparing normal and glaucomatous eyes [1]. It is important to note that most of the studies cited in this section used the older version of the device with fixed corneal compensation.

At two institutions, the utility of the SLP in glaucoma screenings was evaluated. Individuals underwent an ophthalmic examination, HVF (24–2 Fastpac program) and imaging with the SLP. Patients were categorized as either normal, ocular hypertensive, glaucoma suspect, or glaucoma based on ophthalmic history, examination, and HVF results. Optic nerve findings deemed suspicious included a large cup to disc ratio measuring 0.6 or greater, cup to disc asymmetry, or characteristic glaucomatous disc changes such as a notch. Specific parameters such as mean retardation values by sector, calculated ratios of mean retardation values, modulation parameters, and the GDx Number were compared between the normal and glaucoma patients. The overall sensitivity for the device when using the modulation parameter ReMod (S +1) with a cutoff of 665 μm was 86% and the specificity was 90%. When the GDx Number was used at a cutoff of 32, the sensitivity was 68% and the specificity was 90%. The maximum area under the receiver operator curve for the modulation parameters was 0.935 [32]. The sensitivity and the specificity of "the number" will certainly vary based on not only the validity of the gold standard for determining the diagnosis of glaucoma, but also the value selected as a cutoff. Other investigators have noted a higher level of sensitivity and specificity measuring 85.5% and 81.5%, respectively, when a cutoff of 23 was selected. These same investigators also noted greater sensitivity of the number when the severity of the glaucoma increased [7]. The demographics of the population must also be considered when comparing studies involving the SLP since there is a large overlap between eyes with large cup to disc ratios such as 0.8 that have normal fields versus similar eyes that have abnormal fields [30]. Given the significant changes that have been imposed on this technology with the introduction of a device with variable corneal compensation, it is important to continue to investigate the utility of this technology in screening protocols.

3.5
The Promise of Teleophthalmology

In areas of the world where an ophthalmologist may not be directly available to screen patients, the transmission of the digital photos of patients to a central reading center would be an important method to detect glaucoma. The potential of teleophthalmology has been explored by the investigators at the University of Texas. These investigators transmitted digital images of the optic nerve of 32 patients to a remote site. These same patients also underwent optic disc photography. The electronic images and the slides were analyzed for indications of glaucomatous disc changes. Of the 32 images and slides, 26 pairs were analyzed. Signs of glaucomatous changes that could be detected in both methods included vertical elongation, barring of vessel, and focal notching of the rim [21]. This pilot study suggests that teleophthalmology may be a potential addition to screening algorithms, particularly in instances when a physician is not available to conduct the screenings. However, future research should concentrate on larger cohorts to fully explore the usefulness and cost-effectiveness of this methodology.

3.6
The Cost-Effectiveness of Screening for Glaucoma

When policy makers consider implementing programs, these officials must consider the cost-effectiveness of any new initiative. The cost-effectiveness of glaucoma screening was assessed by Gottlieb and coworkers in 1983 [12]. This publication was written prior to the introduction of FDP and SLP in the screening environment and before the completion of major glaucoma clinical trials such as the EMGT and OHTS. Thus, the methods of screening were less precise and the benefits of treatment had not been well established. Furthermore, prostaglandin analogs had not yet been introduced into the clinical environment and the use of laser trabeculoplasty as a clinical therapeutic option had not yet reached

its peak. Nevertheless, it is helpful to review the salient points of this study.

Essentially, the authors [12] note that the "cost-effectiveness is the ratio of the net increase in costs associated with screening, diagnosis, and treatment to the net effectiveness of those activities in terms of years of vision saved." Not only must the direct health costs be considered such as the cost of the equipment, the cost of treatment, and other parameters, but also the cost associated with potential side effects associated with the therapy. Since screenings can be conducted without a physician, and the cost of the equipment such as the FDT and SLP is relatively less expensive than devices considered in the 1980s, this expense has been significantly reduced in the last 20 years. Furthermore, newer medications such as the prostaglandin analogs are associated with fewer side effects compared to timolol, pilocarpine, and systemic carbonic anhydrase inhibitors which were more commonly prescribed in the 1980s. However, one must still consider expenses incurred in following up patients once they have been screened. These costs must then be considered against the cost of caring for blind individuals in a community and the value to an individual to live one more year of life without visual impairment. Interestingly, the authors adjusted their quality years of vision to account for living those additional years with the side effects of therapy. The ratio can be expressed therefore as follows:

$$C/E = Crx + Cse / QAYV$$

where Crx refers to cost of therapy, Cse refers to cost of side effects and the denominator refers to the quality of adjusted years of vision. In the literature, sensitivity and specificity estimates were assigned to various screening protocols such as tonometry 21 mmHg, tonometry 24 mmHg, ophthalmoscopy, perimetry, as well as the initiation and augmentation of therapy. The authors applied their model to a virtual cohort of one million individuals in eight age groups ranging from 40 to 79 years of age. Figure 3.3 illustrates the total costs and benefits when screening was performed based on either tonometric measurements 21 mmHg or ophthalmoscopy. Thus, less sensitive algorithms

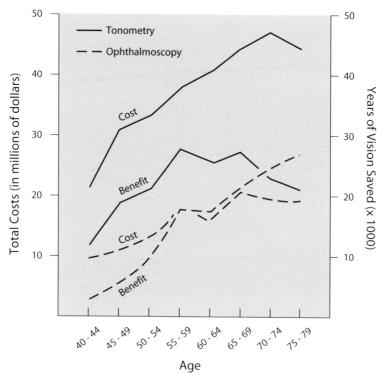

Fig. 3.3. Total costs and benefits associated with two scenarios for screening a virtual population of 1 million individuals: scenario 1 – tonometry only with an IOP of 21 mmHg as a cutoff or ophthalmoscopy only. Note the significant higher costs for tonometry only and declining benefit for screening for ocular hypertension among older individuals. (Reprinted from [12], with permission)

such as tonometry are more costly than more sensitive protocols such as ophthalmoscopy. When screening is targeted to include high risk groups such as family members, then there are much greater benefits at a lower cost (Fig. 3.4). The authors suggested that tonometry may be more beneficial in younger age groups since there is a greater benefit if ocular hypertension is determined earlier in life. On the other hand, ophthalmoscopy is more effective in the later age groups since it is more important at that point to detect true glaucoma patients. However, follow-up and compliance with therapy are persistent issues that need to be addressed and certainly may detract from the initial benefits of identifying individuals.

In a more recent publication in 1996, the Canadians reconsidered the cost effectiveness of screening for primary open angle glaucoma in the province of Quebec. This analysis was completed prior to the release of EMGT [14] and OHTS [18], but did consider newer treatments such as beta blockers and argon laser trabeculoplasty compared to the Gottlieb analysis. Several scenarios were considered such as a screening every 3 years among individuals aged 40–79, which consisted of ophthalmoscopy and tonometry followed by perimetry if there were initial abnormalities noted. Their assumption regarding participation is probably high at 75 % and treatment efficacy at 50 % may have been a reasonable estimate. Nevertheless, the cost, $C100,000 per year of blindness prevented was still considered to be high, particularly when one compares this cost to $C4,500 per year of life gained from breast cancer screening among women aged 50–69. Even when these authors considered more targeted screening scenarios

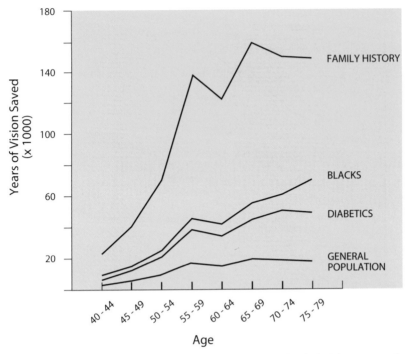

Fig. 3.4. Total years of vision saved when screening is targeted to high risk groups such as those with a family history. (Reprinted from [12], with permission)

that may include individuals aged 65–79, the cost was modestly reduced only to a level of $C42,000 per year of blindness prevented. Thus, the authors concluded that screening for glaucoma is not cost-effective [2].

Although the analysts may consider glaucoma screening too costly, there are issues related to glaucoma and screening that can be considered as "priceless." To some individuals, moderate to severe visual impairment has an equivalent "systemic health state value" that is equivalent to states such as home dialysis for 8 years or moderate to severe stroke [3]. Moreover, a higher prevalence of glaucoma has been reported in specific minority groups such as African Americans and Hispanics. Finally, any screening activity has the powerful indirect benefit of educating individuals as well. This last benefit is certainly difficult to measure but must be considered in any future assessment of this screening activity. Despite the doubts of analysts, in December 2000, President Clinton signed a bill which gave birth to the Glaucoma Detection Benefit which provides coverage for tonometry and a dilated ophthalmoscopy for individuals who are at high risk for glaucoma and who are covered by Medicare [4]. The introduction of this benefit occurred prior to the release of the EMGT [14] and OHTS [18]. Thus it appears that the improvements in perimetric testing, effective, well tolerated therapeutic interventions, and an underlying fear of blindness, likely contributed to reversing conclusions drawn by the OTA in the late 1980s.

Acknowledgments. Supported in part by an unrestricted grant from the Research to Prevent Blindness, New York, NY.

References

1. Bagga H, Greenfield DS, Feiurer W, Knighton RW (2003) Scanning laser polarimetry with variable compensation and optical coherence tomography in normal and glaucomatous eyes. Am J Ophthalmol 135:521–529
2. Bolvin JF, McGregor M, Archer C (1996) Cost effectiveness of screening for primary open angle glaucoma. J Med Screen 3:154–163
3. Brown MM, Brown GC, Sharma S et al. (2003) Quality of life associated with visual loss. Ophthalmol 110:1076–1081
4. Centers for Medicare and Medicaid Services, Program Memorandum Transmittal (2001) Instructions for billing for claims for screenings for glaucoma services, Publication No. CMSPub60B.
5. Chandrasekhar G, Kunjam V, Rao VS et al. (2003) Humphrey visual field and frequency doubling perimetry in the diagnosis of early glaucoma. Ind J Ophthalmol 51:35–38
6. Chen PP (2003) Blindness in patients with treated open angle glaucoma. Ophthalmol 110:726–733
7. Colen TP, Lemij HG (2003) Sensitivity and specificity of the GDx: clinical judgement of standard printouts versus the number. J Glaucoma 12:129–133
8. Eddy DM, Sanders LE, Eddy JF (1983) The value of screening for glaucoma with tonometry. Surv Ophthalmol 28:194–205
9. Ellish NJ, Higginbotham EJ (2002) Differences between screening sites in a glaucoma screening program. Ophthalmic Epidemiol 9:225–237
10. Gasch AT, Wang P, Pasquale LR (2000) Determinants of glaucoma awareness in a general eye clinic. Ophthalmol 107:303–308
11. Gordon MO, Beiser JA, Brandt JD et al. (2002) The Ocular Hypertension Treatment Study. Baseline factors that predict the onset of primary open-angle glaucoma. Arch Ophthalmol 120:714–720
12. Gottlieb LK, Schwartz B, Pauker SG (1983) Glaucoma screening. A cost-effectiveness analysis. Surv Ophthalmol 28:206–226
13. Grodum K, Heijl A, Bengtsson B (2002) A comparison of glaucoma patients identified through mass screening and in routine clinical practice. Acta Ophthalmol Scand. 80:627–631
14. Heijl A, Leske MC, Bengtsson B et al. (2002) Reduction of intraocular pressure and glaucoma progression: results from the Early Manifest Glaucoma Trial. Arch Ophthalmol 120:1371–1372
15. Huang JT, Rhemtulla F, Huang PT (2003) Glaucoma screening by primary care physicians in southern Alberta: patterns, methods, and deficiencies. Can J Ophthalmol 38:279–284
16. Johnson CA, Samuels SJ (1997) Screening for glaucomatous visual field loss with frequency-doubling perimetry. Invest Ophthalmol Vis Sci 38:413–425
17. Joson PJ, Kamantigue ME, Chen PP (2002) Learning effects among perimetric novices in frequency doubling technology perimetry. Ophthalmol 109:757–760
18. Kass MA, Heuer DK, Higginbotham EJ et al. (2003) The Ocular Hypertension Treatment Study: a randomized trial determines that topical ocular hypertensive medication delays or prevents the onset of primary open-angle glaucoma. Arch Ophthalmol 120:701–713
19. Kogure S, Toda Y, Crabb D, Kashiwagi K et al. (2003) Agreement between frequency-doubling perimetry and static perimetry in eyes with high tension and normal tension glaucoma. Br J Ophthalmol 87:604–608
20. Landers JA, Goldberg I, Graham SL (2002) Factors affecting awareness and knowledge of glaucoma among patients presenting to an urban emergency department. Clin Experiment Ophthalmol 30:104–109
21. Li HK, Tang RA, Oschner K et al. (1999) Telemedicine screening for glaucoma. Telemed J 5:283–290
22. Nguyen RL, Raja SC, Traboulsi EI (2000) Screening relatives of patients with familial chronic open angle glaucoma. Ophthalmol 107:1294–1297
23. Pfeiffer N, Krieglstein GK, Wellek S (2002) Knowledge about glaucoma in the unselected population: a German survey. J Glaucoma 11:458–463
24. Power EJ, Wagner JL, Duffy BM (1988) Screening for open-angle glaucoma in the elderly. Congress of the United States. Office of Technology Assessment, October
25. Quigley HA, Park CK, Tracey PA, Pollack IP (2002) Community screening for eye disease by laypersons: the Hoffberger program. Am J Ophthalmol 133:386–392
26. Quigley HA, West SK, Rodriguez J et al. (2001) The prevalence of glaucoma in a population-based study of Hispanic subjects: Proyecto VER Arch Ophthalmol 119:1819–1826
27. Ramakrishnan R, Nirmalan PK, Krishnadas R et al. (2003) Glaucoma in a rural population of southern India: the Aravind comprehensive eye survey. Ophthalmol 8:1484–1490
28. Schoff EO, Hattenhauer MG, Ing HH et al. (2001) Estimated incidence of open-angle glaucoma in Olmsted County, Minnesota. Ophthalmol 5:882–886
29. Singalavanija A, Metheetrairut A, Ruangvaravate N et al. (2001) Ocular diseases and blindness in elderly Thais. J Med Assoc Thai 84:1383–1388

30. Tannenbaum DP, Sangwill LM, Bowd C et al. (2001) Relationship between visual field testing and scanning laser polarimetry in patients with a large cup to disk ratio. Am J Ophthalmol 132:501–506

31. Yamada N, Chen PP, Millis RP et al. (1999) Screening for glaucoma with frequency-doubling technology and Damato campimetry. Arch Ophthalmol 117:1479–1484

32. Yamada N, Chen PP, Mills R et al. (2000) Screening for glaucoma using the scanning laser polarimeter. J Glaucoma 2:254–261

Semi-automated Kinetic Perimetry for Assessment of Advanced Glaucomatous Visual Field Loss

ULRICH SCHIEFER, K. NOWOMIEJSKA, J. PAETZOLD

Core Messages

- Kinetic perimetry is especially useful and efficient for delineating advanced visual field defects via "edge detection"
- Moving targets seem to be much more predictive than static ones for exploring consequences of visual impairment in regard to activities of daily living
- Manual kinetic perimetry depends to a great extent on examiners' skill and experience
- Semi-automated kinetic perimetry (SKP) enhances standardisation and reproducibility of visual field examination with moving targets of defined angular velocity
- Repeated presentation of moving targets along a given "vector" enables estimation of individual local scatter of kinetic thresholds
- Assessment of individual reaction time helps to compensate for systematic shift of scotoma borders
- Intensive training is necessary for learning how to track down and delineate scotomas with moving targets

4.1 Introduction

Kinetic perimetry may nowadays be regarded as an anachronism in glaucoma diagnostics. Manual kinetic perimetry – the basis of visual field examination – was abandoned in routine glaucoma diagnostics many years ago for several reasons: First of all, the procedure crucially depends on examiners' experience, skill and performance. Digital storage and recall of perimetric records in manually driven perimeters is also not possible and there are no auto-calibration routines available for kinetic instruments, such as the Goldmann perimeter, and the Tübingen Manual Perimeter. Furthermore, due to its pantograph mechanism, the spatial resolution of the Goldmann instrument is comparatively poor within the central visual field.

Automation of the examination procedure and digital documentation of the perimetric results was considered to be difficult. The potential realisation of automation has been demonstrated in only few publications [7, 29–31]. Instead of "old fashioned" kinetic techniques, Fankhauser's publication [6] pointed the way for the triumphant advance of computer-based, automated threshold estimating static perimetry.

Nevertheless, the latter technique critically depends on the choice of an adequate grid of test locations and is extremely inefficient and exhausting in cases of advanced visual field loss. Kinetic procedures are very well suited for these patients, since this technique is mainly based on features like edge detection and pattern recognition, which works considerably more efficiently when the scotoma has a definite (steep) border. This may also be the reason for its better acceptance by elderly and/or neurologically impaired patients, compared to static grid perimetry. Moreover, in cases of advanced glaucomatous neuropathy, morphometric examinations are rather inefficient due to subtotal neuronal loss. However, even subtle morphological changes will result in considerable functional deterioration, manifesting in a shift of borders

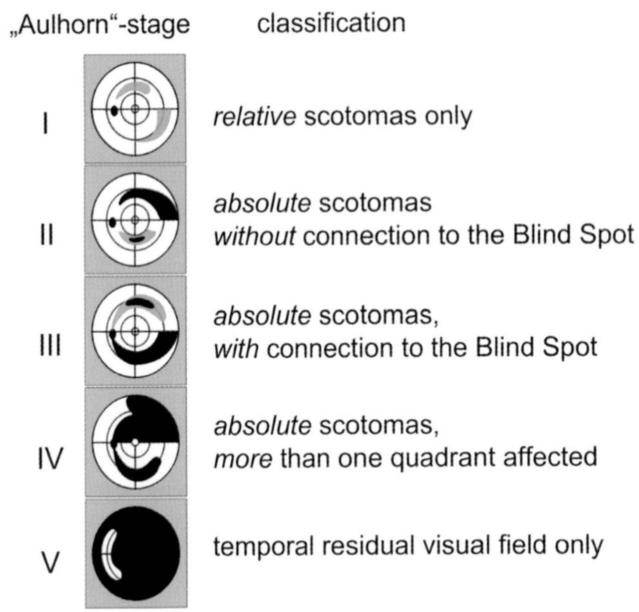

„Aulhorn"-stage classification

I		*relative* scotomas only
II		*absolute* scotomas *without* connection to the Blind Spot
III		*absolute* scotomas, *with* connection to the Blind Spot
IV		*absolute* scotomas, *more* than one quadrant affected
V		temporal residual visual field only

Fig. 4.1. Scotoma classification in cases of (glaucomatous) visual field loss due to retinal nerve fibre layer defects, according to Aulhorn et al. [1]

of the already advanced scotomas. This is yet another diagnostic domain of kinetic perimetry.

Kinetic targets seem to be much closer to reality than static test points in exploring or defining the consequences of visual impairment to daily activities. These facts may explain why kinetic perimetry has maintained its function of providing the final decision in expert opinion and ability tests in many countries.

Kinetic perimetry has undergone further developments to make it less subject to examiner skill, and to increase reliability of digital documentation and processing in the form of semi-automated kinetic perimetry (SKP), which – among other terms – was formerly known as computer-assisted automatic kinetic perimetry (CAKP) [16, 18–20, 21–23, 25–27]. This technique is especially useful in cases of advanced visual field loss, like hemianopia, concentric constriction of the visual field or advanced retinal nerve fibre bundle defect due to glaucomatous or ischemic optic neuropathy, i.e. stage III or more (see Fig. 4.1), according to the Aulhorn classification [1].

Summary for the Clinician

- Manual kinetic perimetry is an efficient and sound method for assessment of advanced (glaucomatous) visual field loss. However, this technique depends on the skill of the examiner to a great extent

4.2
Methods/Methodological Aspects

Fully automated kinetic perimetry seems to be unrealistic due to the variety of potential scotoma patterns in clinical routine. *Semi*-automated techniques nowadays offer a feasible compromise: "scotoma edge detection" is interactively scheduled by the examiner with immediate consideration of the patient's responses. The examination procedure itself is maintained and surveyed by the computer and is routinely carried out as described below.

The origin and direction of kinetic targets are chosen and defined by the examiner with the help of so-called vectors. These are usually directed from non-seeing regions towards intact areas of the visual field, crossing the pre-

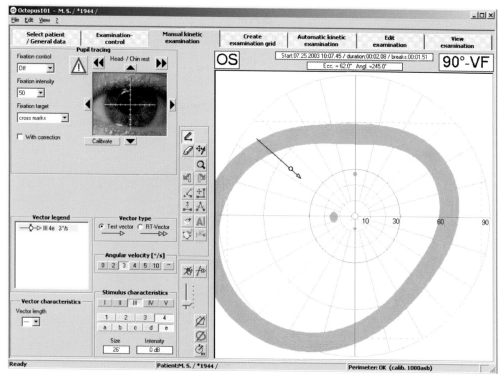

Fig. 4.2. User-guided interface of the OCTOPUS 101 perimeter (Interzeag/Haag-Streit Inc., Koeniz, Switzerland) used for operating the perimeter in the semi-automated kinetic perimetry (SKP) mode. The examination can be carried out with a computer mouse or an electronic pen on a combined graphic tablet/touch screen (see also Fig. 4.3). The *dashed lines* indicate the maximum stimulus eccentricities due to technical limitations. The location of the age-related isopter is described by the broad red band, which represents the predicted mean ± 1 SD

Fig. 4.3. OCTOPUS 101 perimeter (Interzeag/Haag-Streit, Koeniz, Switzerland) with semi-automated kinetic perimetry (SKP) option: attached is a specially-designed projection unit. The examination is carried out on the combined graphic tablet/touch screen unit which, in this case, is positioned on the right side of the perimeter (see also Fig. 4.2)

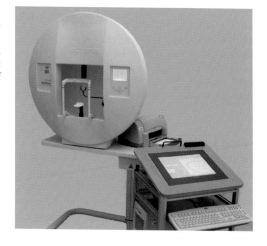

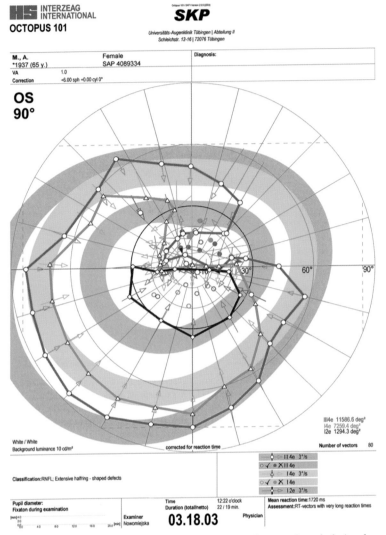

Fig. 4.4. Glaucomatous visual field defect, stage III, corresponding to the Aulhorn classification [1], affecting predominantly the *upper* region of the visual field. Stimulus characteristics (size, luminance) and stimulus angular velocity of the kinetic targets are coded by colours and symbols (see legend). Records were obtained with the OCTOPUS 101 perimeter (Interzeag/Haag-Streit, Koeniz, Switzerland), using the SKP option with single presentation of kinetic targets

sumed scotoma/visual field border almost perpendicularly. The stimulus size and luminance levels can be varied according to the Goldmann classification. Angular velocity can be chosen by the examiner and is kept constant by the computer. The examiner determines the position and length of each vector by means of a computer mouse or a combined graphic display tablet/touch screen unit (Fig. 4.2), which are also used for "electronic drawing" of the isopters and further analyses (e.g. interactive quantitative assessment of the scotoma area). Stimulus characteristics, vector locations, patient responses, and isopters are (optionally) displayed on the monitor or in the printout and can be stored in a database. Each examination

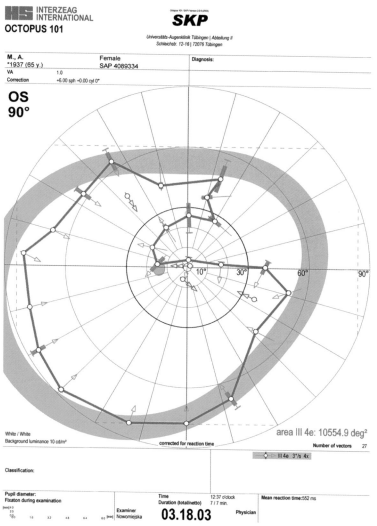

INTERZEAG INTERNATIONAL
OCTOPUS 101

SKP

Universitäts-Augenklinik Tübingen | Abteilung II
Schleichstr. 12-16 | 72076 Tübingen

M., A.	Female	Diagnosis:
*1937 (65 y.)	SAP 4089334	
VA 1.0		
Correction +6.00 sph +0.00 cyl 0°		

OS
90°

10°   30°   60°   90°

White / White
Background luminance 10 cd/m²

corrected for reaction time

area III 4e: 10554.9 deg²

Number of vectors   27

III 4e 3°/s 4x

Classification:

Pupil diameter:
Fixaton during examination

Time   12:37 o'clock
Duration (total/netto)   7 / 7 min.

Mean reaction time:552 ms

Examiner
Nowomiejska

03.18.03

Physician

Fig. 4.5. The same glaucomatous visual field defect as in Fig. 4.4, obtained with the OCTOPUS 101 perimeter using the SKP option, but with repeated (4×) presentation of kinetic targets (III4e, angular velocity: 3°/s). The remaining visual field area can be interactively quantified and is indicated in square degrees (deg²). The variation of local scatter bars is shown along the isopter. The location of the age-related normative isopter is indicated by the broad *red band*, which represents the predicted mean ±1 SD. In principle, other indices, defining the location parameter (e.g. median) and the shape parameter (e.g. 5%–95% reference interval) could be applied alternatively. (For further details, see legend to Fig. 4.4)

record and its related set of vectors serves as an individual baseline for follow-up examinations. This data set is electronically retrievable allowing the entire examination procedure to be repeated in an identical manner.

The software is implemented in a modified version of the OCTOPUS 101 perimeter (In-

terzeag/Haag-Streit, Koeniz, Switzerland), which at the moment seems to be best suited for this purpose (Fig. 4.3). It is equipped with a specially designed projection unit for realising continuous, smooth target movement for any desired stimulus direction with target angular velocities up to 25°/s, and for any given Goldmann stimu-

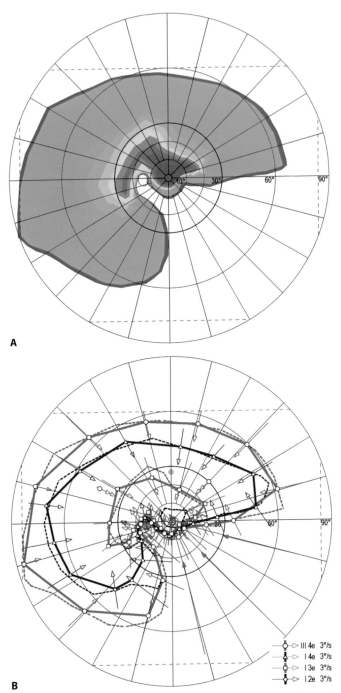

A

B

III 4e 3°/s
I 4e 3°/s
I3e 3°/s
I2e 3°/s

Fig. 4.6 A,B. SKP training program. **A** Glaucomatous visual field defect, which is "carved" into the age-related normative "three-dimensional", colourcoded hill of vision. **B** Actual result of a trainee with super- imposed two-dimensional view of the original scotoma. *Solid lines* represent the results of the trainee, whereas *dashed lines* show the related original isopters

lus condition (size 0–V, i.e., approx. 3' to approx. 100', and luminance level 1a–4e, i.e. 4–320 cd/m²). Stimulus presentation is possible within an eccentricity ("radius") of up to 84° in each horizontal direction, and up to 60° and 78° within the superior and inferior hemifields, respectively. This area is indicated by dashed lines in the related graphics (Figs. 4.4–4.6).

Summary for the Clinician

• Semi-automated kinetic perimetry (SKP) enhances standardisation and repro-ducibility of visual field examination with moving targets of defined angular velocity

4.3
Assessment and Definition of "Local Kinetic Threshold" and Local Scatter

With single presentations, the patient's response for each presented vector is defined as local kinetic threshold (Fig. 4.4). Alternatively or additionally, stimulus presentation per vector may be repeated (usually four times): In this case, the related local threshold is defined as the mean of the single values. Additionally, local scatter is defined as standard deviation (SD) of the single values (Fig. 4.5). The extent of scatter depends on the one hand on the individual patient, which should have an effect on all SD values. On the other hand, local SD is also influenced by slope of the scotoma border in this region: Steep slopes should result in small local scatter, whereas broad scatter bars indicate either a shallow gradient of the scotoma border or short-term variation in its localisation. Variation in eyelid position during examination procedure is responsible for increase of scatter in the upper region of the visual field, whereas ceiling effects due to technical limitations result in an artificially small local dispersion, e.g. in the temporal region.

Summary for the Clinician

• Repeated presentation of moving targets along a given "vector" enables estimation of the individual local scatter of kinetic thresholds

4.4
Assessment and Importance of Individual Reaction Time

Reaction time has an influence on the results of automated *static* grid perimetry only if a given time span is exceeded. This will result in the stimulus being classified as not seen.

However, reaction time is a critical issue in *kinetic* perimetry, since target movement continues within the time interval of subjects' perception and the related reaction (of the subject and the examiner), resulting in a systematic shift of the scotoma and/or visual field border in the direction of the stimulus movement. This displacement increases with target velocity and is mainly influenced by individual reaction time. Thus, an assessment of reaction time is essential to be able to differentiate whether the increased latency of response is due to pathology of the visual pathways or whether it is attributable to impaired co-operability on behalf of the patient.

For clinical purposes, reaction time during SKP is assessed by presenting kinetic stimuli of defined size and luminance (mostly III4e) moving with identical angular velocity along at least two centripetal (so-called reaction time) vectors, which are individually placed in obviously intact visual field regions. In this way, scotoma borders can be optionally corrected for this systematic shift by considering the mean of the assessed reaction time values and thereby determining the average distance covered by the target.

In a normative SKP study, reaction time values were comparatively small: 400–700 ms for an 80% reference interval, and 390–890 ms for a 90% reference interval. This range did not show a relevant age dependency and was graded clinically negligibly [15]. However, the latency was prolonged and more inhomogeneously distributed in patients suffering from advanced visual field loss. In an SKP study on 31 patients with advanced glaucomatous visual field defects, i.e. ≥ Aulhorn stage III [1], reaction times were 391–1614 ms (95% reference interval) [13]. Locations of four RT vectors were distributed within an intact visual field area depending on the character of the defect. We found that RT values increased significantly with eccentricity of the RT vector. This increase of RT was about 1% every 1° of eccentricity.

4.5
Selection of Optimum Target Angular Velocity

Target angular velocity does not only indirectly influence spatial resolution but also has an impact on examination duration. Johnson et al. found a target velocity of 4°/s to be an optimum compromise in kinetic perimetry [10]. Wabbels and Kolling stated that angular velocities exceeding 4°/s would result in a substantial displacement of scotoma borders [26]. However, they did not consider individual reaction time. If individual latency is taken into account, the influence of target angular velocity is negligible [13, 23]. In routine clinical examination target angular velocity in SKP is routinely set to 3°/s. It is reduced to 2°/s if the area of the scotoma is equal to or less than the size of the blind spot.

Summary for the Clinician

- Consideration of individual reaction time reduces the impact of angular velocity on the kinetic threshold location

4.6
Age-Related Normative Values

Normal values are essential for delineating pathological findings in any given age group. This is not only important for the current "status quo", but also for follow-up purposes. Due to the practical relevance of kinetic perimetry, age-related normative values are an indispensable prerequisite for forming an expert opinion on the visual ability and its consequences on daily-life activities. These normative data, taking individual reaction time into consideration, have been assessed for SKP [13, 23]. A smooth model of the normative "kinetic" hill of vision could be created, which allows prediction of age-related isopters for any arbitrary target size and luminance combination. Figure 4.5 shows an example of SKP assessment of advanced glaucomatous visual loss with repeated (4×) target presenta-

tions along each vector. The age-related normative isopter is superimposed.

Summary for the Clinician

- Age-related normative values are an essential pre-requisite for evaluating kinetic perimetric results within the scope of expert opinions

4.7
Comparability of SKP Results with Those of Conventional Manual Kinetic Perimetry Using the GOLDMANN Instrument

In many countries, the GOLDMANN instrument is still considered as the "gold standard" of kinetic perimetry for cases of advanced glaucomatous visual field loss, despite its above-mentioned shortcomings. We therefore compared the visual field records obtained in random sequence, using the OCTOPUS 101 SKP mode (without reaction time correction), with those obtained using the classical manual GOLD-MANN kinetic perimeter in 36 patients suffering from advanced RNFL defect [12]. The area of corresponding isopters (I2e, I3e, I4e, III4e and V4e) was electronically measured using the available option of SKP. However, if only the visual field area is taken as a basis for comparison, the topography of the isopters and scotomas would be completely neglected. In order to enhance the comparability, the ratio of intersection area and union area, related to the isopters, obtained with GOLDMANN manual kinetic perimetry and OCTOPUS 101-SKP, respectively, was calculated. Intersection areas were expressed as a percentage of union areas. The resulting preliminary values of this ratio were approximating 76%–82% depending on isopter, which indicates that SKP indeed leads to results that are well comparable to those obtained using the conventional manual kinetic techniques [12].

Summary for the Clinician

- Results of semi-automated kinetic perimetry (SKP) seem to be comparable to those obtained with conventional manual kinetic perimetry

4.8
Evaluation of Individual
Functional Impairment/Expert Opinion

A quantification of visual (field) loss is essential for kinetic perimetry to enable any assessment of scotoma progression and/or the patient's visual performance ability. The interactive assessment of the area of scotoma (see Fig. 4.5) via a computer-assisted triangulation routine, is one option for this task, which can be performed with the OCTOPUS 101 instrument for any relevant stimulus condition.

Superimposition of a grid for scoring purposes has been introduced by Esterman in order to avoid any kind of complicated planimetry [2–5, 9]. Modification of this grid has recently been proposed by Weber et al. in order to adapt this score form for the special needs, according to German expert opinion, based on kinetic perimetry [28]. The extension of the remaining intact visual field may also be quantified by the so-called MRD (mean radial degrees) assessed by the average length of the meridians (i.e. radial distance of the scotoma borders from the visual field centre) [11], or by adding up triangles aimed toward the visual field centre [8]. However, these methods are mainly applicable in cases of concentric visual field constriction and clearly do not work well with arcuate scotomas.

The course of the intersection–/union–area ratio (see also Sect. 4.7) over time, related to previous or baseline perimetric sessions, may also serve as a valid procedure for quantitative evaluation of progression for kinetic perimetry.

Summary for the Clinician

- There are several options with regard to quantification of kinetic perimetric results

4.9
Training, Education and Learning

In recent decades, the increasing popularity of automated static grid perimetry has resulted in a decrease in experience with kinetic techniques. Therefore, intensive training is necessary to learn this "elaborate craft" of tracking down and delineating scotomas. By means of a specially designed software, various kinds of visual field defects can be "carved" into a three-dimensional, age-related normative hill of vision. In the same way, typical SKP findings can be transferred into this 3D view [14]. This kind of three-dimensional presentation is necessary to provide realistic scotoma borders for any kind of chosen stimulus size and luminance combination. Additionally, "psychophysical habits" of the "dummy" or "artificial" patient, such as individual response characteristics and reaction times, can be varied. Each exercise case is presented with a concise chart presenting essential data about patient history and ophthalmological findings. The training session is performed using exactly the same user-guided interface, which also records the duration of each session. Each vector presented is documented and can be discussed afterwards. Each SKP result, obtained by the trainee with any chosen stimulus size and luminance combination, can be directly compared with the actual finding, which is derived from the "originally carved" hill of vision (Fig. 4.6a). The quality of each presented result can be evaluated by comparing each isopter obtained with that of the actually carved hill of vision, using again the intersection–/union–area ratio (see also Sect. 4.7).

Summary for the Clinician

- Intensive training of kinetic perimetry is mandatory. Recently developed software is helpful in this regard

4.10
Outlook

Follow-up examinations using semi-automated kinetic perimetry should be based on identical sets of kinetic vectors, thereby visualising and quantitatively evaluating systematic shifts of local kinetic thresholds. Additionally, the course of the intersection–/union–area ratio (see also chapters Sects. 4.7 and 4.8) over time, should be analysed.

SKP is implemented in the same instrument as that routinely used for automated static grid perimetry. It should be easy, therefore, to combine these methods within one and the same session, i.e. regions with advanced scotomas are examined with SKP, whereas for other areas with presumably normal differential luminance sensitivity or subtle defects automated static threshold estimating grid perimetry is applied.

Even in the current SKP version, manual static stimuli can be presented in any visual field region by simply setting target velocity to 0°/s. Static stimuli can also be arranged in any desired spacing along the original (kinetic) vectors, thus allowing the assessment of local statokinetic dissociation (SKD) in one and the same instrument within two subsequent sessions [17, 24].

Summary for the Clinician

- Combining various perimetric procedures may even further enhance diagnostic capabilities of visual field examination

Acknowledgement. The authors are gratefully indebted to Dipl.-Ing.(BA) Elke Krapp and Dipl.-Ing. Wilhelm Durst for their help in preparing the manuscript and the figures. They would also like to thank Dr. rer. pol. Reinhard Vonthein for his biometric support, and Priv.-Doz. Dr. rer. nat. Anne Kurtenbach for her linguistic assistance.

References

1. Aulhorn E, Karmeyer H (1977) Frequency distribution in early glaucomatous visual field defects. Doc Ophthalmol Proc Ser 14:17–83
2. Esterman B (1967) Grid for scoring visual fields. I. Tangent screen. Arch Ophthalmol 77:780–786
3. Esterman B (1968) Grid for scoring visual fields. II. Perimeter. Arch Ophthalmol 79:400–406
4. Esterman B (1982) Functional scoring of the binocular field. Ophthalmology 89:1226–1234
5. Esterman B (1983) Functional scoring of the binocular visual field. In: Greve EL, Heijl A (eds) Fifth international visual field symposium. Dr W. Junk, The Hague, the Netherlands, pp 187–192
6. Fankhauser F, Koch P, Roulier A (1972) On automation of perimetry. Albrecht Von Graefes Arch Klin Exp Ophthalmol 184:126–150
7. Gandolfo E, Zingirian M, Capris P (1985) The automated program 'Genoa Glaucoma Screening'. In: Heijl A, Greve EL (eds) Proceedings of the 6th international visual field symposium. Dr. W. Junk, Dordrecht, Netherland, pp 103–107
8. Hardus P, Verduin WM, Engelsman M, Edelbroek PM, Segers JP, Berendschot TT, Stilma JS (2001) Visual field loss associated with vigabatrin: quantification and relation to dosage. Epilepsia 42:262–267
9. Harris ML, Jacobs NA (1995) Is the Esterman binocular field sensitive enough? In: Mills RP, Wall M (eds) Perimetry update 1994/1995. Kugler, pp 403–404
10. Johnson CA, Keltner JL (1987) Optimal rates of movement for kinetic perimetry. Arch Ophthalmol 105:73–75
11. Newman WD, Tocher K, Acheson JF (2002) Vigabatrin associated visual field loss: a clinical audit to study prevalence, drug history and effects of drug withdrawal. Eye 16:567–571
12. Nowomiejska K et al (in preparation) Comparison of semi-automated kinetic perimetry (SKP) using the INTERZEAG OCTOPUS 101 instrument with manual GOLDMANN kinetic perimetry (MKP) in patients with advanced visual field loss.
13. Nowomiejska K et al (in preparation) The reaction time during semi-automated kinetic perimetry (SKP) in patients with advanced visual field loss.
14. Paetzold J, Schiller J, Rauscher S, Schiefer U (2003) A computer application for training kinetic perimetry. In: Wall M, Mills RP (eds) Perimetry update 2002/2003. Kugler, The Hague, The Netherlands, in press
15. Rauscher S et al (in preparation) Reaction times in semi-automated kinetic perimetry (SKP) – a normative study in 84 normal subjects.
16. Rauscher S, Vonthein R, Sadowski B, Erdmann B, Krapp E, Schiefer U (2002) Computer-assisted kinetic perimetry (CAKP) using the Octopus 101 Perimeter: age related normal values of local thresholds using various stimulus conditions and considering individual reaction times. Invest Ophthalmol Vis Sci 43:3810
17. Riddoch G (1917) Dissociation of visual perceptions due to occipital injuries with especial reference to appreciation of movement. Brain 40:15–57
18. Schiefer U, Witte A (1996) Patent: Perimetrisches Untersuchungsverfahren – Autokinetische Perimetrie II. Deutsches Patentamt München, DE 196 21 960 C2, Az.196 21 960.4 1–18
19. Schiefer U, Witte A (2003) Patent: Perimetrisches Untersuchungsverfahren – Autokinetische Perimetrie unter Berücksichtigung und Korrektur der individuellen Reaktionszeit. Deutsches Patentamt München, DE 100 13 682 C2, Az.100 13 682.6–35

20. Schiefer U, Schiller J, Paetzold J, Dietrich TJ, Von-thein R, Besch D (2001) Evaluation ausgedehnter Gesichtsfelddefekte mittels computerassistierter kinetischer Perimetrie. Klin Monatsbl Augenheilkd 218:13–20

21. Schiefer U, Rauscher S, Sadowski B, Hermann A, Nowomiejska KE, Vonthein R, Schiller J (2002) Alterskorrelierte Normwerte für die semi-automatisierte kinetische Perimetrie (SKP) mit dem Interzeag Octopus 101 Instrument. Ophthalmologe 99:106–107

22. Schiefer U, Paetzold J, Rauscher S, Vonthein R, Hermann A, Nowomiejska KE (2003) Semi-automatisierte kinetische Perimetrie (SKP) – ein Verfahren zur weitgehend Untersucher-unabhängigen Evaluation und Verlaufskontrolle fortgeschrittener Skotome. 87. Tagung der Württembergischen Augenärztlichen Vereinigung 26

23. Schiefer U, Rauscher S, Hermann A, Nowomiejska KE, Sadowski B, Vonthein R, Paetzold J, Schiller J (2003) Age dependence of normative values in semi-automated kinetic perimetry (SKP). Invest Ophthalmol Vis Sci 44:E-abstract 1957

24. Schiller J, Paetzold J, Vonthein R, Schiefer U (2003) Evaluation of stato-kinetic dissociation using (examiner-independent) automated perimetric techniques. In: Wall M, Mills RP (eds) Perimetry update 2002/2003. Kugler Publications, The Hague, The Netherlands, in press

25. Wabbels B, Kolling G (1999) Automatische kinetische Perimetrie mit dem Twinfield-Perimeter. Zeitschrift für praktische Augenheilkunde 20:401–406

26. Wabbels B, Kolling G (2001) Automatische kinetische Perimetrie mit unterschiedlichen Prüfgeschwindigkeiten. Ophthalmologe 98:168–173

27. Wabbels BK, Dingeldey C, Kolling G (2001) Age-related influence of different stimulus velocities in automated kinetic perimetry. Invest Ophthalmol Vis Sci 42:852

28. Weber J, Schiefer U, Kolling G (2003) Vorschlag für die funktionelle Bewertung von Gesichtsfeldausfällen mit einem Punktesystem. Ophthalmologe, accepted for publication

29. Zingirian M, Gandolfo E, Orciuolo M (1983) Automation of the Goldmann Perimeter. Doc Ophthalmol Proc Ser 42:103–107

30. Zingirian M, Dorigo MT, Gandolfo E (1990) Contribution of manual and computerized perimetry to the differential diagnosis of optic neuropathies. Metab Pediatr Syst Ophthalmol 13:50–54

31. Zingirian M, Gandolfo E, Capris P, Mattioli R (1991) Computerized system for static and kinetic automatic perimetry. Eur J Ophthalmol 1:181–186

Optic Nerve Imaging: Recent Advances

Linda M. Zangwill, Felipe A. Medeiros,
Christopher Bowd, Robert N. Weinreb

Core Messages

- The HRT, GDx, OCT and RTA provide reproducible, real-time quantitative information on the optic disc and RNFL
- Recent hardware and software advances have improved their ability to detect and monitor glaucomatous damage over time
- The HRT, GDx, OCT and RTA can differentiate between normal and glaucoma eyes, and show promise for detecting change over time
- It is important that the clinician understand the strengths and limitations of each technique, so that the best quality information will be used for glaucoma management decisions
- These techniques should be utilized in conjunction with careful clinical examination and visual function testing

5.1 Introduction

5.1.1 Background

Detecting optic disc and retinal nerve fiber layer (RNFL) damage and change is the cornerstone of glaucoma management. Until recently, evaluation of the optic disc and RNFL has been subjective, with descriptions of change primarily qualitative. With the development of optical imaging instruments, objective and quantitative measurements of the optic nerve head and RNFL are now possible.

Although clinical examination and fundus photography remain the "gold standard" for assessing glaucomatous optic disc and RNFL damage, they are limited by their need for maximal pupil dilation, and subjective, qualitative assessment. A written description or optic disc drawing is necessary to summarize information from the clinical examination, making detection of change over time difficult. Photography provides objective documentation for comparison over time, but requires subjective assessment, and variation in interpretation of photographs is well documented. In addition, photographs require processing and are therefore not available at the time of the patient visit.

In contrast to clinical examination and photography, computer-based imaging instruments provide real-time quantitative information on the optic disc and RNFL, with reduced need for pupil dilation and clear media. For these reasons, in many clinical practices, imaging instruments are the standard method used for documenting optic nerve head and RNFL appearance.

Table 5.1. Summary of HRT, GDx, and OCT, and RTA specifications and changes

	CSLO		SLP		OCT		RTA2
	HRT	HRTII	GDx NFA	GDx VCC	OCT	Stratus OCT	
Year commercially introduced	1992	1999	NFA, 1992; GDx NFA, 1996	2002	1997	2001	2002
Pixels	65,000	147,456	65,000	36,600	100 A-scans, each of 500 data points	128, 256, or 512 A-scans, each of 1024 data points	2560 for macular thickness, 3072 for disc topography
Pupil dilation necessary?	No	No	No	No	Yes	In some eyes	For macular scans
Real-time feedback on image quality	Yes	Yes	Yes	Yes	No	In progress	No
Measures RNFL?	Indirectly, with reference plane	Indirectly, with reference plane	Yes, with fixed corneal compensation	Yes, with variable corneal compensation	Yes	Yes	Indirectly, with reference plane
Measures optic disc topography?	Yes	Yes	No	No	No	Yes	Yes
Normative database (number of eyes)	100	112	1200	540	150	328	105 For regression analysis, 400+ for retinal thickness
Change detection with probability algorithm	Yes, recent software upgrade	Yes	No	In progress	No	No	Yes
Automated image quality assessment	Yes	Yes	Yes	Yes	No	No	Yes
Limitations	Reference plane for some diagnostic parameters, IOP dependent	Reference plane for some diagnostic parameters, IOP dependent	Fixed corneal compensation	Macular pathology can effect corneal compensation	Dilation needed, only 100–A scans	Limited number of data points	Reference plane for some topography parameters, dilation needed for macular scans

Specifications are subject to change by the manufacturer.

For a new diagnostic tool to be useful in clinical practice, the measurements should be reproducible, and provide information that has the potential to change management practice so that patients will be better off as a result of the test. That is, the test should produce consistent measurements, and provide information to assist in detecting the disease, and monitoring its progression over time. The number of published articles evaluating the ability of imaging instruments to detect glaucoma has increased dramatically in recent years. However, as the number of manuscripts increases, it becomes more difficult to synthesize the results of these studies in order to determine how these instruments can be used to help detect glaucomatous optic disc and RNFL damage. Furthermore, as highlighted in Table 5.1, each of these instruments has undergone significant hardware and software improvements in the last few years, so that issues that were once limitations for a given technique may no longer be relevant.

The objective of this chapter is to highlight recent hardware and software improvements for four commercially available diagnostic imaging instruments, a confocal scanning laser ophthalmoscope (Heidelberg Retina Tomograph [HRT and HRT II], Heidelberg Engineering, Dossenheim, Germany), a scanning laser polarimeter (GDx Nerve Fiber Analyzer and GDx VCC, Laser Diagnostics Technologies, San Diego, CA), the Optical Coherence Tomograph (OCT and Stratus OCT, Carl Zeiss Meditec, Dublin, CA), and the Retinal Thickness Analyzer (RTA, Talia Technology Ltd., Neve-Ilan, Israel). Each instrument makes use of different properties of light and different characteristics of retinal tissue to obtain their measurements. Brief descriptions of the operating principles and analysis features of the four imaging instruments will be provided with case examples, and with a summary of what is known about each technique's image quality, reproducibility, ability to detect glaucoma and to monitor its progression, and correlation with functional indices. The chapter will supplement recent reviews [24, 44, 69] by summarizing relevant, good quality publications that evaluate how recent advances in these technologies can assist in monitoring glaucomatous optic disc and RNFL damage. Based on guidelines for interpreting articles about diagnostic testing adapted from evidence-based medicine assessment techniques [36], emphasis will be placed on: (1) studies that used a masked comparison with an independent gold standard, applied similarly to all study participants regardless of whether they have glaucoma or not; (2) studies in which the results of the diagnostic test under investigation did not influence the decision to perform the reference standard; (3) studies in which the investigators faced diagnostic uncertainty. In addition, the strengths and limitations of each technique will be outlined so that the structural information they provide can be applied appropriately to the management of glaucoma patients. To facilitate this review, the chapter begins with a brief discussion of theoretical issues related to image quality, measurement reproducibility, detection of glaucomatous damage and progression, and correlation of structural and functional damage.

5.1.2
Image Quality

Image quality is important. Clinicians know that at best, limited information can be obtained from poor quality optic disc photographs, and unreliable visual fields. Similarly, caution should be used when interpreting poor quality images from optical imaging instruments. Several imaging instruments currently provide automated image quality assessment and feedback to the operator during or immediately after image acquisition. Although this feedback facilitates the acquisition of high quality images, there will likely be some patients for whom good quality scans are very difficult or impossible to obtain. It is therefore important to evaluate the quality of the scan before using the measurements derived from it. Unfortunately, the proportion of patients with usable scans is rarely reported in the scientific literature.

5.1.3
Reproducibility

The first test of a new instrument is to determine whether the measurements it produces are reproducible and consistent across operators and time. Poor reproducibility can result from problems with the test measurements, and/or with its interpretation. In general, the instruments described in this chapter have been shown to provide reproducible measurements in clinical settings. It is important to acknowledge that the reproducibility studies available to date were performed by taking several images of patients over a relatively short period of time, and studies evaluating the long-term reproducibility of instrument measurements are still lacking. Moreover, there is a paucity of information on the reproducibility of the interpretation of the information provided by these instruments.

5.1.4
Detecting Glaucoma

The large variability in the number of optic nerve axons in healthy eyes, ranging from 750,000 to 1,500,000, results in considerable overlap in RNFL thickness and optic disc topography measurements of healthy and glaucoma eyes. This limits the ability of any measurement obtained at one point in time, to differentiate between healthy eyes and eyes with early to moderate glaucoma.

There are several ways to describe and summarize the ability of a diagnostic test to detect disease. The most common measures of diagnostic accuracy include sensitivity, specificity and area under receiver operating characteristic (ROC) curves. In brief, sensitivity is the proportion of persons with the disease who test positive for the test under evaluation or the proportion correctly identified as having the disease. Specificity is the proportion of persons without the disease whose test results are negative for the disease, or the proportion of persons correctly identified as not having the disease. The area under the ROC represents, in one number, the diagnostic accuracy of a test. The ROC curve is plotted with the x-axis as "1-specificity", and the y-axis as "sensitivity". An area under the ROC curve of 1.0 represents perfect discrimination, while a value of 0.5 represents random discrimination.

Estimates of the ability of an instrument to detect glaucoma are influenced by characteristics of the study population. Studies that include mostly advanced glaucoma will often have better sensitivity and specificity than studies that restrict their patient population to those with early to moderate disease. For this reason, and to facilitate comparison across studies, this chapter will focus on studies that include early to moderate glaucoma in their patient population.

5.1.5
Association Between Structure
and Function

Ideally, detectable glaucomatous structural damage will correspond topographically to visual field damage. However, there is consistent evidence that optic disc and RNFL damage can be detected before the development of glaucomatous visual field damage using standard automated perimetry [37]. As a result, in eyes with early to moderate glaucoma damage, detectable structural damage is often more extensive than detectable standard automated perimetry functional damage. Therefore, at any given point in time, a strong correlation between structural and functional damage in eyes with early to moderate glaucoma damage is not expected.

5.1.6
Detecting Change Over Time

An advantage of imaging instruments is the large amount of data available for analysis. This data is particularly important for developing analysis strategies for detecting change over time. For a change in the optic disc or RNFL to be important clinically, at the very least the change should be greater than the variability of the measurement. With the imaging instruments discussed in this chapter, three scans are usually obtained at each imaging session, so that measurement variability can be calculated, both globally and regionally. It is therefore possible to identify regions of the optic disc and RNFL that have changed significantly (greater than the variability of the measurements) over time. Furthermore, as the repeatability of change is important to document, these instruments have the potential to automatically identify regions of the optic disc and RNFL that have significant and consistent change over several consecutive imaging sessions.

5.2
Confocal Scanning Laser Ophthalmoscopy

5.2.1
Background

5.2.1.1
Principles of Operation

Two commercially available confocal scanning laser ophthalmoscopes (CSLO) are currently available for imaging the posterior segment of the eye: the Heidelberg Retina Tomograph (HRT), and the newer Heidelberg Retina Tomograph II (HRT II), both instruments from Heidelberg Engineering, Dossenheim, Germany. Both instruments utilize the same technology and similar software, and data presumably are compatible between the two, although this has not been well tested. The HRT II, designed specifically for imaging in glaucoma, is more compact and image acquisition is almost completely automatic.

These instruments employ a diode laser (670 nm wavelength) to sequentially scan the retinal surface in the x and y directions at multiple focal planes. Using confocal scanning principles, a three-dimensional topographic image is constructed from a series of optical image sections at consecutive focal planes (a variable number at 16/mm, depending on desired scan depth, for HRT II compared to a total of 32 for HRT). The depth of scanning range is 0.5 mm to 4 mm, in increments of 0.5 mm. The topography image determined from the acquired three-dimensional image consists of 384×384 (147,456 total) for HRT II and 256×256 picture elements (pixels) (65,536 total) for HRT, each of which is a measurement of retinal height at its corresponding location. The field of view for HRT II is set at 15° and is variable (10°, 15°, or 20°) for HRT.

For HRT II, three topographical images are obtained in succession in approximately 2 s, compared to 1.6 s for a single topographic image for HRT. In both cases, the three topographic images are combined and automatically aligned to make a single mean topography used for analysis. For both instruments, magnification error can be corrected using patients' corneal curvature measurements. Acquired images are stored and analyzed using a standard personal computer.

5.2.1.2
Information and Analyses

Both HRTs include a comprehensive software package that facilitates image acquisition, storage, retrieval and quantitative analysis. Stereometric parameters provided by the HRT include disc area, neuroretinal rim area and volume, cup area and volume, cup depth, cup disc area ratio, RNFL thickness, and cup shape. These and other topographic parameters have been described in detail elsewhere [69]. Some stereometric parameters are calculated relative to a reference plane automatically defined as 50 μm posterior to the mean retinal height between 350° and 356° (temporal) along an operator drawn contour line outlining the disc margin. This segment corresponds to the location of the papillomacular nerve fiber bundle, which is assumed to change only late in the course of progressive glaucoma. In addition, both HRTs include a classification analysis (Moorfields Regression Analysis [66]) that compares rim area (adjusted for disc area) from a particular examination, to a normative database. Using this technique, eyes are classified as within normal limits, borderline, or outside normal limits. Classification results are available both globally (360°) and in each of six rim sectors. To assist in interpretation, normal ranges for these measurements are provided. Three-dimensional and cross-sectional two-dimensional representations of the topography also are viewable for subjective evaluation.

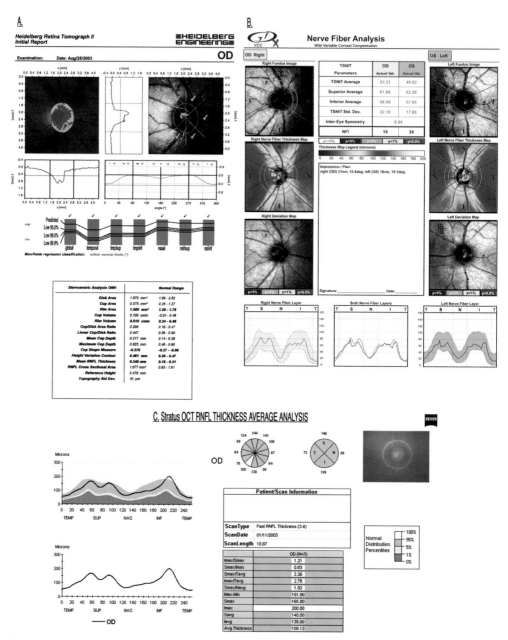

Fig. 5.1 A–C. A 42-year-old healthy female. **A** HRT II report (*OD*) indicates that the Moorfields regression classification and stereometric parameters are within normal limits. **B** GDx VCC standard printout (*OU*) shows that the deviation map, TSNIT graph and TSNIT parameters are all within normal limits. **C** The Stratus OCT RNFL thickness average analysis (*OD*) indicates that the TSNIT graph and parameter measurements are all within normal limits

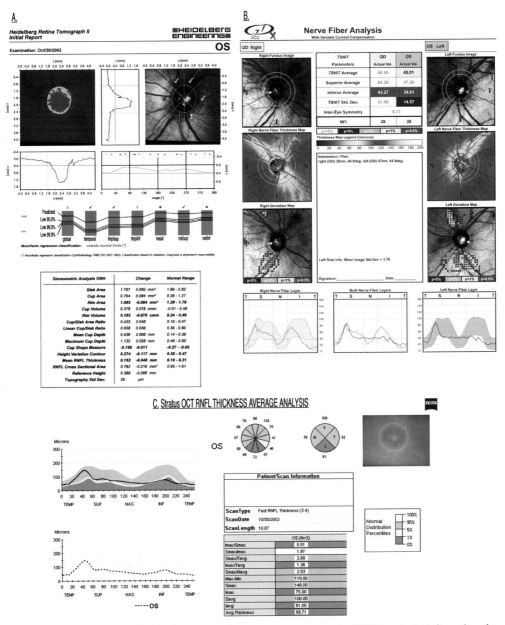

Fig. 5.2 A–C. A 55-year-old female glaucoma patient with optic disc and RNFL damage consistent with early visual field damage (MD –2.1 dB) [see Fig. 5.5 for the 2002 visual field (*OS*)]. **A** HRT II report (*OS*) shows the overall Moorfields regression classification, as well as the nasal and nasal inferior region as "outside normal limits." The stereometric analysis ONH results are consistent with the Moorfields analysis; rim area and volume, mean and maximum cup depth, height variation contour, and RNFL cross sectional area are outside the normal range. **B** GDx VCC Nerve Fiber Analysis indicates more extensive RNFL loss in the left eye than the right. Specifically, in the left eye, a larger area of the inferior and superior deviation maps is outside normal limits than in the right eye. Similarly, more TSNIT parameters in the left eye are outside normal limits (*p*<5%) than in the right eye. **C** Stratus OCT RNFL thickness analysis report highlights the extensive loss of RNFL in the inferior region; The TSNIT graph, inferior quadrant, and inferior clock hours are all outside normal limits. Several RNFL parameters, including average thickness, are also outside of normal values

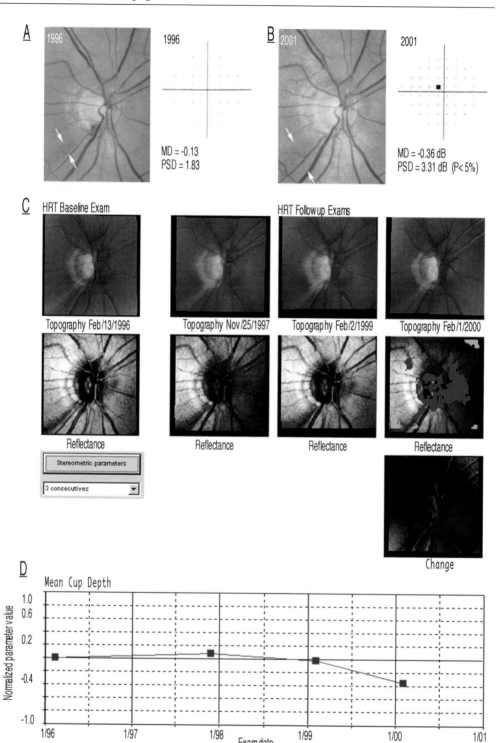

The HRT printout of a healthy eye (Fig. 5.1 A) shows all regions of the Moorfields Regression Analysis to be within normal limits. In contrast, the Moorfields Regression Analysis of a glaucomatous eye (Fig. 5.2 A) shows nasal and nasal inferior regions outside of normal limits.

HRT software includes automated methods for describing change over time. The Stereometric Progression Chart diagrams the change over time of parameters that have been normalized to zero at the baseline examination. With this analysis, a contour line is imported from the baseline examination to follow-up examinations and images are automatically aligned. The normalized change of any parameter is zero if that parameter is stable over time, negative if the parameter worsens (becomes more similar to the values in glaucoma eyes) over time, and positive if the parameter improves over time.

Another means of determining change over time is called "change probability map analysis", and is not dependent on a contour line/reference plane. Using this method, the resolution of the full-field image is reduced by constructing 4 pixel × 4 pixel (16 HRT pixels) "super-pixels". At each super-pixel, an F-test compares the within-test variability of the baseline and follow-up examinations to the between-test variability of the baseline and follow-up examinations. If this difference is significant, with an error probability of less than 5%, the super-pixel is flagged as red for decrease in retinal height and green for increase in retinal height [16]. Because of non-disease related variability in consecutive HRT examinations, repeatable change is required in at least two consecutive examinations to be flagged. HRT software automatically determines whether change is repeatable in two or three consecutive imaging sessions, and superimposes the location of the change detected

by the probability map analysis on the reflectance images. Figure 5.3 illustrates both the change probability map analysis and normalized increase in mean cup depth of an eye with glaucomatous progression.

5.2.2
Image Quality

The HRT II and HRT provide feedback to the operator on image quality during the image acquisition process. Text messages state whether the image quality is acceptable and provide suggestions on how to change scan parameters to improve image quality. During image acquisition, the HRT II quality control system automatically determines whether three good quality scans have been obtained. If one or more of the images cannot be used, additional scans are obtained automatically. The HRT II also visually displays the quality of the image with a moving blue bar. A numerical measure of sensitivity is also displayed. In addition, the standard deviation of the mean topography image has been suggested as a measure of image quality with values of <50 µm as acceptable.

5.2.3
Reproducibility

The reproducibility of HRT optic disc topography measures is generally good with average standard deviations of pixel height measurements of approximately 25–30 µm, with variability slightly higher in glaucomatous eyes compared to healthy eyes. Reported coefficients of variation (standard deviation/mean) for topographic parameters of 2%–10% also have

Fig. 5.3 A–D. Longitudinal follow-up of a 65-year-old female glaucoma patient with HRT exams. **A** Optic nerve head photograph and pattern deviation (PD) plot from 1996. **B** Optic nerve head photograph and PD plot from the same patient in 2001. There is progression of glaucomatous damage to the RNFL compared to 1996, notably an increase in size of an in-ferior-temporal wedge defect (*arrows*) corresponding to the appearance of a superior arcuate visual field defect in the PD plot. **C** Change Probability Map Analysis showing repeatable decrease in RNFL thickness in the inferior-temporal region and elsewhere. **D** Stereometric progression chart showing increase over time of mean cup depth

been reported [69]. Similar coefficients of variation have been reported for HRT II topographic parameters [35, 57].

With respect to interpreting HRT clinical printouts, good interobserver reproducibility for differentiating between normal and glaucoma eyes has been reported, with kappas between 0.67 and 0.73 for agreement among graders [55].

5.2.4
Detecting Early to Moderate Glaucoma

Despite the large individual differences in optic disc characteristics in healthy eyes, sensitivity and specificity of HRT parameters for detecting glaucomatous eyes are good (Table 5.2). Studies using glaucomatous visual fields as the gold standard for a glaucoma diagnosis report sensitivities and specificities for standard HRT topographic parameters ranging from 63%–88% and 73%–90%, respectively [23, 30, 68]. Studies using classifiers included in HRT software (HRT Classification, and Moorfields Regression Analysis) report sensitivities and specificities ranging from 58% to 84% and 65% to 96%, respectively [7, 22, 49, 50]. Finally, studies using novel approaches such as complicated geometric analyses [33], and machine learning classifiers [10] report sensitivities and specificities ranging from 80% to 85% and 90% to 100%, respectively.

5.2.5
Relationship Between Structure and Function

As summarized previously [37], the relationship between HRT topographic parameter measurements and standard automated perimetry global indices (i.e., mean deviation, MD; and pattern standard deviation, PSD) in eyes with glaucoma is generally fair to good, with the best R^2 values ranging from 20% to 42% (all correlations in the predicted direction).

Studies have also shown regional relationships between specific areas of the optic disc and specific areas of the visual field. Correlations as high as $r=-0.52$ were reported when comparing inferior optic disc topography measurements with superior standard automated perimetry MD. In another study, 84% of 26 eyes with inferior focal rim defects also had superior focal visual field defects on standard automated perimetry.

Other studies have demonstrated significant relationships between HRT topography measurements and ganglion cell-specific visual function tests such as short-wavelength (blue-on-yellow) perimetry and motion perimetry.

5.2.6
Detecting Change Over Time

Because glaucoma is a slowly progressing disease, especially when treated, studies investigating change over time require extensive follow-up. Therefore, all studies of this type have been conducted using HRT, not HRT II. In glaucoma research, there is no consensus definition of glaucomatous progression, so although change may be noted in topographic parameters or Change Probability Map Analysis, there is no one existing gold standard with which to confirm it. Figure 5.3 illustrates repeatable optic nerve head changes identified by the Change Probability Map Analysis.

In one study, using change probability map analysis, significant retinal height changes (requiring change on three consecutive tests) were detected in 69% of 77 eyes followed for approximately 5 years [17]. A total of 27% of the same eyes showed significant standard automated perimetry changes based on the Glaucoma Change Probability Analysis. In 16 of these 77 eyes, comparable photographic documentation also was available. Agreement between repeatable Change Probability Map results and subjective assessment of stereoscopic photographs for change was found in 80% of the 16 eyes. This result suggests that HRT can detect change over time in glaucomatous eyes undergoing change documented by visual fields and photographs. Another study measured the variability of HRT parameters in healthy eyes between multiple visits, and used this variability to define significant changes in ocular hypertensive eyes [38]. In this study, 13 of 21 eyes that converted to glaucomatous visual fields showed concurrent changes in HRT parameters. Finally, in a third study,

Table 5.2. Ability to detect glaucoma using confocal scanning laser ophthalmoscopy according to selected recently published studies

Reference number	Study population			Best parameter[a]	Detecting glaucoma	
	Healthy eyes (*n*)	Glau-coma eyes (*n*)	VF MD in glaucoma eyes(dB)		Area under ROC curve	Sensitivity/ specificity (%)
[10]	189	108	−6.08±5.77	Support vector machine classifier using HRT parameters	0.96	85/90
[22]	48	104	−4.83 (median) 90% C.I.=−2.2 to −12.17	Moorfields regression analysis	Not reported	78/81
[23]	39	50	−3.9±2.2	Rim area	0.92	84/90
[30]	153	75	−8.2 (range: 0 to −31)	Vertical CDR	Not reported	85/95
[43]	98	98	7.6±4.7 (Octopus G1)	Bagging classification tree analysis using HRT parameters	Not reported	82/89
[49]	55	95	Not reported	HRT software 2.01 linear discriminant function	Not reported	80/61
[50]	193	113	−9.73±7.13	Moorfields regression analysis	Not reported	74/94
[55]	50	39	−5.04±3.32	Evaluation of standard printouts	Not reported	75/80
[60]	100	100	−4.9±2.7	Mathematical model of optic nerve head morphology	Not reported	88/89
[66]	80	51	−3.6±1.7	Rim area corrected for disc area compared to normative data	Not reported	84/96
[68]	50	41	−5.14, 95% C.I.=−3.47 to −6.81	Mean height of contour line in nasal inferior sector	0.86	63/90

[a]All available sensitivity and specificity combinations are included for best parameter reported.

the baseline variability of sectorial neuroretinal rim area measurements (30° rim sectors, dependent on an eye-specific reference plane) in individual eyes was determined and compared to rim area measurements from follow-up examinations [61]. If the rim area measurements changed by an amount exceeding the baseline variability in two of three consecutive examinations, significant rim area change was assumed. This technique successfully identified 18/20 ocular hypertensive eyes that converted to glaucomatous visual fields during 3 years of follow-up. Seven of 20 longitudinally studied healthy eyes also were identified as changed.

5.2.7
Strengths and Limitations

HRT imaging provides a large amount of objective, quantitative, reproducible, data. These data, coupled with analyses comparing patient results with those from a normative database, provide an unprecedented amount of information on optic disc topography. A strength of the HRT is its analysis of the optic disc, a structure with characteristics likely more familiar to the ophthalmologist than the retinal nerve fiber layer. In addition, HRT measurements are theoretically not affected by anterior segment birefringence.

The reliance on an operator drawn contour line to define the optic disc margin and reference plane can affect the accuracy of HRT measurements. To address this issue, the HRT II and HRT (software version 3.0, Heidelberg Eye Explorer) have included built-in features to assist the operator in accurate contour line placement.

Another possible limitation of HRT is the significant influence of IOP [11].

Summary for the Clinician

- Improvements with the HRT II enable image acquisition with minimal operator input
- HRT II image quality control system modifies scanning parameters during image acquisition and provides real-time feedback on image quality to the operator
- HRT clinical printouts include identification of regions and measurements that are outside the range of normal values
- Sophisticated probability-based analysis of change over time is available
- Some HRT measurements are determined based on a subjectively placed contour line, so some expertise in identifying the optic disc margin is required
- HRT measurements are influenced by fluctuations in IOP. Users should consider possible IOP related change when assessing progression

5.3
Scanning Laser Polarimetry

5.3.1
Background

5.3.1.1
Principles of Operation

Scanning laser polarimetry provides objective and quantitative measures of the RNFL by measuring the change in polarization (retardation) that occurs when light illuminates birefringent tissue, such as the RNFL. The light source for the scanning laser polarimeter is a polarization modulated laser beam (wavelength 780 nm). The parallel arrangement of the microtubules in the RNFL produces linear birefringence that changes the state of polarization (retardation) of light passing through it. The thicker the birefringent structure, the greater the retardation of transmitted light.

However, the RNFL is not the only birefringent media in the eye; the cornea and to a lesser extent the lens also have polarizing properties that contribute to ocular retardation. The accuracy of scanning laser polarimetry RNFL measurements depends on its ability to extract RNFL retardance from total ocular retardance. The scanning laser polarimeter (GDx Nerve Fiber Analyzer, Laser Diagnostic Technologies, San Diego, CA) included a corneal polarization compensator with a fixed corneal polarization axis (CPA) of 15° nasally downward and corneal polarization magnitude (CPM) of 60 nm. Recent studies have shown that there is variation in the axis and magnitude of corneal polarization, so that in approximately 30% of eyes, fixed corneal compensation may not adequately take into account retardation from the anterior segment [28, 63]. In order to address this issue, the GDx VCC (Laser Diagnostic Technologies, San Diego, CA) has been designed to measure the axis and magnitude of corneal polarization for each eye, to individually compensate for corneal birefringence in order to provide more accurate measurements of the RNFL. Details of this method have been described elsewhere [64, 73].

In brief, compensation for corneal birefringence is based on measurements of the macula. Because of the radial arrangement of the Henle fibers, the macula exhibits minimal, fairly uniform birefringence. First, uncompensated GDx VCC images of the macula are obtained. The resulting retardation profile reflects the combined retardance of both the cornea and the Henle layer. The axis and magnitude of corneal polarization are then calculated from this signal, and the instrument automatically adjusts to compensate for them. A fully compensated macular SLP image exhibits little retardance. Next, compensated images of the RNFL are obtained using the measured axis and magnitude of corneal polarization values. The difference between the total signal and the corneal signal then represents the RNFL retardation. This automated image acquisition process is completed for both eyes by experienced operators in less than 5 min.

Pupil dilation is not required, and measurements are independent of a reference plane and magnification effects of the eye. For follow-up imaging, the instrument automatically uses the previously calculated axis and magnitude of corneal polarization for its corneal compensation, thereby reducing image acquisition time.

5.3.1.2
Information and Analyses

The GDx VCC includes a comprehensive software package that facilities image acquisition, storage, retrieval and quantitative summary information on the RNFL. As illustrated in Fig. 5.1 B (healthy eye) and Fig. 5.2 B (glaucoma eye), the standard GDx printout shows the fundus image, retardation or thickness map, deviation (from normal values) map, TSNIT graph, and RNFL parameters. The fundus image can be used in the assessment of image quality, to determine whether the image is focused, evenly illuminated and whether the optic disc is adequately centered in the image. The retardation or thickness map uses a color scale to depict RNFL thickness, with thicker areas as yellow, orange and red, and thinner areas as blue and green. The deviation map is based on a "super pixel" analysis that identifies the locations and

magnitude of the RNFL defect by comparing each scan to the normative database. The super pixel is the average of a 4×4 pixel region. The different colors in the deviation map represent different probabilities (p-values) of the measured RNFL thickness being outside normal limits, with red having the greatest probability ($p<0.5\%$), followed by yellow ($p<1\%$), light blue ($p<2\%$) and dark blue ($p<5\%$). The TSNIT graph displays the RNFL thickness values along the calculation circle beginning with temporal measurements followed by superior, nasal, inferior and temporal again. Normal values are within the shaded area, whereas abnormal values are below the shaded area. The RNFL summary parameters measured on the calculation circle include TSNIT average, superior average, inferior average, TSNIT standard deviation measures the modulation (peak to trough difference of the double-hump pattern; high modulation is normal, low modulation is not), inter-eye symmetry (values of 1 represent good symmetry, values near 0 represent poor symmetry). Values are color-coded by the probability of being outside normal limits. In addition, the printout includes the nerve fiber indicator (NFI), a measure calculated from a neural network trained to differentiate between normal and glaucoma. The higher the NFI, the more likely the eye has glaucoma.

The GDx VCC retardation map of the healthy eye (Fig. 5.1 B) shows thick RNFL in the superior and inferior region (yellow) with no areas outside of normal limits on the deviation map and TSNIT plot. RNFL parameters are also all within the normal range of values. In contrast to the healthy eye, the deviation map, TSNIT graph and RNFL parameters of the glaucoma eye (Figs. 5.2 B and 5.5) show values outside normal limits. In addition, the NFI values for the glaucoma eyes are larger (28 and 38) than the values for the normal eyes (19 and 24).

Changes in RNFL thickness over time are summarized in the serial analysis report. Analysis includes digital subtraction of follow-up images from baseline images to obtain the absolute change in RNFL thickness over time. The RNFL thickness for each examination is plotted on the retardation map, deviation map, and TSNIT graph, so that consistent changes can be easily identified. Analysis that identifies change that is outside the variability of the measurement is under development for the GDx VCC.

5.3.2
Image Quality

5.3.2.1
GDx Nerve Fiber Analyzer with Fixed Corneal Compensation

Feedback on image quality is available immediately after image acquisition by reviewing the "image check" screen. Good quality images can be obtained in the majority of eyes; 93% of 249 eyes from the population-based Baltimore Eye Follow-up Study had usable images [62].

5.3.2.2
GDx VCC

Immediately after image acquisition, feedback on image quality is available to the operator by reviewing the "image check" screen. This screen shows the image quality scores resulting from automated assessment of alignment, fixation, and refraction. There are currently no published estimates of the number of eyes with unusable images. Estimates of the proportion of usable images should include estimates of the number of eyes for which compensation for corneal birefringence is adequate, and on the number of eyes with good quality RNFL scans.

5.3.3
Reproducibility

5.3.3.1
GDx Nerve Fiber Analyzer with Fixed Corneal Compensation

RNFL measurements have been shown to be reproducible in clinical settings, with good inter- and intra-operator reproducibility; coefficients of variation ranging between 3.5% and 10% in glaucoma and normal eyes [24, 69]. With respect to interpreting GDx Nerve Fiber Analyzer clinical printouts, good interobserver repro-

ducibility for differentiating between normal and glaucoma eyes has been reported, with kappas between 0.55 and 0.66 for agreement among graders in one study [55], and kappas of 0.42 for normal eyes and 0.48 for glaucoma eyes in another [18]. However, slight agreement (kappa of 0.09) among observers was found for identifying glaucoma suspects [18].

5.3.3.2
GDx VCC

To date, no reproducibility studies have been published using the GDx VCC. Estimates of the reproducibility of the GDx VCC RNFL measurements should include assessment of the reproducibility of the axis and magnitude of corneal polarization values, as well as the resulting RNFL measurements.

5.3.4
Detecting Early to Moderate Glaucoma

5.3.4.1
GDx Nerve Fiber Analyzer with Fixed Corneal Compensation

Due to the variability in the number of retinal nerve fibers in the healthy eye, there is considerable overlap in scanning laser polarimetry RNFL measures in healthy and glaucoma eyes. Despite this overlap, significant differences between normal eyes and eyes with early to moderate glaucoma have been reported. In studies that included early to moderate glaucoma defined using visual field criteria, sensitivities of discriminant functions of GDx parameters had the best diagnostic accuracy; at a high fixed specificity of 90%, sensitivity ranged from 33% to 81%, while area under the ROC curve ranged from 0.79 to 0.94 [12, 23, 68].

5.3.4.2
GDx VCC

Correction for the axis of corneal polarization reduces the range of values in the healthy eyes [27]. This results in a narrower range of RNFL thickness values that fall within normal limits.

Table 5.3. Ability to detect glaucoma using scanning laser polarimetry according to selected recently published studies

CDx type[a]	Reference number	Study population			Best parameter[b]	Detecting glaucoma	
		Healthy eyes (n)	Glau - coma eyes (n)	VF MD in glaucoma eyes(dB)		Area under ROC curve	Sensitivity/specificity (%)
FCC	[12]	38	42	–6.08±5.77	LDF	0.81	71/71 32/92
FCC	[18]	29	42	Not reported	Printout	Not reported	79/80
FCC	[23]	39	50	–3.9±2.3	LDF	0.94	89/87
FCC	[47]	53	48 (Focal defects)	–5.3±3.8	LDF Fourier	0.93	71/91
FCC	[51]	32	82[c] (14 A, 46 L, 22 M)	A, –21.5; L, –5.1; M, –6.3	Evaluation of standard printout	Not reported	68/97
FCC	[53]	68	91	–8.2±5.7	Number >27	Not reported	62/96
FCC	[55]	50	39	–5.0±3.3	Evaluation of standard print out	Not reported	72–82/ 56–82
FCC	[58]	34	34	–8.7±7.2	Amplitude and hemiretina symmetry	Not reported	94/91
FCC	[62]	149	100	–5.3±7.9	Number >20	Not reported	72/82
FCC	[67]	122	22	–8.2±7.1	Modulation superior and inferior	0.94	68/90
FCC	[68]	50	41	–5.1 (–3.5, –6.8)	LDF	0.84	66/86 54/90 32/96
FCC and VCC	[64]	40	54	–6.5±4.9	RNFL thickness	FCC, 0.62–0.68 VCC, 0.75–0.83	F, 46/90 V, 67/90
VCC	[48]	52	55	–5.9	Fourier LDF	VCC, 0.95	V, 84/92

[a] FCC, GDx Nerve Fiber Analyzer with fixed corneal compensation; VCC, GDx Nerve Fiber Analyzer modified to measure with variable corneal compensation.
[b] All available sensitivity and specificity combinations are included for best parameter reported.
[c] A, advanced glaucoma; L, local defect only; M, mixed defect.

Several investigators, all defining glaucoma based on visual field criteria, have reported a reduction in global and regional RNFL thickness values with the GDx VCC compared to the GDx Nerve Fiber Analyzer with fixed corneal compensation [19, 64]. These and other studies reported improvement in the sensitivity and specificity of RNFL thickness measures obtained with a prototype GDx with variable corneal compensation (Table 5.3). At a fixed specificity of 90%, sensitivity improved from approximately 37%–46% using fixed compensation, to 48%–67% using variable corneal compensation. It should be noted that the ratio and modulation parameter values obtained using the GDx VCC are similar to those obtained with using GDx Nerve Fiber Analyzer with fixed compensation [19, 64]. Similarly, there is little improvement in the ability to discriminate between glaucoma and healthy eyes of ratio and modulation parameters obtained with the GDx VCC compared to those obtained using scanning laser polarimetry with fixed corneal compensation [64].

5.3.5
Relationship Between Structure and Function

5.3.5.1
GDx Nerve Fiber Analyzer with Fixed Corneal Compensation

The association between RNFL measurements and visual field indices (mean deviation and corrected pattern standard deviation) has been studied both globally and regionally, with results showing weak to moderate correlations with R^2 values ranging between 8% and 26% [5, 13, 24, 69].

5.3.5.2
GDx VCC

Compared to scanning laser polarimetry with fixed corneal compensation, RNFL thickness measurements obtained with the GDx VCC are more strongly associated with visual field indices [5, 13]. However, the correlation between RNFL thickness values and visual field indices remains modest (R^2 values ranging from 12% to 36%).

5.3.6.
Detecting Change Over Time

5.3.6.1
GDx Nerve Fiber Analyzer with Fixed Corneal Compensation

Although there are two case reports describing longitudinal RNFL loss in patients with non-glaucomatous optic neuropathies [20, 46], there are currently no published reports documenting the ability of the GDx Nerve Fiber Analyzer to detect change over time in a large group of glaucoma patients. In a small study of 17 patients with optic disc hemorrhage, 10 of the 17 eyes developed visual field progression, but a significant change in the SLP image was not seen [9].

5.3.6.2
GDx VCC

The serial analysis report documents RNFL thickness change over time (Fig. 5.4). Probability-based analysis that evaluates whether the change is greater than the measurement variability is currently under development. Although the axis of corneal polarization has been shown to be stable for a period of a year [26], long-term stability of the axis and magnitude of corneal polarization is unknown. Longitudinal studies documenting change in GDx VCC RNFL measurements are not yet available.

It is important to note that compensation for corneal retardation should be reassessed after corneal laser refractive procedures, ocular surface disease or other conditions that may cause a change in corneal architecture. Recent studies have shown that LASIK changes the axis and magnitude of corneal polarization. However, GDx VCC RNFL measurements are similar before and after LASIK, once the corneal compensation has been reassessed post-operatively [1].

5.3.7
Strengths and Limitations

Scanning laser polarimetry strengths include its ability to measure the RNFL throughout the parapapillary retina without the need for pupil dilation, a reference plane, or magnification correction. The introduction of the GDx VCC has addressed several of the limitations of the GDx Nerve Fiber Analyzer with fixed corneal compensation. Compared to scanning laser polarimetry measurements with fixed corneal compensation, RNFL thickness measurements obtained with the GDx VCC can better discriminate between healthy and glaucoma eyes [64], and are more strongly associated with visual field indices [5, 13]. Furthermore, correction for the axis of corneal polarization reduces the variance of normal retardation measurements [27].

It is important to note that as neutralization of corneal retardation is based on macular measurements of Henle's layer, macular pathologies can influence the ability to ade-

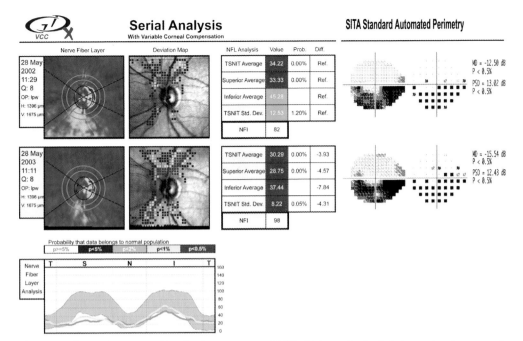

Fig. 5.4. Left eye of a 61-year-old male glaucoma patient with progressive RNFL loss. The GDx VCC Serial Analysis deviation map highlights a reduction in RNFL thickness in the inferior region from 2002 to 2003. A corresponding progression of superior visual field damage in the same time period is also apparent

quately compensate for corneal retardation in some patients [6]. Alternative techniques are under development to effectively compensate for corneal retardation in eyes with macular pathologies. Furthermore, compensation for corneal retardation should be reassessed after corneal laser refractive procedures or other conditions that may cause a change in the corneal architecture. Recent studies report that although LASIK causes a measurable change in corneal retardation [1] by simply reassessing corneal compensation after laser refractive procedures, RNFL measurements remain stable after surgery.

Summary for the Clinician

- Improvements with the new commercially available GDx VCC are likely to enhance its utility in clinical practice
- GDx VCC clinical printouts include identification of regions and measurements that are outside the range of normal RNFL thickness values
- GDx VCC corneal compensation should be reassessed after laser refractive procedures, ocular surface disease, or other conditions that may cause a change in corneal architecture
- Techniques to automatically compensate for corneal retardation in eyes with macular pathologies are under development

---

5.4
Optical Coherence Tomography

5.4.1
Background

5.4.1.1
Principles of Operation

Optical coherence tomography (OCT) uses optical technology that is analogous to ultrasound B mode imaging, but utilizing light instead of sound to acquire high resolution images of ocular structures, using the principles of low coherence interferometry [32]. In brief, interferometry uses information from interference fringes to precisely determine small distances or thicknesses of structures. In OCT, a low coherence near infrared (840 nm) light beam is directed onto a partially reflective mirror (beam splitter), that creates two light beams: a reference and a measurement beam. The measurement beam is directed onto the subject's eye, and is reflected from intraocular microstructures and tissues according to their distance, thickness, and different reflectivity. The reference beam is reflected from the reference mirror at a known, variable position. Both beams travel back to the partially reflective mirror, recombine, and are transmitted to a photosensitive detector. The use of low coherence light allows only the reflections from a narrow region of the retina to interfere with the reference beam, giving the high resolution of the instrument. The pattern of interference is used to provide information regarding distance and thickness of retinal structures. Bi-dimensional images are created by successive longitudinal scanning in transverse direction.

OCT is capable of scanning the peripapillary retina, optic nerve head (ONH), and macular region. The peripapillary scan is a continuous circular scan centered on the ONH with a default diameter of 3.4 mm. The ONH and macular scanning are composed of six radial scans in a spoke like pattern centered on the ONH or the fovea with each radial scan spaced 30° from one to another. To fill the gaps between the scans, OCT utilizes interpolation. For each of these scan types, a "fast" scan option, in which three scans are obtained at once, is available.

The final image provided by the OCT appears in a color-coded map that is artificially produced by the OCT software (Fig. 5.1C). Dark colors (black and blue) represent regions of minimal optical reflectivity, whereas bright colors (red and white) represent regions of high reflectivity. To obtain thickness measurements, OCT first determines the retinal boundaries, constituted by the vitreoretinal interface and the retinal pigment epithelium (RPE) which defines the inner and outer retinal boundaries, respectively. These two boundaries are associated with the sharpest edges in each OCT scan because of the high contrast in optical reflectivity between the relatively non-reflective vitreous and the reflective neurosensory retina and between the minimally reflective photoreceptor outer segments and the highly reflective retinal pigment epithelium/choriocapillaris. The RNFL corresponds to the high reflective layer (red) underneath the inner retinal boundary. The posterior boundary of the RNFL is determined by evaluating each scan for a threshold value chosen to be 15 dB greater than the filtered maximum reflectivity of the adjacent neurosensory retina. There is evidence that the current OCT algorithm to detect the boundaries of RNFL is still imperfect. Previous work has demonstrated that the current algorithm tends to falsely determine the RNFL borders in some situations, especially when the RNFL reflectivity is low, as may occur in glaucomatous patients [34]. A new algorithm has been proposed, based on a search and evaluation of peaks of reflectivity of the OCT image, which provided a better detection of RNFL borders than the currently employed algorithm [34].

The Stratus OCT includes several improvements over the original OCT, including better resolution, increased number of A-scans, and reduced need for pupil dilation. For the Stratus OCT the in vivo resolution is estimated to be between 8–10 µm, whereas for the original OCT the in vivo resolution is 10–12 µm. The Stratus OCT provides 128–512 lateral pixel retinal tomograms (A-scans) throughout a 360°-RNFL circular scan, each consisting of 1024 data points with a depth of 2–3 mm. Good quality Stratus OCT scans can often be obtained without pupil dilation. The OCT obtains only 100 measurements (A-scans) in the same region, and requires pupil dilation of greater than 5 mm.

5.4.1.2
Information and Analyses

The Stratus OCT includes a comprehensive software package that facilities image acquisition, storage, retrieval, and quantitative summary information on the RNFL, macula, and optic nerve head.

5.4.1.2.1
RNFL Scan

A printout of the Stratus OCT RNFL thickness analysis of a normal patient is shown in Fig. 5.1 C. The curve of distribution of RNFL thickness values around the optic disc is shown as a black line. The green shaded area indicates the 95 % confidence limits of normal, whereas the red shaded area indicates values below 99 % of the normal population. Borderline values are indicated by the yellow shaded area. The probability of abnormality is calculated based on an age-matched normal group. Fig. 5.2 C shows a glaucoma eye with inferior RNFL thickness values outside the normal range of values.

The printout also provides RNFL thickness values in clock hours and in quadrants. The same color code indicates the probability of abnormality for each sector/quadrant. Summary parameters are also provided including average thickness, ratios, and maximum RNFL thickness values in the superior and inferior quadrants.

5.4.1.2.2
Macula Scan

The macula scan displays two maps, centered on the macula, showing retinal thickness and volume. Three concentric circles divide each map into three zones: fovea, inner macula, and outer macula. The inner and outer zones are further divided in four quadrants by two diagonal lines. Thus, a total of nine areas (fovea, superior outer, superior inner, inferior outer, inferior inner, temporal outer, temporal inner, nasal outer, and nasal inner) are available for analysis. In one map, a color code represents the retinal thickness (or volume) in each area, whereas in the other map, the actual values of thickness (or volume) are given for each area. The user can select the diameters of the three concentric circles and change the area to be analyzed. Two options are available. One with concentric circles of 1 mm, 3 mm and 6 mm; and the other with concentric circles of 1 mm, 2.22 mm, and 3.45 mm.

5.4.1.2.3
Optic Nerve Head Scan

The ONH scan consists of six radial scans in a spoke-like pattern centered on the ONH. The OCT interpolates between the scans to provide measurements throughout the ONH. In optic nerve head scans, the device automatically determines the disc margin as the end of the retinal pigment epithelium/choriocapillaris layer. A straight line connects the edges of the retinal pigment epithelium/choriocapillaris, and a parallel line is constructed 150 µm anteriorly. Structures below this line are defined as the disk cup and above this line as the neuroretinal rim. Several topographic optic disc parameters are automatically calculated including disk area, cup area, rim area, cup/disk area ratio, cup/disk horizontal ratio, cup/disk vertical ratio, cup volume and rim volume.

A recent study compared optic nerve head measurements obtained by OCT and HRT in glaucoma patients, glaucoma suspects, and normal individuals. A fair to moderate correlation was found between the results obtained by the two instruments for disc area, cup/disc area ratio, cup area, cup volume and rim volume, with R^2 ranging from 12 % to 72 % [56]. It is important to emphasize that, although significant correlations were obtained, the absolute values for the optic nerve head parameters were generally different between the two instruments.

5.4.2
Image Quality

The OCT and Stratus OCT currently do not provide real-time feedback on image quality. Good quality images should have a focused fundus image and centered optic disc. The signal-to-noise ratio should also be acceptable. There are no reports on the proportion of patients with usable scans.

5.4.3
Reproducibility

5.4.3.1
OCT

RNFL thickness measurements obtained with OCT have good reproducibility with intraclass correlation coefficients of approximately 0.55 and coefficients of variation of approximately 10% [8, 15]. Also, the intra-operator reproducibility was demonstrated to be good, indicating that longitudinal measurements taken for the same patient over a period of time may be compared even when image acquisition is performed by different experienced operators. Part of the variability in OCT RNFL measurements may be due to the small number of sample points obtained in each image acquisition. Increasing the sampling density of OCT scans seems to increase the reproducibility of OCT RNFL measurements [31].

With respect to interpreting OCT clinical printouts, good interobserver reproducibility for differentiating between normal and glaucoma eyes has been reported, with kappas of 0.51 and 0.73 for agreement among graders [55].

5.4.3.2
Stratus OCT

Stratus OCT reproducibility data have not yet been reported. As mentioned above, the Stratus OCT is able to obtain a larger number of RNFL measurements around the optic nerve than the OCT, and therefore may have better reproducibility than the OCT.

5.4.4
Detecting Early to Moderate Glaucoma

5.4.4.1
RNFL Measurements

Several studies have provided evidence that RNFL measurements obtained with OCT are able to differentiate glaucomatous from normal subjects with relatively good sensitivity and specificity (Table 5.4), although a considerable amount of overlap exists. The areas under the ROC curves have been reported to range from 0.79 to 0.94, depending on the parameter and characteristics of the population evaluated [12, 23, 29, 40, 65, 68]. In studies evaluating the diagnostic ability of several OCT parameters, the RNFL thickness in the inferior region often had the best performance to discriminate healthy eyes from eyes with early to moderate glaucoma with sensitivities between 67% and 79% for specificities $\geq 90\%$ [12, 40, 68]. In another approach, a discriminant analysis function combining RNFL thickness measurements obtained from four different 30° sectors around the optic disc had a sensitivity of 67% for specificity set at 90% [23].

5.4.4.2
Macular Thickness

Recent attention has been directed to the role of OCT macular thickness measurements for glaucoma diagnosis. Loss of retinal ganglion cells in glaucoma is also known to occur in the posterior pole, where these cells may constitute 30%–35% of the retinal thickness in the macular region [71]. The mean macular thickness of glaucomatous eyes has been shown to be significantly lower than that of normal control eyes [25]. Also, a significant correlation was found between OCT macular thickness and visual field mean defect in glaucomatous eyes [25]. Although macular thickness values have been reported to be lower in glaucomatous eyes [25, 29, 42], the ability of these measurements to discriminate glaucomatous from normal eyes does not seem to be better than RNFL peripapillary measurements. A maximum ROC curve area of 0.77 for macular thickness parameters was obtained for the discrimination between early glaucoma and normal subjects, whereas peripapillary RNFL thickness parameters had maximum ROC curve area of 0.94 in the same situation [29]. It is also important to emphasize that macular thickness measurements have limited use for monitoring or evaluating glaucoma in patients with macular comorbidity. It is possible that advances in the software designed to extract data from the macular area will improve

Table 5.4. Ability to detect glaucoma using optical coherence tomography according to selected recently published studies

Reference number	Study population			Detecting glaucoma		
	Healthy eyes (n)	Glaucoma eyes (n)	VF MD in glaucoma eyes (dB)	Best parameter[a]	Area under ROC curve	Sensitivity/specificity (%)
[12]	38	42	−4.0±4.2	Inferior thickness	0.91	88/71 79/92
[23]	39	50	−3.9±2.13	Discriminant function	0.88	82/84 67/90
[29]	33	35	−3.01±2.88	Global average RNFL thickness	0.94	N/A
[39]	160	237	−3.13±1.77	Inferior temporal	0.87	67/90 81/80
[55]	50	39	−5.04±3.32	Evaluation of standard printout	not reported	76–79/ 68–81
[59]	25	42	−4.3±3.3	Global average RNFL thickness	0.87	not reported
[68]	50	41	−5.14	Inferior temporal	0.87	76/86 71/94 68/96

[a]All available sensitivity and specificity combinations are included for best parameter reported.

detection of retinal ganglion cell loss in the posterior pole.

5.4.4.3
Optic Nerve Head

Stratus OCT optic nerve head topographic parameters were able to discriminate between patients with glaucomatous visual field defects and healthy eyes with ROC curve areas ranging from 0.54 to 0.76 [56]. The areas under the ROC curves were comparable to those obtained with the HRT optic nerve head topographic parameters [56].

The utility of the topographic evaluation of the optic nerve head with OCT for glaucoma diagnosis and monitoring still needs to be further evaluated. As the automatic algorithm for detection of the disc margin is based on the determination of the end of the RPE/choriocapillaris layer, it is possible that disc margin evaluation will be influenced by changes in these layers as it may occur in progressive peripapillary atrophy in glaucoma. Although the Stratus OCT also provides a manual disc margin determination

option, the influence of progressive optic disc changes on disc margin and reference plane determination with this instrument still needs to be addressed.

5.4.5
Relationship Between Structure and Function

Previous studies have shown good correlation between RNFL loss detected by semi-quantitative analysis of red-free photographs and OCT RNFL thickness in glaucoma, with R^2 ranging from 30% to 52% [59, 70].

Correlations of OCT RNFL measurements and standard automated perimetry mean deviation and pattern deviation have also been reported with R^2 values of 35%–43% [70]. Localized OCT RNFL thinning at 6, 7 and 8 o-clock hours (inferior region), was topographically related to decreased localized SAP sensitivity in the superior arcuate and nasal step areas in glaucomatous patients [21].

5.4.6
Detection of Longitudinal Change over Time

No studies are currently available demonstrating the ability of OCT RNFL measurements to monitor glaucomatous progression over time. Figure 5.5 illustrates a reduction in RNFL thickness in the inferior region of a glaucoma patient during a 4-year follow-up period. Evidence for the ability of OCT to detect longitudinal RNFL loss over time was provided by the analysis of sequential OCT exams in a patient that was fol-

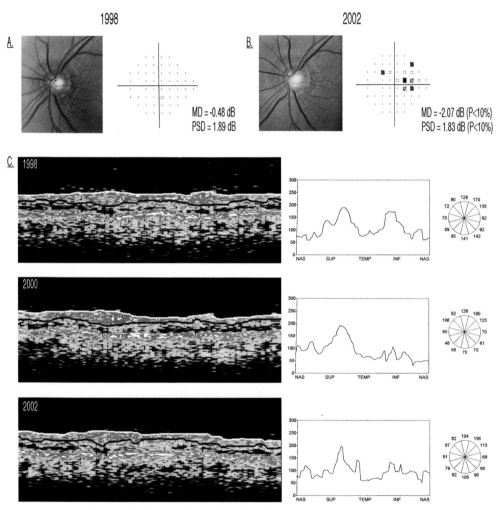

Fig. 5.5 A–C. Left eye of the 55-year-old female glaucoma patient included in Fig. 5.2, with progressive RNFL loss detectable with optical coherence tomography. **A** Optic nerve photograph and standard automated perimetry pattern deviation (PD) plot from 1998. **B** Optic nerve head photograph and standard automated perimetry PD plot from the same patient in 2002. There is progression of glaucomatous damage to the optic nerve compared to 1998, notably an increase in the inferior rim thinning corresponding to the appearance of a superior arcuate visual field defect in the PD plot. **C** Sequence of OCT exams obtained in 1998, 2000, and 2002. Observe the progressive loss of the inferior RNFL, as indicated by the color-coded map (decrease in the thickness of the inner red layer), blunting of the inferior hump as shown by the curve of distribution of RNFL thickness, and decrease in the inferior RNFL thickness values as indicated by the clock-hour map

lowed after an episode of severe traumatic optic neuropathy. The OCT exams demonstrated progressive loss of RNFL in agreement with the ophthalmoscopic and photographic evaluation [45]. Changes in OCT RNFL thickness measurements over time were also demonstrated after IOP reduction in glaucoma patients. A significant increase in overall mean RNFL thickness after trabeculectomy, related to the magnitude of IOP reduction, was demonstrated in glaucoma patients [4].

5.4.7
Strengths and Limitations

Strengths of the OCT include its ability to measure peripapillary RNFL thickness without the need for a reference plane or magnification correction. Also, with the Stratus OCT it is possible to obtain images without pupillary dilation. However, the OCT does not provide objective immediate feedback regarding image quality, and many patients still need pupillary dilation for the acquisition of good quality images, even with Stratus OCT. Another potential advantage of the OCT is that the same equipment incorporates the ability to measure peripapillary RNFL thickness, optic nerve head topographic parameters and macula thickness measurements. It still needs to be determined, however, whether a combination of all the information from the OCT including RNFL thickness, ONH topography, and macula measurements will provide a better assessment of a patient than the use of each of the analyses alone.

One of the limitations of the peripapillary RNFL thickness evaluation with the OCT is that only 100 data points are obtained around the optic disc. This limitation was addressed by the Stratus OCT that is able to obtain up to 512 measurements in the same region. However, this number of points is still considerably lower than that obtained by other imaging instruments. Whether the increase in the number of data points acquired with OCT will further increase its diagnostic ability still needs to be determined. Currently, both the OCT and Stratus OCT lack a normative database for evaluation of optic nerve head and macula thickness meas-

urements. For RNFL thickness measurements, a proprietary software that compares a patient's exam with a normative database has recently been released and still needs further validation.

Summary for the Clinician

- Improvements with the Stratus OCT include an increase in the number of scan points, and a reduced need for pupillary dilation
- Stratus OCT is able to assess peripapillary RNFL thickness, optic nerve head topography, and macula thickness using the same instrument
- Stratus OCT RNFL thickness printouts include identification of regions and measurements that are outside normal limits
- Pupillary dilation is needed to obtain good quality Stratus OCT images in some eyes

5.5
Scanning Retinal Thickness Analyzer

The commercially available scanning Retinal Thickness Analyzer (Talia Technology, Neve-Ilan, Israel) is based on the principals of slit-lamp biomicroscopy. The RTA has primarily been used for retinal thickness analysis of macular pathologies, but has been recently modified (RTA Version 2) to include analyses of optic disc topography.

5.5.1
Background

5.5.1.1
Principles of Operation

A laser (543-nm helium-neon) slit is projected obliquely and scanned, in steps, across the retina, and retinal thickness is defined as the separation between the reflection from the vitreo-retinal interface and the chorioretinal interface (two reflective peaks that result from the oblique beam projection and the transparency of the retina). Each 0.3-s scan results in a 3-mm² image composed of 16 optical sections (one section each 0.1875 mm). Interpolation is used to depict a continuous surface. A large portion of the retina including the macula, parapapillary region, and optic disc can be imaged with multiple scans by changing fixation position between each scan in a single imaging session. To determine optic disc topography, an operator drawn contour line is placed, outlining the optic disc margin.

Acquired images are stored and analyzed using a standard personal computer. The RTA 2 includes a comprehensive software package that facilitates image acquisition, storage, retrieval and quantitative analysis. Stereometric optic disc parameters and a classification analysis provided by the RTA 2, some of which rely on an operator drawn contour line outlining the disc margin, are similar to those provided by the HRT software. These parameters are compared to normative data and resulting probabilities are shown. Other reports include color-coded deviation-from-normal-thickness maps, covering parapapillary and posterior pole regions. These reports include color-coded associated probabilities for each region.

5.5.1.2
Information and Analyses

For detecting retinal thickness change over time, the RTA 2 provides a color-coded two-dimensional map depicting thickness deviation from baseline measurements. A color-coded map depicting thickness deviation, in *p*-values relative to two standard deviations of reproducibility in normal eyes, is also shown. For detecting changes in optic disc topography over time, regions with significant change defined as greater than 2.2 standard deviations from normal variability are shown on a two-dimensional deviation map.

5.5.2
Image Quality

The RTA 2 provides feedback on image quality immediately after image acquisition with text messages that state whether the image quality is acceptable and provide suggestions on how to change scan parameters to improve image quality. In a study of 55 eyes, only 34 (62%) had us-

able RTA scans available for analysis, with poor quality scans primarily due to media opacities [54]. Information is not available on the proportion of usable scans with RTA 2.

5.5.3
Reproducibility

The reproducibility of RTA retinal thickness measurements is generally good with average standard deviations of approximately 15–20 μm [3, 41, 72]. Coefficients of variation of 5%–20% also have been reported [3, 41, 52]. No published information is available on the reproducibility of RTA 2 measurements.

5.5.4
Discriminating Between Healthy Eyes and Eyes with Early to Moderate Glaucoma

Reported sensitivity for detecting known glaucomatous eyes (defined by standard automated perimetry) using retinal thickness values was as high as 88% when specificity was 57% [14]. However, some eyes in this study had advanced glaucoma, likely increasing the sensitivity compared to when glaucoma is early to moderate. In another study, maps depicting deviation from normal retinal thickness values were shown to masked readers who were instructed to divide them into glaucoma, normal, and questionable groups. Sensitivity and specificity in this study were 91% and 97%, respectively. The questionable group made up 17% of the total and was composed of 80% healthy eyes. No study has compared optic disc topography measurements using RTA 2 between healthy and glaucoma eyes.

5.5.5
Relationship Between Structure and Function

One study, using RTA, showed a good relationship between superior versus inferior asymmetry of macular thickness loss (compared to healthy eyes) and superior versus inferior asymmetry of central visual field sensitivity loss (standard automated perimetry, loss relative to healthy eyes) (r=0.72) [71]. In another study, subjective scoring of RTA retinal thickness map defects (six-point scale) was significantly associated (r=0.58) with subjective scoring of visual field defects (seven-point scale) in glaucoma and glaucoma suspect eyes [2].

5.5.6
Detecting Change Over Time

No studies have evaluated the ability of the RTA or RTA 2 to detect glaucomatous changes over time.

5.5.7
Strengths and Limitations

RTA imaging provides a large amount of objective, quantitative, reproducible, data. These data, coupled with analyses comparing patient results with those from a normative database, provide a large amount of information on retinal thickness and optic disc topography. One advantage of RTA compared to some of the other optical imaging modalities described in this chapter is its analysis of retinal thickness coupled with optic disc topography (although this aspect has not been investigated). RTA measurements are theoretically not affected by anterior segment birefringence. The reliance on an operator drawn contour line to define the optic disc margin and reference plane can affect the accuracy of some parameters. The effect of IOP change on RTA has not been determined.

Pupil dilation is required to obtain acceptable RTA images in most eyes, although optic disc imaging without dilation is possible. This is a limitation not present with HRT and GDx VCC, and present to a lesser degree with the Stratus OCT. In addition, the RTA is more affected by media opacities than OCT [58].

Finally, interpolation is required to reproduce a continuous retinal thickness map with RTA. It is possible that focal defects in retinal thickness or disc topography could be overlooked because of this.

Summary for the Clinician

- Improvements with the new RTA Version 2 include non-mydriatic optic disc imaging and three-dimensional interactive presentation of optic disc topography
- RTA clinical printouts include identification of regions and measurements that are outside the range of normal values
- Sophisticated probability-based analysis of change over time is available
- Pupil dilation is required for macular scans
- Some RTA measurements are determined based on a subjectively placed contour line, so some expertise in identifying the optic disc margin is required

5.6
Conclusions

Optic nerve imaging instruments provide reproducible, objective measurements of the optic disc and RNFL in glaucoma. Recent hardware and software advances have improved their ability to detect and monitor glaucomatous damage over time. Each technique has specific strengths and limitations so that one instrument may not be best for all patients and for all clinical situations. Furthermore, each instrument is at a different stage of development, so that current limitations may not be relevant in the near future. Because of the limited ability of any one test, at one point in time, to diagnose glaucoma, these techniques should be utilized in conjunction with careful clinical examination and visual function testing. In addition, it is important that the clinician understand the strengths and limitations of each technique, so that the best quality information will be used for glaucoma management decisions.

As the reproducibility of imaging instruments is good, these techniques are particularly well suited for detecting small, subtle changes in the optic disc and RNFL. To detect these changes, improved methods for identifying glaucomatous progression, based on recognition of change outside of measurement variability, are needed. It should be noted that the technique most useful for detecting glaucoma may not be the best for monitoring glaucomatous progression. In summary, these instruments show considerable promise for providing measurements of the optic disc and RNFL that can assist the clinician in detecting glaucomatous optic disc and RNFL damage.

Acknowledgments. Supported in part by NIH grant EY11008 (LMZ). Financial Disclosure: Dr. Weinreb has received research support from Heidelberg Engineering, Laser Diagnostic Technologies, Carl Zeiss Meditec Inc and Talia Technologies. RNW is a consultant or has received honorarium from Carl Zeiss Meditec, Laser Diagnostic Technologies, and Heidelberg Engineering.

References

1. Abunto T, Angeles R, Zangwill LM, Bowd C, Schanzlin D, Weinreb RN (2003) Retinal nerve fiber layer thickness measurements after laser assisted in situ keratomileusis (LASIK). Association for Research in Vision and Ophthalmology Annual Meeting. Ft. Lauderdale, Florida: E-Abstract 3399
2. Asrani S, Challa P, Herndon L, Lee P, Stinnett S, Allingham RR (2003) Correlation among retinal thickness, optic disc, and visual field in glaucoma patients and suspects: a pilot study. J Glaucoma 12:119–128
3. Asrani S, Zou S, d'Anna S, Vitale S, Zeimer R (1999) Noninvasive mapping of the normal retinal thickness at the posterior pole. Ophthalmology 106:269–273
4. Aydin A, Wollstein G, Price LL, Fujimoto JG, Schuman JS (2003) Optical coherence tomography assessment of retinal nerve fiber layer thickness changes after glaucoma surgery. Ophthalmology 110:1506–1511
5. Bagga H, Greenfield DS, Feuer W, Knighton RW (2003) Scanning laser polarimetry with variable corneal compensation and optical coherence tomography in normal and glaucomatous eyes. Am J Ophthalmol 135:521–529
6. Bagga H, Greenfield DS, Knighton RW (2003) Scanning laser polarimetry with variable corneal compensation: identification and correction for corneal birefringence in eyes with macular disease. Invest Ophthalmol Vis Sci 44:1969–1976
7. Bathija R, Zangwill L, Berry CC, Sample PA, Weinreb RN (1998) Detection of early glaucomatous structural damage with confocal scanning laser tomography. J Glaucoma 7:121–127
8. Blumenthal EZ, Williams JM, Weinreb RN, Girkin CA, Berry CC, Zangwill LM (2000) Reproducibility of nerve fiber layer thickness measurements by use of optical coherence tomography. Ophthalmology 107:2278–2282
9. Boehm MD, Nedrud C, Greenfield DS, Chen PP (2003) Scanning laser polarimetry and detection of progression after optic disc hemorrhage in patients with glaucoma. Arch Ophthalmol 121:189–194
10. Bowd C, Chan K, Zangwill LM, Goldbaum MH, Lee TW, Sejnowski TJ, Weinreb RN (2002) Comparing neural networks and linear discriminant functions for glaucoma detection using confocal scanning laser ophthalmoscopy of the optic disc. Invest Ophthalmol Vis Sci 43:3444–3454
11. Bowd C, Weinreb RN, Lee B, Emdadi A, Zangwill LM (2000) Optic disk topography after medical treatment to reduce intraocular pressure. Am J Ophthalmol 130:280–286
12. Bowd C, Zangwill LM, Berry CC, Blumenthal EZ, Vasile C, Sanchez-Galeana C, Bosworth CF, Sample PA, Weinreb RN (2001) Detecting early glaucoma by assessment of retinal nerve fiber layer thickness and visual function. Invest Ophthalmol Vis Sci 42:1993–2003
13. Bowd C, Zangwill LM, Weinreb RN (2003) Association between scanning laser polarimetry measurements using variable corneal polarization compensation and visual field sensitivity in glaucomatous eyes. Arch Ophthalmol 121:961–966
14. Brusini P, Tosoni C, Miani F (2000) Quantitative mapping of the retinal thickness at the posterior pole in chronic open angle glaucoma. Acta Ophthalmol Scand Suppl:42–44
15. Carpineto P, Ciancaglini M, Zuppardi E, Falconio G, Doronzo E, Mastropasqua L (2003) Reliability of nerve fiber layer thickness measurements using optical coherence tomography in normal and glaucomatous eyes. Ophthalmology 110:190–195
16. Chauhan BC, Blanchard JW, Hamilton DC, LeBlanc RP (2000) Technique for detecting serial topographic changes in the optic disc and peripapillary retina using scanning laser tomography. Invest Ophthalmol Vis Sci 41:775–782
17. Chauhan BC, McCormick TA, Nicolela MT, LeBlanc RP (2001) Optic disc and visual field changes in a prospective longitudinal study of patients with glaucoma: comparison of scanning laser tomography with conventional perimetry and optic disc photography. Arch Ophthalmol 119:1492–1499
18. Choplin NT, Lundy DC (2001) The sensitivity and specificity of scanning laser polarimetry in the detection of glaucoma in a clinical setting. Ophthalmology 108:899–904

19. Choplin NT, Zhou Q, Knighton RW (2003) Effect of individualized compensation for anterior segment birefringence on retinal nerve fiber layer assessments as determined by scanning laser polarimetry. Ophthalmology 110:719–725

20. Colen TP, van Everdingen JA, Lemij HG (2000) Axonal loss in a patient with anterior ischemic optic neuropathy as measured with scanning laser polarimetry. Am J Ophthalmol 130:847–850

21. El Beltagi TA, Bowd C, Boden C et al. (2003) Retinal nerve fiber layer thickness measured with optical coherence tomography is related to visual function in glaucomatous eyes. Ophthalmology 110:2185–2191

22. Ford BA, Artes PH, McCormick TA, Nicolela MT, LeBlanc RP, Chauhan BC (2003) Comparison of data analysis tools for detection of glaucoma with the Heidelberg Retina Tomograph. Ophthalmology 110:1145–1150

23. Greaney MJ, Hoffman DC, Garway-Heath DF, Nakla M, Coleman AL, Caprioli J (2002) Comparison of optic nerve imaging methods to distinguish normal eyes from those with glaucoma. Invest Ophthalmol Vis Sci 43:140–145

24. Greenfield DS (2002) Optic nerve and retinal nerve fiber layer analyzers in glaucoma. Curr Opin Ophthalmol 13:68–76

25. Greenfield DS, Bagga H, Knighton RW (2003) Macular thickness changes in glaucomatous optic neuropathy detected using optical coherence tomography. Arch Ophthalmol 121:41–46

26. Greenfield DS, Knighton RW (2001) Stability of corneal polarization axis measurements for scanning laser polarimetry. Ophthalmology 108:1065–1069

27. Greenfield DS, Knighton RW, Feuer WJ, Schiffman JC (2003) Normative retardation data corrected for the corneal polarization axis with scanning laser polarimetry. Ophthalmic Surg Lasers Imaging 34:165–171

28. Greenfield DS, Knighton RW, Huang XR (2000) Effect of corneal polarization axis on assessment of retinal nerve fiber layer thickness by scanning laser polarimetry. Am J Ophthalmol 129:715–722

29. Guedes V, Schuman JS, Hertzmark E, Wollstein G, Correnti A, Mancini R, Lederer D, Voskanian S, Velazquez L, Pakter HM, Pedut-Kloizman T, Fujimoto JG, Mattox C (2003) Optical coherence tomography measurement of macular and nerve fiber layer thickness in normal and glaucomatous human eyes. Ophthalmology 110:177–189

30. Gundersen KG, Heijl A, Bengtsson B (2000) Comparability of three-dimensional optic disc imaging with different techniques. A study with confocal scanning laser tomography and raster tomography. Acta Ophthalmol Scand 78:9–13

31. Gurses-Ozden R, Ishikawa H, Hoh ST, Liebmann JM, Mistlberger A, Greenfield DS, Dou HL, Ritch R (1999) Increasing sampling density improves reproducibility of optical coherence tomography measurements. J Glaucoma 8:238–241

32. Huang D, Swanson EA, Lin CP, Schuman JS, Stinson WG, Chang W, Hee MR, Flotte T, Gregory K, Puliafito CA et al (1991) Optical coherence tomography. Science 254:1178–1181

33. Iester M, De Ferrari R, Zanini M (1999) Topographic analysis to discriminate glaucomatous from normal optic nerve heads with a confocal scanning laser: new optic disk analysis without any observer input. Surv Ophthalmol 44[Suppl 1]:S33–40

34. Ishikawa H, Piette S, Liebmann JM, Ritch R (2002) Detecting the inner and outer borders of the retinal nerve fiber layer using optical coherence tomography. Graefes Arch Clin Exp Ophthalmol 240:362–71

35. Itai N, Tanito M, Chihara E (2003) Comparison of optic disc topography measured by Retinal Thickness Analyzer with measurement by Heidelberg Retina Tomograph II. Jpn J Ophthalmol 47:214–20

36. Jaeschke R, Guyatt G, Lijmer J (2002) Diagnostic tests. In: Rennie D (ed) Users' guides to the medical literature: essentials of evidence-based clinical practice. AMA Press, Chicago, pp 187–217

37. Johnson CA, Cioffi GA, Liebmann JR, Sample PA, Zangwill LM, Weinreb RN (2000) The relationship between structural and functional alterations in glaucoma: a review. Sem Ophthalmol 15:221–233

38. Kamal DS, Garway-Heath DF, Hitchings RA, Fitzke FW (2000) Use of sequential Heidelberg retina tomograph images to identify changes at the optic disc in ocular hypertensive patients at risk of developing glaucoma. Br J Ophthalmol 84:993–998

39. Kanamori A, Escano MF, Eno A, Nakamura M, Maeda H, Seya R, Ishibashi K, Negi A (2003) Evaluation of the effect of aging on retinal nerve fiber layer thickness measured by optical coherence tomography. Ophthalmologica 217:273–278

40. Kanamori A, Nakamura M, Escano MF, Seya R, Maeda H, Negi A (2003) Evaluation of the glaucomatous damage on retinal nerve fiber layer thickness measured by optical coherence tomography. Am J Ophthalmol 135:513–520

41. Konno S, Akiba J, Yoshida A (2001) Retinal thickness measurements with optical coherence tomography and the scanning retinal thickness analyzer. Retina 21:57–61

42. Lederer DE, Schuman JS, Hertzmark E, Heltzer J, Velazques LJ, Fujimoto JG, Mattox C (2003) Analysis of macular volume in normal and glaucomatous eyes using optical coherence tomography. Am J Ophthalmol 135:838–843

43. Mardin CY, Hothorn T, Peters A, Jünemann AG, Nguyen NX, Lausen B (2003) New glaucoma classification method based on standard Heidelberg Retina Tomograph parameters by bagging classification trees. J Glaucoma 12:340–346

44. Mardin CY, Jünemann AG (2001) The diagnostic value of optic nerve imaging in early glaucoma. Curr Opin Ophthalmol 12:100–104

45. Medeiros FA, Moura FC, Vessani RM, Susanna R (2003) Axonal loss after traumatic optic neuropathy documented by optical coherence tomography. Am J Ophthalmol 135:406–408

46. Medeiros FA, Susanna R (2001) Retinal nerve fiber layer loss after traumatic optic neuropathy detected by scanning laser polarimetry. Arch Ophthalmol 119:920–921

47. Medeiros FA, Susanna R (2003) Comparison of algorithms for detection of localised nerve fibre layer defects using scanning laser polarimetry. Br J Ophthalmol 87:413–419

48. Medeiros FA, Zangwill LM, Bowd C, Bernd AS, Weinreb RN (2003) Fourier analysis of scanning laser polarimetry measurements with variable corneal compensation in glaucoma. Invest Ophthalmol Vis Sci 44:2606–2612

49. Miglior S, Casula M, Guareschi M, Marchetti I, Iester M, Orzalesi N (2001) Clinical ability of Heidelberg retinal tomograph examination to detect glaucomatous visual field changes. Ophthalmology 108:1621–1627

50. Miglior S, Guareschi M, Albe' E, Gomarasca S, Vavassori M, Orzalesi N (2003) Detection of glaucomatous visual field changes using the Moorfields regression analysis of the Heidelberg retina tomograph. Am J Ophthalmol 136:26–33

51. Nicolela MT, Martinez-Bello C, Morrison CA, LeBlanc RP, Lemij HG, Colen TP, Chauhan BC (2001) Scanning laser polarimetry in a selected group of patients with glaucoma and normal controls. Am J Ophthalmol 132:845–854

52. Oshima Y, Emi K, Yamanishi S, Motokura M (1999) Quantitative assessment of macular thickness in normal subjects and patients with diabetic retinopathy by scanning retinal thickness analyser. Br J Ophthalmol 83:54–61

53. Paczka JA, Friedman DS, Quigley HA, Barron Y, Vitale S (2001) Diagnostic capabilities of frequency-doubling technology, scanning laser polarimetry, and nerve fiber layer photographs to distinguish glaucomatous damage. Am J Ophthalmol 131:188–197

54. Polito A, Shah SM, Haller JA, Zimmer-Galler I, Zeimer R, Campochiaro PA, Vitale S (2002) Comparison between retinal thickness analyzer and optical coherence tomography for assessment of foveal thickness in eyes with macular disease. Am J Ophthalmol 134:240–251

55. Sanchez-Galeana C, Bowd C, Blumenthal EZ, Gokhale PA, Zangwill LM, Weinreb RN (2001) Using optical imaging summary data to detect glaucoma. Ophthalmology 108:1812–1818

56. Schuman JS, Wollstein G, Farra T, Hertzmark E, Aydin A, Fujimoto JG, Paunescu LA (2003) Comparison of optic nerve head measurements obtained by optical coherence tomography and confocal scanning laser ophthalmoscopy. Am J Ophthalmol 135:504–512

57. Sihota R, Gulati V, Agarwal HC, Saxena R, Sharma A, Pandey RM (2002) Variables affecting testretest variability of Heidelberg Retina Tomograph II stereometric parameters. J Glaucoma 11:321-8

58. Sinai MJ, Essock EA, Fechtner RD, Srinivasan N (2000) Diffuse and localized nerve fiber layer loss measured with a scanning laser polarimeter: sensitivity and specificity of detecting glaucoma. J Glaucoma 9:154–162

59. Soliman MA, Van Den Berg TJ, Ismaeil AA, De Jong LA, De Smet MD (2002) Retinal nerve fiber layer analysis: relationship between optical coherence tomography and red-free photography. Am J Ophthalmol 133:187–195

60. Swindale NV, Stjepanovic G, Chin A, Mikelberg FS (2000) Automated analysis of normal and glaucomatous optic nerve head topography images. Invest Ophthalmol Vis Sci 41:1730–1742

61. Tan JC, Hitchings RA (2003) Approach for identifying glaucomatous optic nerve progression by scanning laser tomography. Invest Ophthalmol Vis Sci 44:2621–2626

62. Vitale S, Smith TD, Quigley T et al (2000) Screening performance of functional and structural measurements of neural damage in open-angle glaucoma: a case-control study from the Baltimore Eye Survey. J Glaucoma;9:346–356

63. Weinreb RN, Bowd C, Greenfield DS, Zangwill LM (2002) Measurement of the magnitude and axis of corneal polarization with scanning laser polarimetry. Arch Ophthalmol 120:901–906

64. Weinreb RN, Bowd C, Zangwill LM (2003) Glaucoma detection using scanning laser polarimetry with variable corneal polarization compensation. Arch Ophthalmol 121:218–224

65. Williams ZY, Schuman JS, Gamell L, Nemi A, Hertzmark E, Fujimoto JG, Mattox C, Simpson J, Wollstein G (2002) Optical coherence tomography measurement of nerve fiber layer thickness and the likelihood of a visual field defect. Am J Ophthalmol 134:538–546

66. Wollstein G, Garway-Heath DF, Hitchings RA (1998) Identification of early glaucoma cases with the scanning laser ophthalmoscope. Ophthalmology 105:1557–1563

67. Yamada N, Chen PP, Mills RP, Leen MM, Stamper RL, Lieberman MF, Xu L, Stanford DC (2000) Glaucoma screening using the scanning laser polarimeter. J Glaucoma 9:254–261

68. Zangwill LM, Bowd C, Berry CC, Williams J, Blumenthal EZ, Sánchez-Galeana CA, Vasile C, Weinreb RN (2001) Discriminating between normal and glaucomatous eyes using the Heidelberg Retina Tomograph, GDx Nerve Fiber Analyzer, and Optical Coherence Tomograph. Arch Ophthalmol 119:985–993

69. Zangwill LM, Bowd C, Weinreb RN (2000) Evaluating the optic disc and retinal nerve fiber layer in glaucoma II: Optical Image Analysis. Seminars in Ophthalmology;15:206–220

70. Zangwill LM, Williams J, Berry CC, Knauer S, Weinreb RN (2000) A comparison of optical coherence tomography and retinal nerve fiber layer photography for detection of nerve fiber layer damage in glaucoma. Ophthalmology 107:1309–1315

71. Zeimer R, Asrani S, Zou S, Quigley H, Jampel H (1998) Quantitative detection of glaucomatous damage at the posterior pole by retinal thickness mapping. A pilot study. Ophthalmology 105:224–231

72. Zeimer R, Shahidi M, Mori M, Zou S, Asrani S (1996) A new method for rapid mapping of the retinal thickness at the posterior pole. Invest Ophthalmol Vis Sci 37:1994–2001

73. Zhou Q, Weinreb RN (2002) Individualized compensation of anterior segment birefringence during scanning laser polarimetry. Invest Ophthalmol Vis Sci 43:2221–2228

New Concepts in the Diagnosis of Angle-Closure Glaucoma: The Role of Ultrasound Biomicroscopy

Celso Tello, Jeffrey M. Liebmann, Robert Ritch

6

Core Messages

- An understanding of the pathophysiology of the several different types of angle-closure glaucoma is critical to insure accurate diagnosis and optimal treatment
- The ultrasound biomicroscope (UBM) can provide high resolution images of anterior segment anatomy that can not be obtained any other way
- The anatomical classification of angle closure into pupillary block, plateau iris, malignant glaucoma, and lens-related glaucoma is aided by UBM. Each has its unique UBM characteristics
- Pupillary block has a variety of time courses that further characterize the clinical picture and response to laser iridotomy
- Plateau iris often responds to laser iridotomy but may need additional laser iridoplasty to open the angle
- Cataract extraction is usually required for phacomorphic glaucoma
- Malignant glaucoma has two varieties: Aqueous misdirection which often responds to disruption of the anterior hyaloid face, and anteriorly rotated ciliary body which usually responds to conservative medical therapy but may require surgical drainage

6.1
Introduction

The angle-closure glaucomas are a diverse group of disorders characterized by mechanical blockage of the trabecular meshwork by the peripheral iris. This alteration in anterior segment anatomy can be caused by changes in the relative or absolute sizes or positions of anterior segment structures or by forces originating in the anterior or posterior segments. An understanding of the pathophysiology of angle-closure glaucoma is critical to ensure accurate diagnosis and optimal treatment.

Assessment of anterior segment structures and their relationships can be performed with complementary techniques including slit-lamp biomicroscopy, gonioscopy and ultrasound biomicroscopy. Slit-lamp biomicroscopy provides a direct view of the cornea, lens, iris, conjunctiva, and sclera. However, slit-lamp biomicroscopy does not allow direct visualization of the anterior chamber angle, which is best achieved in the clinical setting with gonioscopy. Indentation gonioscopy permits dynamic evaluation of the angle and the assessment of appositional or synechial closure, but only reveals inferential knowledge regarding the structures posterior to the iris. Provocative testing can also be used to diagnose potentially occludable anterior chamber angles. This review will emphasize the role of ultrasound biomicroscopy in the diagnosis and management of the angle-closure glaucomas.

6.2
Ultrasound Biomicroscopy

Ultrasound biomicroscopy (UBM, Paradigm Medical Industries, Inc., Salt Lake City, Utah), developed by Pavlin et al. [13–16] is a non-invasive diagnostic technique that uses high frequency transducers to provide high resolution, in vivo imaging of the anterior segment [7, 10, 12, 15–17]. The structures surrounding the posterior chamber, including the ciliary body, iridolenticular relationship, and zonular apparatus of Zinn, previously hidden from clinical observation, can be imaged and their normal anatomic relationships assessed. The development of pathologic changes involving anterior segment architecture can be qualitatively and quantitatively evaluated.

Current UBM technology is based on research initially conducted by Pavlin, Sherar and Foster [13, 16]. Their technique incorporated 50- to 100-MHz transducers in a B-mode echography clinical scanner. Different transducer frequencies can be utilized depending on the ocular tissue to be imaged. In general, increasing the transducer frequency improves the image resolution but limits the depth of tissue penetration. Conversely, a decrease in transducer frequency increases the penetration depth but decreases tissue resolution.

The UBM unit used to obtain the images presented in this review operates at 50 MHz and provides lateral and axial resolution of approximately 50 µm and 25 µm, respectively. Tissue penetration is approximately 4–5 mm. The scanner produces a 5×5-mm field with 256 vertical image lines (or A-scans) at a scan rate of eight frames per second. Increasing the transducer frequency to 100 MHz increases the tissue resolution to approximately 20 µm. However, the resulting decreased penetration depth limits scanning to the cornea but may be useful in evaluating the effects of refractive surgery. The increased penetration depth afforded with a 34-MHz transducer permits visualization of the ciliary body and the zonules and has proved useful in studies of accommodation [9].

The technique of performing UBM has been reported in detail elsewhere and is similar to traditional immersion B-scan ultrasonography [12, 13]. The probe is suspended from an articulated arm to diminish motion artifacts. Utilizing a linear scan format minimizes lateral distortion. Scanning is performed in the supine position. An eye cup, measuring 18, 20 or 22 mm in diameter, is inserted between the lids and holds methylcellulose or normal saline as the coupling agent [27]. After insertion of the probe into the coupling medium, the real-time image is displayed on a video monitor and can be stored on videotape for later analysis. Inexperienced examiners with minimal practice can typically obtain good qualitative information. However, ultrasonography is an art, and acquisition of highly reproducible distance measurements is strongly dependent on examiner technique and experience. The distance from the center of the anterior chamber, plane of section, and the orientation of the probe with respect to the perpendicular may affect the apparent structural configuration of the anterior segment.

Quantitative assessment of anterior segment relationships using the information contained in UBM scans requires a more sophisticated approach. Pavlin [12] described and quantified normal values for anterior segment anatomy. However, interobserver error partially limits their application [26, 30]. Factors which contribute to the variability of UBM image acquisition include room illumination, fixation, and accommodative effort [7], each of which affects anterior segment anatomy by altering pupillary size, ciliary body architecture, or probe orientation. These variables should be held constant, particularly when quantitative information is being gathered [26]. In our laboratory, patients are asked to fixate with the fellow eye at a ceiling mounted target to minimize changes in accommodation and eye position. Room illumination is held constant. Since the probe is in constant motion during scanning, a soft contact lens may be used to prevent potential corneal injury [28].

Summary for the Clinician

- Ultrasound biomicroscopy uses high frequency transducers to provide high resolution, in vivo imaging of the anterior segment structures
- In general, increasing the transducer frequency improves the image resolution but limits the depth of tissue penetration

Fig. 6.1. Ultrasound biomicroscopy of normal eye. The anterior chamber (*AC*), posterior chamber (*PC*), cornea (*C*), iris (*I*), lens capsule (*LC*), angle (*white arrow*), scleral spur (*thin black arrow*), Schwalbe's line (*thick black arrow*) sclera (*S*), and ciliary body (*CB*) are visible

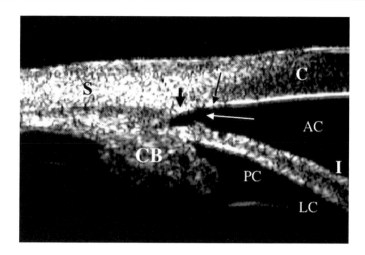

Fig. 6.2. A Anatomically narrow angle (*arrows*) under normal room illumination. **B** Same angle showing significant appositional closure (*arrows*) during dark-room testing

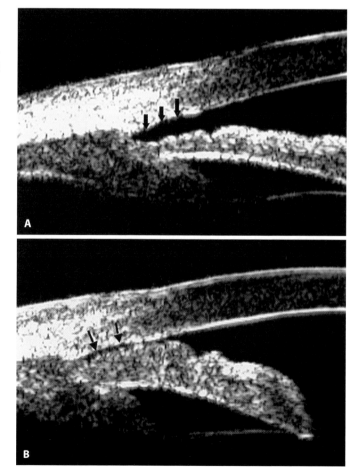

6.3
The Normal Eye

Knowledge of the ultrasound biomicroscopic appearance of normal ocular anatomy is important for recognizing pathologic changes. In the normal eye, the cornea, anterior chamber, posterior chamber, iris, ciliary body, and anterior lens surface can be easily recognized (Fig. 6.1). Identification of Schwalbe's line, trabecular meshwork, scleral spur, and the zonular apparatus requires more precision and attention to technique on the part of the examiner.

The anatomic relationships of the structures of the anterior segment are extremely important when interpreting pathology involving the angle. In many normal individuals, the iris has a roughly planar configuration; however, a variety of physiologic stimuli, including accommodation and pupillary reaction to the amount of ambient light [11], can change the configuration of the anterior segment (Fig. 6.2 A,B) and this should be considered when interpreting UBM images.

6.4
Anatomical Classification
of the Angle-Closure Glaucomas

Based on the anatomical level where forces act to change the angle configuration, the angle-closure glaucomas can be classified as: pupillary block, plateau iris, phacomorphic glaucoma, and aqueous misdirection or malignant glaucoma [19,22]. This classification facilitates an understanding of the various mechanisms involved in the disease process and permits treatment to be directed at the underlying pathophysiology. It is important to realize that these forms of angle-closure are not mutually exclusive. For example, pupillary block may be a contributing factor in each type of angle closure.

6.4.1
Pupillary Block

Pupillary block is the most common form of angle-closure glaucoma and is responsible for more than 90% of cases. In relative pupillary block, flow of aqueous from the posterior chamber, to the anterior chamber, is limited by resistance through the pupil at the level of iridolenticular contact. The accumulation of aqueous in the posterior chamber forces the peripheral iris anteriorly, causing anterior iris bowing, narrowing of the angle, and acute or chronic angle-closure glaucoma (Fig. 6.3 A). The central anterior chamber depth and the anatomic relationships of other anterior segment structures appear otherwise normal. Pupillary block may be absolute, as when the iris is completely bound down to the lens by posterior synechiae, but most often is a functional block, termed relative pupillary block. The physiologic processes which convert relative pupillary block to an acute attack of angle-closure glaucoma are unknown. Although predisposing factors have been repeatedly described (i.e., fatigue, anxiety, excitement, close work, or upper respiratory illness) the actual mechanisms still remain unclear [23].

Relative pupillary block usually causes no signs or symptoms. However, if the pupillary block is sufficient to cause appositional closure of a portion of the angle without sudden elevation of the intraocular pressure, peripheral anterior synechiae may gradually form, leading to chronic angle-closure glaucoma (Fig. 6.4). If the pupillary block becomes absolute, the pressure in the posterior chamber increases and pushes the peripheral iris farther forward to cover the trabecular meshwork, thereby closing the angle with an ensuing rise of IOP and acute angle-closure glaucoma.

In acute angle-closure glaucoma, the IOP may rise high enough to cause corneal edema. As a result, patients may experience a decrease in visual acuity, halos around lights, intense pain, conjunctival injection, secondary lacrimation, and lid edema. Patients may also present with anxiety, fatigue, and vasovagal responses such as bradycardia and diaphoresis. On exam-

Fig. 6.3. **A** Pupillary block angle-closure is characterized by a convex iris configuration (*white arrows*). The angle is closed (*black arrows*). **B** Laser iridotomy, allows aqueous access to the anterior chamber and the pressure gradient is eliminated. The iris assumes a flat (planar) configuration and the angle opens

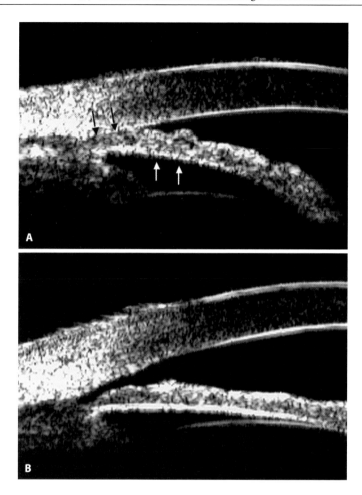

Fig. 6.4. Chronic angle-closure glaucoma is characterized by the formation of peripheral anterior synechiae (*arrows*)

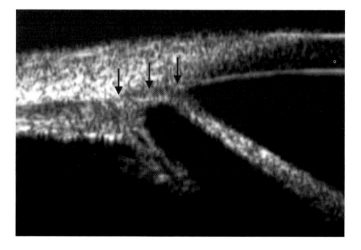

ination, corneal edema may limit the view of the anterior and posterior segment, even after the topical application of glycerin. The anterior chamber may appear moderately shallow and the pupil fixed and mid-dilated. Examination of the fellow eye usually demonstrates a shallow anterior chamber and narrow angle and is useful in differentiating acute angle-closure glaucoma from uveitic, neovascular or phacolytic glaucoma. During the attack, the optic nerve head may be edematous and hyperemic. Spontaneous termination of an acute angle-closure attack can occur as a result of suppression of aqueous secretion caused by the high intraocular pressure or when aqueous from the posterior chamber percolates through areas of newly formed iris atrophy and necrosis, effectively bypassing the pupillary block.

In chronic angle-closure glaucoma, there is a gradual elevation of IOP that can lead to glaucomatous disc damage and subsequent visual field loss. The progressive elevation of IOP does not result in corneal endothelial decompensation and the development of corneal edema is rare. Symptoms are usually absent until peripheral anterior synechiae have progressed enough to impair aqueous outflow, leading to a rise in IOP that causes corneal endothelial dysfunction. In other cases, patients may present with elevated IOP, glaucomatous optic neuropathy, and a silent, progressive decrease of peripheral vision.

Intermittent angle-closure glaucoma is characterized by repeated, brief episodes of iridotrabecular contact, with or without elevated IOP. Patients may present with mild symptoms and elevated IOP during attacks, but the process is usually asymptomatic. Examination often reveals a narrow angle, shallow anterior chamber, and occasionally, an enlarged pupil caused by ischemia of the pupillary sphincter which may occur during attacks. Intermittent angle-closure glaucoma can result in the progressive formation of peripheral anterior synechiae, leading to chronic angle-closure glaucoma and elevated IOP, or it can suddenly convert to an acute angle-closure attack.

When assessing a patient with a narrow angle for occludability, it is important to perform indentation gonioscopy in a completely darkened room, using the smallest amount of slit-lamp illumination possible to avoid stimulating the pupillary light reflex. In the absence of peripheral anterior synechiae formation, indentation gonioscopy shows the iris to move posteriorly across its entire length and the angle to open uniformly. The angle is relatively easy to open as aqueous is displaced from the posterior chamber. Ultrasound biomicroscopy is always performed in lighted and darkened conditions to assess the anterior chamber angle configuration during miosis and pupillary dilation associated with and without light stimulation, respectively. In fact, our current provocative test of choice utilizes UBM under light and dark room conditions [11, 18].

Laser iridotomy is the procedure of choice to treat pupillary block. Since nearly all cases of angle-closure glaucoma have some component of pupillary block, all of these eyes should be treated with laser iridotomy. However, this procedure is contraindicated in angle-closure glaucoma secondary to anterior mechanisms of closure, such as proliferating anterior segment membranes in neovascular glaucoma or iridocorneal endothelial syndrome since pupillary block is not contributing to the development of disease in these conditions.

Laser iridotomy eliminates the pressure differential between the anterior and posterior chambers and relieves the iris convexity. This results in several changes in anterior segment anatomy. The iris assumes a flat or planar configuration and the iridocorneal angle widens (Fig. 6.3 B). The region of iridolenticular contact actually increases after this procedure as aqueous flows through the iridotomy rather than the pupillary space [2]. With current techniques and equipment, laser iridotomy is now able to achieve success at penetration of the iris in virtually 100% of eyes in a single session [21]. The techniques, indications and complications of this procedure have been described in detail elsewhere [21].

Fig. 6.5. A In plateau iris syndrome, the ciliary body is anteriorly positioned forcing the peripheral iris into the angle. Iridotomy relieves the pupillary block component but not the closure related to the abnormal ciliary body position. The scleral spur is visible (*arrow*). **B** Laser iridoplasty (*arrows*) may relieve appositional angle closure

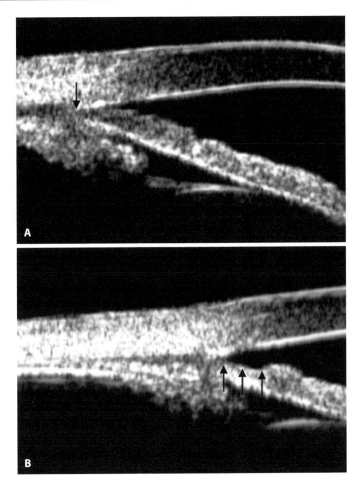

6.4.2
Plateau Iris

Plateau iris configuration results from a large or anteriorly positioned ciliary body that mechanically holds the peripheral iris against the trabecular meshwork (Fig. 6.5 A). The iris root is inserted anteriorly on the ciliary face so that the angle appears crowded and narrow. The anterior chamber is usually not shallow and the iris surface appears flat or slightly convex. On indentation gonioscopy the "double-hump" sign will be seen.

The most peripheral "hump" is determined by the ciliary body propping up the iris root and the most central "hump" represents the central third of the iris resting over the anterior lens surface. The space between the "humps" represents the space between the ciliary processes and the end point of contact of the iris to the anterior lens capsule. Plateau iris syndrome is most commonly seen in women. Patients are younger and less hyperopic than those with pupillary block and there is often a family history of glaucoma.

Since a component of pupillary block may exist in patients with plateau iris, laser iridotomy should always be performed as the first intervention. If persistent iridotrabecular apposition is present, the diagnosis is consistent with plateau iris syndrome and peripheral laser iridoplasty is indicated (Fig. 6.5 B).

Argon laser peripheral iridoplasty is the procedure of choice to effectively open an angle that remains occluded following successful laser iridotomy. The procedure consists of placing contraction burns on the surface of the peripheral iris to contract the iris stroma between the site of burn and the angle. The result is iris stromal tissue contraction and compaction that physically widens the angle. The technique, indications and complications have been described in detail elsewhere [20].

6.4.3
Pseudoplateau Iris

In pseudoplateau iris, the clinical appearance of the anterior chamber angle is similar to that seen in plateau iris syndrome. The difference between these conditions is determined by the underlying mechanism that results in the typical appearance of the peripheral iris. In pseudoplateau iris, the anterior displacement of the peripheral iris is not caused by an enlarged or anteriorly positioned ciliary body. Cysts of the iris and/or ciliary body neuroepithelium are most often responsible [1].

The conditions responsible for pseudoplateau iris are usually easily diagnosed, as the angle is closed either in one quadrant or, if cysts are multiple, at several, focal loculations. However, when angle-closure mimicking pupillary block occurs in association with these conditions, a high index of suspicion and careful gonioscopic evaluation is required to confirm this diagnosis (Fig. 6.6).

Other disease processes, including enlargement of the ciliary body due to inflammation or tumor infiltration, and air or gas bubbles after intraocular surgical procedures may be confused with plateau iris configuration. UBM is extremely helpful in making the diagnosis in these patients [6].

Treatment of pseudoplateau iris depends on the underlying mechanism, and both, laser iridotomy and argon laser peripheral iridoplasty may be indicated to modify the anterior chamber angle configuration [3, 20, 21].

6.5
Lens-Related Angle-Closure

Abnormalities in the size or position of the lens can alter the anatomic relationship of the anterior segment structures leading to angle-closure glaucoma. These abnormalities may occur as part of the normal aging process, in association with other anterior segment pathology or as a result of trauma. The end result is a mechanical compression of the iris against the trabecular meshwork and subsequent acute or chronic angle closure. These conditions are collectively termed phacomorphic glaucoma.

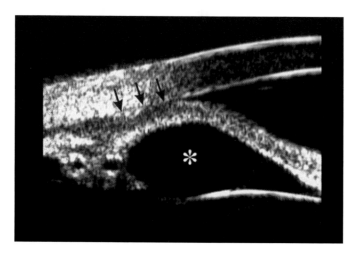

Fig. 6.6. Iridociliary cysts (*asterisk*) are thinned-walled echolucent lesions that may displace the peripheral iris against the trabecular meshwork (*arrows*)

Fig. 6.7. A Phacomorphic
glaucoma is characterized by
shallow anterior chamber angle.
Lens intumescence or anterior
subluxation, can increase pupillary block (*arrowheads*).
B In some cases of phacomorphic glaucoma, acute angle-
closure glaucoma may develop
due to mechanical compression
of the iris against the trabecular
meshwork (*black arrows*)

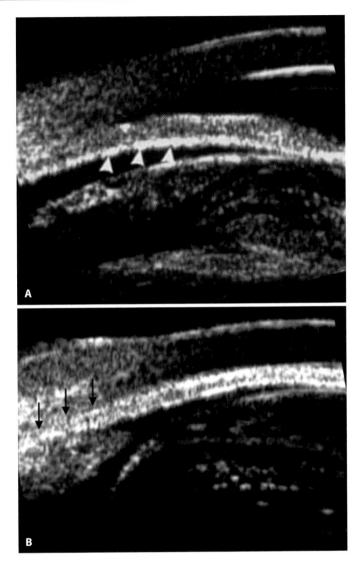

Anterior subluxation of the lens may occur as a result of the increasing zonular laxity seen in many pathologic conditions involving the eye including Marfan's syndrome, homocystinuria, Weill-Marchesani syndrome, acquired syphilis, hyperlysinemia, and sulfite-oxidase deficiency. It can also occur, to a less exaggerated degree, in patients with high myopia, chronic inflammation and pseudoexfoliation syndrome. Miotic-induced ciliary muscle constriction relaxes the zonules, producing anterior lens movement and increased lens thickness and curvature, all of

which augment pupillary block. Most common-ly, anterior subluxation occurs as a result of blunt ocular trauma and zonular dehiscence.

Intumescence results in an increase in the axial length of the lens. There is increased irido-lenticular contact and increased resistance to aqueous flow from the posterior to the anterior chamber, consistent with pupillary block. Accumulation of aqueous in the posterior chamber will cause bowing of the peripheral iris and narrowing of the anterior chamber angle (Fig. 6.7 A). In cases where the subluxation or swelling of the lens is severe, the iris may be mechanically pushed against the trabecular meshwork (Fig. 6.7 B).

Laser iridotomy is not likely to be successful in relieving most forms of phacomorphic glaucoma since pupillary block is not the main feature. Although peripheral iridoplasty may transiently relieve the iridotrabecular contact, cataract extraction may be required.

6.6
Malignant Glaucoma

Malignant glaucoma, also known as ciliary block glaucoma or aqueous misdirection glaucoma, is a secondary angle-closure glaucoma characterized by normal or elevated IOP, shallow anterior chamber, patent iridectomy, and normal posterior segment anatomy by ophthalmoscopy and B-scan ultrasonography. This condition is a relatively rare but serious complication of intraocular surgery.

Although the majority of these cases develop after filtration surgery in eyes with chronic angle-closure glaucoma, it has also been seen after extracapsular cataract extraction with posterior chamber intraocular lens implantation, intracapsular cataract extraction, Nd:YAG transscleral cyclophotocoagulation, laser iridotomy, laser release of scleral flap sutures, diode laser cyclophotocoagulation, central retinal vein occlusion, retinopathy of prematurity, and the use of pilocarpine in eyes with previous filtering procedures [5, 24].

The anatomy and pathophysiology of malignant glaucoma remain unclear. Shaffer [24] proposed that aqueous flow is diverted into the vitreous cavity. He attributed this misdirection of aqueous to an abnormal vitreociliary relationship and later coined the descriptive term "ciliary block glaucoma."

We have identified at least two distinct mechanisms that may be responsible for what is usually called postoperative malignant glaucoma. In the first group, the ciliary body is detached

Fig. 6.8. **A** In one form of malignant glaucoma the ciliary body (*CB*) is detached (*D*) and rotated anteriorly. The anterior chamber (*asterisk*) is flat and the lens–iris diaphragm (*large, white arrow*) is rotated forward causing mechanical angle closure (*short, white arrows*). **B** In other forms of aqueous misdirection, there is no ciliary body (*CB*) detachment. The anterior chamber (*asterisk*) is flat and the lens–iris diaphragm (*curved arrow*) is rotated forward causing mechanical angle closure (*white arrowheads*)

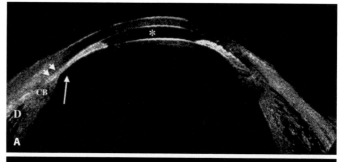

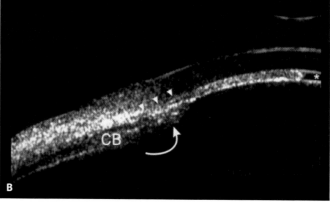

and rotated anteriorly causing angle-closure (Fig. 6.8 A). In the second group the anterior chamber angle is closed but the ciliary body is not detached or anteriorly rotated.(Fig. 6.8 B). It is possible that in this group of patients a true misdirection of aqueous to the vitreous cavity occurs, increasing the posterior segment pressure which will force the lens and iris against the trabecular meshwork.

Treatment of malignant glaucoma depends upon the underlying mechanism. If the ciliary body is detached and rotated anteriorly, the treatment of choice consists of conservative medical therapy including intensive cycloplegia, topical steroids and systemic steroids if appropriate. Resistant cases may require surgical drainage of the suprachoroidal effusion [8]. If the malignant glaucoma is due to aqueous misdirection, the treatment consists of rupture of the anterior hyaloid face (Nd:YAG laser or surgical) to eliminate the vitreociliary block when medical therapy has failed [29].

6.7
Conclusion

The angle-closure glaucomas are a group of disorders characterized by the final common endpoint pathway of iridotrabecular contact, elevated intraocular pressure, optic nerve damage, and loss of peripheral visual field. Early diagnosis and adequate treatment is crucial for the long-term retention of visual function. Ultrasound biomicroscopy has been instrumental in enhancing our understanding of the underlying pathophysiology of the various forms of angle closure glaucomas, in addition to its practical applications in clinical practice.

Note. The authors do not have a financial interest in any technique or device described in this manuscript.

References

1. Azuara-Blanco A, Spaeth GL, Araujo SV, Augsburger JJ, Terebuh AK (1996) Plateau iris syndrome associated with multiple ciliary body cysts. Report of three cases. Arch Ophthalmol 114: 666–668
2. Caronia RM, Liebmann JM, Stegman Z et al. (1996) Iris-lens contact increases following laser iridotomy for pupillary block angle-closure. Am J Ophthalmol 122:53–57
3. Caronia RM, Liebmann JM, Stegman Z, Sokol J, Ritch R (1996) Increase in iris-lens contact after laser iridotomy for pupillary block angle closure. Am J Ophthalmol 122:53–57
4. DiSclafani M, Liebmann JM, Ritch R (1989) Malignant glaucoma following argon laser release of scleral flap sutures after trabeculectomy. Am J Ophthalmol 108:597–598
5. Duy TP, Wollensak J (1987) Ciliary block (malignant) glaucoma following posterior chamber lens implantation. Ophthalmic Surg 18:741–744
6. Gentile RC, Stegman Z, Liebmann JM, Dayan AR, Tello C, Walsh JB, Ritch R (1996) Risk factors for ciliochoroidal effusion after panretinal photocoagulation. Ophthalmology 103:827–832
7. Liebmann JM, Tello C, Chew SJ, Cohen H, Ritch R (1995) Prevention of blinking alters iris configuration in pigment dispersion syndrome and in normal eyes. Ophthalmology 102:446–455
8. Liebmann JM, Weinreb RN, Ritch R (1998) Angle-closure glaucoma associated with occult annular ciliary body detachment. Arch Ophthalmol 116: 731–735
9. Ludwig K, Wegscheider E, Hoops JP, Kampik A (1999) In vivo imaging of the human zonular apparatus with high-resolution ultrasound biomicroscopy. Graefes Arch Clin Exp Ophthalmol 237: 361–371
10. Marigo FA, Finger PT, McCormick SA, Iezzi R, Esaki K, Ishikawa H, Seedor J, Liebmann JM, Ritch R (1998) Anterior segment implantation cysts. Ultrasound biomicroscopy with histopathologic correlation. Arch Ophthalmol 116: 1569–1575
11. Pavlin CJ, Foster FS (1999) Plateau iris syndrome: changes in angle opening associated with dark, light, and pilocarpine administration. Am J Ophthalmol 128:288–291
12. Pavlin CJ, Harasiewicz K, Foster FS (1992) Ultrasound biomicroscopy of anterior segment structures in normal and glaucomatous eyes. Am J Ophthalmol 113:381–389

13. Pavlin CJ, Harasiewicz K, Sherar MD, Foster FS (1991) Clinical use of ultrasound biomicroscopy. Ophthalmology 98:287–295

14. Pavlin CJ, McWhae JA, McGowan HD, Foster FS (1992) Ultrasound biomicroscopy of anterior segment tumors. Ophthalmology 99:1220–1228

15. Pavlin CJ, Ritch R, Foster FS (1992) Ultrasound biomicroscopy in plateau iris syndrome. Am J Ophthalmol 113:390–395

16. Pavlin CJ, Sherar MD, Foster FS (1990) Subsurface ultrasound microscopic imaging of the intact eye. Ophthalmology 97:244–250

17. Potash SD, Tello C, Liebmann J, Ritch R (1994) Ultrasound biomicroscopy in pigment dispersion syndrome. Ophthalmology 101:332–339

18. Ritch R (1996) Angle-closure glaucoma. Treatment overview. In:Ritch R, Shields MF, Krupin T (eds) The glaucomas. CV Mosby Co., St Louis

19. Ritch R, Liebmann J, Tello C (1995) A construct for understanding angle-closure glaucoma: the role of ultrasound biomicroscopy. Ophthalmol Clin N Amer 8:281–293

20. Ritch R, Liebmann JM (1996) Argon laser peripheral iridoplasty. Ophthalmic Surg Lasers 27:289-300

21. Ritch R, Liebmann JM (1996) Argon laser peripheral iridoplasty. Ophthalmic Surg Lasers 27:289–300

22. Ritch R, Liebmann JM (1998) Role of ultrasound biomicroscopy in the differentiation of block glaucomas. Curr Opin Ophthalmol 9:39–45

23. Ritch R, Lowe RF (1996) Angle-closure glaucoma: clinical types. In:Ritch R, Shields MF, Krupin T (eds) The glaucomas. CV Mosby Co., St. Loius, pp 821–840

24. Shaffer RN (1954) The role of vitreous detachment in aphakic and malignant glaucoma. Trans Am Acad Ophthalmol Otolaryngol 58:217–231

25. Tello C, Chi T, Shepps G, Liebmann J, Ritch R (1993) Ultrasound biomicroscopy in pseudophakic malignant glaucoma. Ophthalmology 100:1330–1334

26. Tello C, Liebmann J, Potash SD, Cohen H, Ritch R (1994) Measurement of ultrasound biomicroscopy images: intraobserver and interobserver reliability. Invest Ophthalmol Vis Sci 35:3549–3552

27. Tello C, Liebmann JM, Ritch R (1994) An improved coupling medium for ultrasound biomicroscopy. Ophthalmic Surg 25:410–411

28. Tello C, Potash S, Liebmann J et al. (1994) Soft contact lens modification of the ocular cup for high resolution ultrasound biomicroscopy. Ophthalmic Surg 24:563–564

29. Tsai JC, Barton KA, Miller MH et al. (1997) Surgical results in malignant glaucoma refractory to medical or laser therapy. Eye 11:677–681

30. Urbak SF, Pedersen JK, Thorsen TT (1998) Ultrasound biomicroscopy. II. Intraobserver and interobserver reproducibility of measurements. Acta Ophthalmol Scand 76:546–549

KARIM F. TOMEY

Core Messages

- Prevalence: 1:10,000 live births
- Sedation with chloral hydrate is helpful for examination of infants
- Most inhalation anesthetics lower IOP significantly
- IOP, corneal diameter, corneal clarity, retinoscopy, gonioscopy, and fundus examination are the parameters for diagnosing congenital glaucoma
- Medical therapy is not advised for long-term treatment
- Best surgical prognosis is present in isolated trabeculodysgenesis (primary congenital glaucoma), the disease appearing during the first year of life and a corneal diameter of less than 14 mm
- Goniotomy (ab interno) and trabeculotomy (ab externo) are the surgical procedures of choice for first-line treatment
- Filtering procedures (including use of MMC) or combined trabeculotomy/trabeculectomy may be considered in refractory congenital glaucomas
- Drainage implants and cyclodestructive procedures are reserved for cases with failure of multiple previous surgeries
- Treatment of amblyopia accounts for half of the success of visual stabilization and rehabilitation
- Anisometropia and corneal opacities are the major causes of amblyopia

7.1
Introduction

Childhood glaucoma is a potentially blinding condition that afflicts infants and young children, either immediately at birth or within the first few months or years of life. In most populations, primary infantile glaucoma is rare, and usually seen in 1:10,000 live births, whereas in other societies where intermarriage is common, the rate could go up to 1:5000 or even 1:2500 [10, 16]. The significance of early diagnosis and prompt treatment cannot be overemphasized. An infant with congenital glaucoma exhibits specific clinical findings, and the diagnosis is thus easily made. Unfortunately, the typical symptoms of glaucoma may occasionally be attributed (usually by non-ophthalmologists) to other, less serious conditions, such as congenital nasolacrimal duct obstruction. Therefore, family practitioners and pediatricians must always keep this serious condition in mind and refer the infant promptly for specialized care.

The terminology used in describing and classifying childhood glaucomas can sometimes be confusing. Terms such as "congenital," "infantile," "juvenile," and "developmental" have all been used, sometimes interchangeably, to describe the same condition [18]. This is, of course, wrong and confusing. To add further confusion, childhood glaucomas have been labeled as *primary* or *secondary*. Therefore, some clarification is in order. *Congenital* glaucoma presents immediately at birth, whereas 80 % of the *infantile* glaucoma cases present within the first year of life; *juvenile* glaucoma is seen between the age of 4 years and up to the teens [10, 18]. *Prima-*

ry childhood glaucomas are not associated with any other ocular or systemic abnormalities, whereas the *secondary* are. The term *developmental* refers to the situation where glaucoma arises "from the development of an ocular abnormality that is not present from birth" [18]. Another anatomical classification has been suggested by Hoskins [10]. *Trabeculodysgenesis* refers to isolated maldevelopment of the trabecular meshwork. "It is the most common glaucoma of infancy, occurring in about 1 in 30,000 live births" [9]. *Iridotrabeculodysgenesis* and *(irido)corneotrabeculodysgenesis* refer to involvement of the iris, or of the iris *and* cornea, respectively, in the faulty development process. This classification has some bearing on prognosis, because the more ocular structures are involved, the worse the response to surgery. Isolated trabeculodysgenesis usually has the best surgical prognosis. Unfortunately, despite all these useful classification systems, most of us keep using the term *congenital glaucoma* to describe childhood glaucoma of any type, presenting at any age. Other terms such as *bupthalmos* (Greek for "ox eye") and *hydrophthalmia* are used less nowadays.

Summary for the Clinician

Terminology Used in Childhood Glaucomas

- *Congenital:* Presentation at birth or soon thereafter
- *Infantile:* Presentation within the first 2 years of life
- *Juvenile:* Presentation between 4 years and teen age
- *Developmental:* Glaucoma arising from maldevelopment of ocular structures
- *Primary:* Glaucoma not associated with ocular or systemic abnormalities
- *Secondary:* Glaucoma associated with ocular or systemic abnormalities

Summary for the Clinician

Anatomic (Hoskins) Classification of Childhood Glaucomas

- *Trabeculodysgenesis:* Isolated maldevelopment of the trabecular meshwork
- *Iridotrabeculodysgenesis:* Involvement of the iris (in addition to the trabecular meshwork) in the maldevelopment process.
- *(Irido)corneotrabeculodysgenesis:* Involvement of the iris as well as the cornea (in addition to the trabecular meshwork) in the maldevelopment process

For a more thorough discussion of issues such as epidemiology, pathophysiology, nomenclature, and classification, the reader is referred to some excellent reviews and textbook chapters that have been written over the years [9, 10, 11, 16, 18].

7.2
Patient Evaluation

7.2.1
Clinical Features

As mentioned earlier, the diagnosis of childhood glaucoma is made mostly on clinical grounds. Proper clinical examination is mandatory, which in infants and uncooperative children necessitates some form of sedation, or even general anesthesia. Nevertheless, a lot can be learned by simple inspection, even without approaching the (usually uncooperative) infant. There is usually a typical triad of corneal enlargement and often clouding, photophobia, and hyperlacrimation (Fig. 7.1).

7.2.2
Examination Under Sedation

Quite often it is possible to examine younger infants without any sedation. For pressure measurement, Quigley [31] and Jaafar [16] recommend the use of the pneumatonograph, because its small tip obviates forceful lid retraction or the need for a speculum, and because it can avoid scarred areas of the cornea [16]. Other tonometers that can be useful include the Schiotz tonometer, the Perkins hand-held applanation tonometer (Kowa Corp. Japan), and the Tonopen (Mentor Corp., Ca.) [11]. I, personally, would use the Schiotz tonometer *only* if no other type is available. Sedation with oral chloral hydrate, in my own experience and according to Jaafar and Kazi [17], provides the closest

Fig. 7.1. A Clinical example of unilateral left congenital glaucoma with corneal enlargement and clouding. **B,C** More advanced cases of corneal scarring, obscuring intraocular details

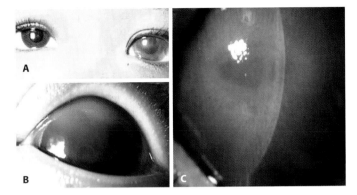

situation to natural sleep, and hence has the least influence on the true pressure level. Previously, ketamine sedation had been advocated [31], but this required the direct supervision of an anesthesiologist in the operating room. On the other hand, chloral hydrate can be easily administered in the clinic, with monitoring by the clinic nurse. The recommended dose ranges from 25–50 mg/kg body weight [11] up to 100 mg/kg for the first 10 kg, then 50 mg/kg for every additional kilogram [16]. It is important to have the child fasting for several hours before administering the sedative, and to monitor vital signs while the child is asleep. Ideally, there should be a special room equipped with the necessary monitoring equipment and supervised by a full-time nurse, who ensures the safety of the babies while they are under sedation. Under chloral hydrate sedation, the examiner can easily measure the pressure, examine the anterior segment, do retinoscopy, and examine the fundus. Sedation may also be deep enough to allow other tests, such as photography, gonioscopy, and ultrasound examination. Following sedation, it is imperative to instruct the parents to maintain an open airway and take special precautions against aspiration in case the child vomits. It is best to have the child lie on his/her side with the neck slightly extended. Food and drink should under no circumstances be resumed before the child is fully awake.

> ### Summary for the Clinician
>
> **Guidelines for Chloral Hydrate Sedation**
> - Suitable for patients between 6 months and 2 years of age
> - Patient must be fasting for at least 3–4 h before receiving oral sedation
> - Patient must be free from any febrile or other illnesses
> - Dosage: 25–50mg, up to 100 mg/kg body weight for the first 10 kg, then 50 mg/kg for additional weight
> - Vital signs must be monitored carefully during sleep. Food and drink must be withheld until infant is fully awake

7.2.3
Examination Under Anesthesia (EUA)

Children between 2 and 5 years of age are usually uncooperative for an office examination, yet too old for chloral hydrate sedation. General anesthesia becomes mandatory in such cases. Ketamine may be sufficient for examination, though it causes a slight rise in intraocular pressure (IOP), but is usually not suitable for surgery [11, 12]. Most inhalation general anesthetics lower IOP significantly, and hence pressure readings obtained under general anesthesia cannot be used reliably [11, 12, 16]. However, several other parameters can be assessed with great accuracy while the child is anesthetized, such as measurement of the corneal diameter, evaluation of corneal clarity, retinoscopy, gonioscopy, fundus examination,

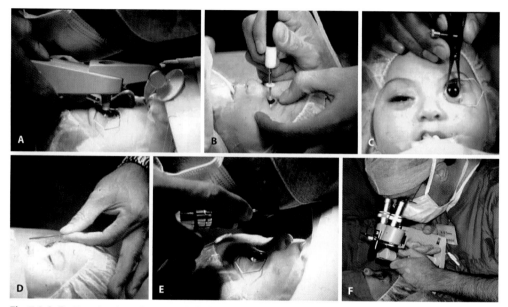

Fig. 7.2 A–F. Examination of a congenital glaucoma patient under general anesthesia: Perkins tonometry (**A**); pneumatonometry (**B**); measurement of corneal diameter (**C**); retinoscopy (**D**); disc examination using the direct ophthalmoscope (**E**); biomicroscopy using the portable slit lamp (**F**)

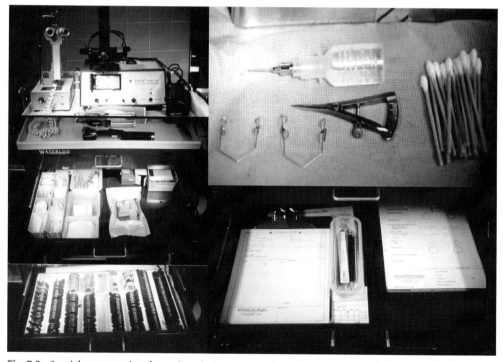

Fig. 7.3. Special cart carrying the various instruments and supplies that are needed for examination under anesthesia

and photography [9, 11, 16, 31] (Fig. 7.2). Axial length measurement by ultrasound may provide some additional information, but it is not an absolute necessity according to Dickens and Hoskins [11]. On the other hand, Dietlein et al. [12] report that an axial length of 24 mm or more is associated with poor surgical success (see Sect. 7.4.4 below). It is very helpful to have a special cart in the operating room containing all the necessary equipment and supplies used in the examination (Fig. 7.3). The cart can thus be wheeled to the room where it is needed. The reader is referred to the excellent description of the examination process by DeLuise and Anderson [9] and by Jaafar [16].

7.2.4
Special Diagnostic Tests

In the presence of a portable fundus camera, disc photography may be helpful in the follow-up of congenital glaucoma patients. Following the growth of the globe by periodic echographic axial length measurements may also be useful [25], though some find repeated cycloplegic refractions [16], or measurement of the corneal diameter [11], simpler, more practical, and even more revealing than ultrasound.

7.3
Medical Management

7.3.1
Indications

The role of medical treatment in childhood glaucomas is limited. There is little justification for keeping an infant or child on life-long medical treatment, in the presence of viable surgical alternatives, particularly when we know that children's response to and compliance with medical treatment are not the best. Given the long life expectancy of a child, it is unacceptable to expose him/her to the side effects of treatment, let alone the prohibitive cost and negative impact on quality of life. However, medical treatment is often needed to lower IOP preoperatively. In addition to its obvious benefits of pre-

venting optic nerve damage and of reducing the risks of sudden decompression of a globe with high IOP, medical treatment can also help clear the cornea for better visualization during diagnostic examination and goniotomy [11]. Long-term medical treatment may be justified in cases where glaucoma procedures fail repeatedly, so that any additional procedures become unlikely to control IOP, and even carry high morbidity.

7.3.2
Efficacy and Safety

Miotics are ineffective in childhood glaucomas in general [22], and their unpleasant side effects can be quite intense in this particular age group. It may be useful, however, to use pilocarpine immediately before surgery, whether goniotomy, trabeculotomy, or trabeculectomy. This keeps the iris taught and decreases the likelihood of its prolapse through the surgical incision. Pilocarpine has also been used for several weeks following 360° trabeculotomy [24] to have the iris pull on the opened area, and hopefully keep it open and functional by the time angle tissues heal. Adrenergic agents are hardly used at all nowadays (even in adults), and, of course, they can also produce serious systemic and local side effects. Beta-blockers are probably the most popular first-choice agents, but in infants, they have to be used with caution; apnea has been reported [30]. Conceivably, the newer gel-forming preparations may be safer insofar as they minimize systemic absorption. If there is any risk of asthma, betaxolol may be the better choice. Alpha-2 adrenergic agonists, such as brimonidine, are absolutely contraindicated in very young infants, because they may cause serious, and even fatal central nervous system depression [7]. Topical carbonic anhydrase inhibitors (CAI) and prostaglandin analogs are probably the safest preparations in infants. It is still not fully known how effective the latter compounds are in the very young age group. Acetazolamide may be used immediately before or after surgery (as an oral suspension, 5–10 mg/kg body weight every 6–8 h [9, 11, 16]), but there is little justification for its long-term usage [22], except in very rare situations: persistent pressure elevation despite multiple glaucoma procedures and maximal topical therapy. However, such treatment regimens should be limited to the older child, with careful, periodic monitoring of serum electrolytes and blood counts. Even though topical CAIs are safer than the systemic preparations for long-term usage, the latter are still more effective and especially useful for preoperative IOP lowering.

Summary for the Clinician

Medical Treatment Guidelines
- *Miotics:* Generally of little benefit
- *Beta blockers:* May cause apnea in infants, in addition to their known respiratory, cardiac, and other side effects
- *Alpha-2 adrenergic agonists:* Can cause fatal central nervous system depression in small infants, and hence perhaps are better avoided altogether in children
- *Systemic CAIs:* Indicated primarily for IOP lowering immediately before surgery. Dosage: 5–10 mg/kg body weight every 6–8 h, as oral suspension or intravenously
- *Topical CAIs and prostaglandin analogues:* Probably less risky than other preparations, but their very long-term efficacy and safety remains to be determined

7.4
Surgical Management

The treatment of glaucoma in infancy and childhood is surgical par excellence. Incision of the anomalous or maldeveloped angle can be achieved either from inside, under direct visualization (goniotomy), or from outside (trabeculotomy ab externum), the latter approach usually being reserved for cases with cloudy corneas. The success rate of either procedure, as far as IOP control, is generally high, in the 80%–90% range [9, 11, 16]. Success depends on the age of onset, the extent of involvement of ocular tissues by the congenital anomaly, and the amount of globe distortion and stretching. Cases that have the best surgical prognosis are those with isolated trabeculodysgenesis, with the disease appearing at between 1 and 12 months of age,

and with corneal diameters less than 14 mm [2, 16, 31]. A good review of the literature in this respect has been presented by DeLuise and Anderson [9]. Trabeculectomy may be another option, but is usually less desirable as a first line procedure. In my own opinion, there is little justification for the general ophthalmologist to resort to trabeculectomy as a first procedure in cases of primary congenital glaucoma (especially newborns and infants), simply because he/she has no experience with goniotomy or trabeculotomy. The treating ophthalmologist must not feel embarrassed referring such cases to the glaucoma specialist or pediatric ophthalmologist. Even in the hands of experienced glaucoma surgeons, the distorted anatomical relationships in buphthalmic globes render trabeculectomy technically demanding and fraught with intra- and postoperative complications. Moreover, the postoperative management of trabeculectomy in children, and more so in infants, can be very difficult. In the uncooperative child, maneuvers and procedures such as ocular massage, manual suture release or laser suture lysis, repeated postoperative 5-fluorouracil (5-FU) injections, and bleb needling may be difficult if not impossible.

7.4.1
Goniotomy

Goniotomy has long been advocated as the procedure of choice for congenital glaucoma, and is especially highly successful in cases presenting at between 1 and 24 months of age [11]. It is beyond the scope of this chapter to go into the extensive literature describing and discussing the procedure. I have chosen a few of the pertinent publications for the reader who is interested in more details [9–11, 16].

I would only like to make a few comments, mostly based on personal experience. Goniotomy may seem like a "simple procedure" to the general ophthalmologist. It is not. Goniotomy is not a procedure for the casual glaucoma surgeon [11]. In inexperienced hands, the results can be catastrophic. Injury to the iris or to the crystalline lens can easily occur if one is not familiar with working under gonioscopic control.

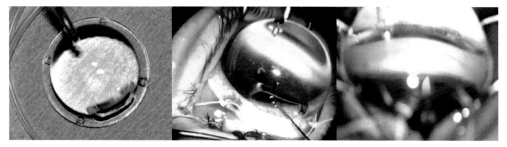

Fig. 7.4. Goniotomy under viscoelastic, using the *Worst* goniotomy lens with built-in irrigation and scleral fixation holes

This is why I nowadays insist on filling the anterior chamber with viscoelastic before introducing the knife. Such practice is especially useful for the surgeon beginning a fellowship training program. (I stress *fellowship* because, in my opinion, with the exception of *experienced* glaucoma surgeons or pediatric ophthalmologists, only glaucoma and pediatric ophthalmology fellows, and *not residents*, should be allowed to do cases of childhood glaucoma.) Another important point pertaining to goniotomy is that one must not insist on goniotomy if the cornea is not clear enough for proper visualization of the angle intraoperatively. Certain measures have been advocated to improve visualization through the cloudy cornea, such as the preoperative administration of oral acetazolamide (up to 25 mg/kg body weight) [16], or scraping of the edematous corneal epithelium [11]. However, epithelial scraping has almost been abandoned nowadays, because the severe pain it causes postoperatively makes the child even less cooperative (MS Jaafar, personal communication). In my own opinion, the surgeon must be able to shift to trabeculotomy (see Sect. 7.4.2.1) if there is any doubt as to whether goniotomy can be performed safely. It is true that before the era of microsurgery and modern instrumentation surgeons used to perform goniotomy "blindly"; however, such practice should be strongly discouraged in this day and age. For similar reasons, the practice of goniopuncture is also not very desirable. Goniotomy may be repeated up to three times. Figure 7.4 illustrates the procedure of goniotomy.

In an attempt to find a safer goniotomy technique, we published a pilot study of neodymium:YAG laser goniotomy, comparing it to the classical knife goniotomy in paired eyes [33]. Our preliminary impression was that both types of incision were equally effective. However, a larger sample and longer follow-up would have been better for more meaningful conclusions. Nevertheless, the idea of being able to incise the angle without actually introducing a knife into the anterior chamber remains quite appealing and deserves further investigation.

Summary for the Clinician

Guidelines For Safe Goniotomy
- To be performed *only* by (or with the assistance of) experienced glaucoma surgeons or pediatric ophthalmologists
- A clear cornea and good visualization of the angle under the operating room microscope are mandatory
- Filling the anterior chamber with viscoelastic prior to introducing the goniotomy knife is *mandatory* to ensure safety and to minimize the chances of injury to vital structures. Prior miosis with pilocarpine and/or acetylcholine also helps protect the crystalline lens

7.4.2
Trabeculotomy

This procedure is especially useful for congenital glaucoma eyes with significant corneal clouding. Success rates between 73% and 100% have been reported [2, 25].

If the surgeon chooses to learn and master only one technique, then trabeculotomy should be the procedure of choice, as it can be done on all eyes, regardless of corneal clarity [22]. Quigley published a detailed description of the surgical steps in 1982 [31]. First of all, the conjunctival flap can be either limbus-based [16, 31] or fornix-based [22]. The latter is easier to fashion and handle, and allows better exposure intraoperatively. Like goniotomy, trabeculotomy should be performed *only* by *experienced* glaucoma surgeons or pediatric ophthalmologists. The surgeon must be perfectly familiar with the surgical anatomy of the corneoscleral limbus, which is often distorted in buphthalmic eyes, and must also be comfortable operating under high magnification, for easier identification of Schlemm's canal. *This is by far the most important step in trabeculotomy.* The procedure may be done with or without [22] dissecting a partial-thickness scleral flap. My own preference is to work under a flap, for two reasons. With part of the scleral thickness removed, identification of Schlemm's canal becomes easier, though great care must be taken in buphthalmic eyes with a thin sclera [16, 31]. The presence of a scleral flap is very useful in case there is inadvertent entry into the anterior chamber, in which case it is easy to convert to trabecu*lectomy*. Identifying Schlemm's canal is the key to the success of trabeculotomy. The first step is to make the proper radial cut across the roof of the canal. This requires high magnification, a steady *pair* of hands (one hand steadying the other), and a few little tips. A 30° super-sharp blade is ideal. The surface of the scleral bed is dried well and irrigation by the assistant is withheld. The initial cut across the canal roof must be made perpendicular to the surface in one, clean, superficial stroke. Additional cuts must be made exactly in the center of the first cut, deepening the level very gradually and gently. The surgeon himself holds a cellulose sponge to dry the site from time to time. Two signs herald the identification of the lumen: a very minimal and slow ooze of aqueous, and a change in the color and direction of scleral fibers. At this stage, tiny perpendicular cuts are made in the sides of the initial radial cut to create a cruciate opening. In order to verify the true course of the canal, a fine (5–0 or 6–0) nylon or polypropylene thread is passed through the lumen. The piece of thread must not have a sharp or barbed tip; this can be blunted easily by approaching it to a hot cautery tip. A fine forceps is used to hold the thread about 3 mm from its tip, and one hand should steady the other, to minimize any tremors. Once the thread tip passes easily into the lumen, it is threaded gently to follow the course of the canal, and pushed through as far as it will go *without any resistance*, usually up to three clock hours on either side of the entry site. Some surgeons may elect to verify the correct position of the thread with the help of intraoperative gonioscopy. (One technique involves threading a 6–0 Prolene suture along the whole circumference of the canal and retrieving it from the other end of the same opening; the two ends of the thread are then pulled simultaneously to open the whole 360° of the canal [24] (see Sect. 7.4.4 below). The surgeon may then proceed with the actual trabeculotomy using the trabeculotomes of his/her choice. As the trabeculotome is swept into the chamber, there should be minimal resistance and no visible pull on the iris root [22]. With experience, the surgeon learns to recognize the correct feeling as to when the amount of resistance is just right. If the trabeculotome is forced into the canal or swept forcefully into the chamber, serious complications can occur: Descemet's detachment, iris dialysis, ciliary body dialysis leading to hypotony, severe intraocular bleeding, and injury to the crystalline lens or vitreous face. After the first sweep, the chamber may be lost. It is therefore useful to inject an air bubble to deepen the chamber momentarily before introducing the trabeculotome in the other direction. Viscoelastic may also be used for the same purpose. Even after completing both sides of the trabeculotomy, it is a good idea to leave a large air bubble in the chamber. This is useful when the (usually uncooperative) child is examined the next day: the size and movement of the air bubble help in evaluating the chamber status, even from a distance, using a simple pen light. Like goniotomy, trabeculotomy may be repeated more than once. The procedure of trabeculotomy is illustrated in Fig. 7.5.

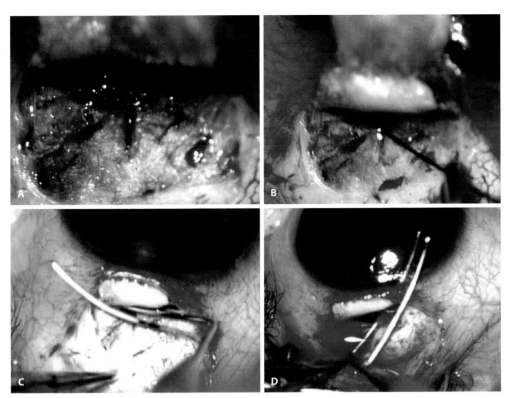

Fig. 7.5 A–D. Trabeculotomy steps: radial incision over Schlemm's canal (**A**); verification of the proper position of the canal using a nylon thread (**B**); left (**C**) and then right (**D**) trabeculotomy using the Harms trabeculotomes

Summary for the Clinician

Guidelines For Safe Trabeculotomy

- To be performed *only* by (or with the assistance of) experienced glaucoma surgeons or pediatric ophthalmologists
- A scleral flap is desirable in the event of conversion to trabeculectomy
- The location of Schlemm's canal must be verified using a nylon thread (5–0 or 6–0) before introducing the trabeculotome
- Forceful entry with the trabeculotome may end up in cyclodialysis, iris dialysis, or Descemet's detachment
- May be performed with or without viscoelastic

7.4.3
Trabeculectomy

Trabeculectomy is a viable alternative to goniotomy and trabeculotomy in childhood glaucomas. However, I believe that it should *not* be the first line of treatment, for more than one reason. The surgical anatomy in buphthalmic eyes is different from that in eyes with normal dimensions [12] (Fig. 7.6). Therefore, the scleral flap, for example, must be dissected at least 2 mm into clear cornea; otherwise, the trabecular opening will lie over the iris root, or even ciliary body, which increases the risk of bleeding and of injury to vital structures when doing the iridectomy. In buphthalmic eyes, it is not uncommon for vitreous to prolapse through posteriorly placed fistulas (as soon as the iris is cut) [12], which automatically dooms the procedure

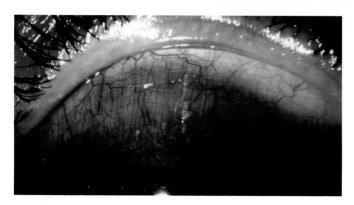

Fig. 7.6. Close-up view of the stretched limbus in a buphthalmic eye

to failure. As mentioned earlier, infants and young children are usually difficult to manage following trabeculectomy. Overfiltering blebs may need to be pressure-patched, and poor filtration may have to be managed by repeated massage, by laser suture lysis or manual release (in case of releasable sutures), and possibly by repeated 5-FU injections. All of these maneuvers are generally not tolerated by most children. In the long term, thin blebs may be especially vulnerable to infections in children, who are usually less attentive to hygiene in the course of their active daily life.

If trabeculectomy has to be performed on a child or infant, some important points and technical details need to be borne in mind. First of all, I recommend a limbus-based conjunctival flap whenever possible, mainly because secure closure can be achieved much easier than with a fornix-based flap. As mentioned earlier, dissection of the scleral flap needs to be carried well into clear cornea, and excision of the "trabecular" window should be strictly corneal. It is my own preference in all cases in general, and in children in particular, to pre-place at least two sutures across the corners of the scleral flap *before* excising the trabecular specimen. It is also essential to do a clear-cornea paracentesis before opening the chamber. One may elect to inject some viscoelastic at this stage. Great care must be exercised while catching and excising the iris. Children have tremendous positive vitreous pressure. As soon as the iridectomy is done, the preplaced sutures are tightened and tied. In children, I use multiple (4–6), *absorbable* sutures (such as 8-0, 9-0, or 10-0

Vicryl) to close the scleral flap really tight. It is also advisable to fill the chamber with viscoelastic after closure of the scleral flap. It is my experience that titration of scleral flap suture tightness by filling the chamber with balanced saline solution (BSS) through the paracentesis is not as useful as it is in adults. Despite all precautionary measures, such as tight flap closure and leaving viscoelastic in the chamber, this latter is usually found shallow or flat on the first postoperative day. Luckily, most shallow chambers in children form spontaneously with little or no intervention. I aim at having a deep chamber as of the first postoperative day, even if the bleb is absent and the pressure is slightly elevated.

With an intensive postoperative regimen of topical corticosteroid treatment, I expect a good filtering bleb to develop and the pressure to normalize with time, as the absorbable flap sutures loosen gradually. Bleb function is enhanced further if mitomycin C (MMC) is used. This highly toxic substance may have to be used in some children, especially those with history of previous ocular surgery. However, if not used carefully and judiciously, MMC is a double-edged sword that can result in serious side effects in the long run, such as hypotony, bleb leaks, and bleb-related infections. When using antimetabolites, meticulous conjunctival closure is a must. My preference is for a two-layer closure technique, Tenon's layer first with a simple running type of closure, followed by running mattress, or "purse string", closure of the conjunctiva (Fig. 7.7). Monofilament 10-0 Vicryl on a round needle is my suture of choice.

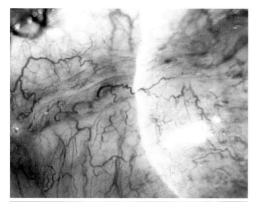

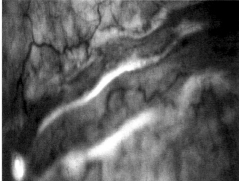

Fig. 7.7. Limbus-based conjunctival flap closed using the running mattress technique. Note the absence of exposed suture material and the water-tight closure

Azuara-Blanco et al. [5] reported their experience with filtration procedures plus MMC (0.4 mg/ml for 1–5 min) in patients who were 17 years or younger. Six patients had isolated trabeculodysgenesis and eight were aphakic. Almost 70 % of the phakic eyes had had glaucoma surgery before. Over a mean follow-up period of 18 months, "absolute success" (IOP <21 mmHg without medication or severe complications, and with a stable clinical picture) was achieved in nearly 77 % of the phakic eyes, but in *none* of the aphakics. Success was not influenced by age. My own experience with filtering procedures in aphakic eyes (even in adults) has been equally frustrating. Even with a thorough anterior vitrectomy, and with an intensive regimen of MMC intraoperatively *plus* 5-FU postoperatively, trabeculectomy in an aphakic eye is doomed to failure. With very rare exceptions, my procedure of choice in all aphakic eyes is implantation of a glaucoma drainage device, without even considering trabeculectomy. If an aphakic eye is not suitable for tube implantation (and especially if the visual potential is poor), then I (reluctantly) resort to cyclodestruction.

In their review of 29 eyes of patients under 18 years of age, who underwent trabeculectomy with MMC (0.5 mg/ml concentration for 1.5–5 min), Sidoti et al. [34] reported a success rate (IOP between 5 and 21 mmHg) of 82 % at 1 year, with the probability dropping to 59 % at 2 and 3 years. They found no difference in success or complications between cases of primary infantile glaucoma and those with secondary glaucoma. In all, 17 % of the cases developed bleb-related infections ("blebitis" in three patients and bleb-related endophthalmitis in two). By life-table analysis, the risk of bleb-related infections increased from 4 % at 1 year to 37 % at 3 years.

Summary for the Clinician

Guidelines for Safe Trabeculectomy
- Limbus-based conjunctival flap allows safer closure in children
- Scleral flap must be dissected 1–2 mm into clear cornea
- At least two scleral flap sutures must be pre-placed to ensure quick closure
- Iridectomy must not be too basal
- Scleral flap must be closed rather tightly, using several, absorbable sutures (8–0, 9–0, or 10–0 Vicryl, or equivalent)
- The anterior chamber must be filled with viscoelastic at the end
- Antifibrotics do enhance filtration in young eyes, especially in re-operations. Although MMC is more effective and practical (than repeated 5-FU injections in uncooperative children), it still predisposes to hypotony and late bleb infections

7.4.4
Goniotomy versus Trabeculotomy versus Trabeculectomy versus Other Procedures

What is the best procedure for childhood glaucoma? The literature is full of articles describing the results of goniotomy and of trabeculotomy, or comparing the two procedures. Some have

Table 7.1. Overview of success rates of some of the childhood glaucoma procedures as reported in the literature

Reference	Surgical procedure	Success rate (%)
[32]	Goniotomy	92
[2]	Trabeculotomy	88
[31]	Trabeculotomy	80
[15]	Trabeculectomy	72
	Trabeculotomy + -ectomy	94
[1]	Trabeculectomy +MMC	39
	Trabeculotomy + -ectomy + MMC	57
[5]	Trabeculectomy + MMC	77
[12]	Trabeculotomy	53
	Trabeculectomy	48
	Trabeculotomy + -ectomy	58
[28]	Trabeculotomy + trabeculectomy	78
[24]	360° trabeculotomy	92
	Goniotomy	58
[25]	Trabeculotomy	93
[34]	Trabeculectomy + MMC	59
[23]	Trabeculotomy + trabeculectomy	72
[21]	Deep sclerectomy	00
[13]	Ahmed valve	64
[26]	Ahmed valve	73
[35]	Cyclocryotherapy	44
[19]	Diode laser cyclophotocoagulation	72
[4]	Diode laser cyclophotocoagulation	79

found no major differences, whereas others favor trabeculotomy over goniotomy [22]. Unfortunately, it is not possible to go into the details of such comparative studies within the scope of this chapter. The reader is referred to the reviews by DeLuise and Anderson [9] and by Jaafar [16]. Table 7.1 lists some of the reported success rates of various procedures in childhood glaucoma.

As mentioned earlier, if the glaucoma specialist were to choose only one technique and master it well, it should be trabeculotomy. This procedure can be performed on all eyes, regardless of corneal clarity [22]. In my opinion, both procedures are preferable to trabeculectomy, insofar as they address the specific anatomic abnormality that underlies congenital glaucoma, namely trabeculodysgenesis. Moreover, both procedures, unlike trabeculectomy, do not carry the risk of significant chamber shallowing postoperatively.

Mendicino et al. [24] compared their technique of 360° trabeculotomy (using a 6–0 Prolene thread) done on 24 eyes, with standard goniotomy done on 40 eyes. All eyes had primary congenital glaucoma, and all procedures were done below 1 year of age. The trabeculotomy group was followed up for a mean of 4 years and the goniotomy group for 9 years. The rate of success (IOP <22 mmHg with or without medications; no progression of nerve damage; no additional surgery) was significantly higher (92%) in the trabeculotomy group than with goniotomy (57.7 %). Also, good vision (20/50 or better) was achieved in a significantly higher percentage (79.2 %) of eyes after trabeculotomy than after goniotomy (52.5%). The authors argue that opening the whole circumference of the angle obviates the need for multiple procedures, as may be required in the case of goniotomy or standard trabeculotomy.

The combination of trabeculotomy and trabeculectomy has been described [15, 23, 25, 28]. Elder [15] reported a 93.5 % cumulative chance of success of such a combination, after 24 months, as compared to 72% for trabeculectomy alone. In their retrospective review of 100 eyes (95 of which had corneal opacification), Mullaney et al. [28] reported 78% success (IOP <21 mmHg) of "combined" surgery in eyes that did not have any associated anterior segment abnormalities, as opposed to only 45% in eyes with anomalies such as ectropion uveae, Peter's, or aniridia. A total of 87% of all eyes received MMC intraoperatively. Al-Hazmi et al. [1] published a review of 254 eyes of 180 pediatric patients (up to 7 years of age) who had undergone either trabeculectomy (150 eyes) or combined trabeculotomy-trabeculectomy (104 eyes). The combined procedure was done only in infants up to 2 years of age. Almost all patients had primary congenital glaucoma, and all received intraoperative MMC (0.2 mg/ml or 0.4 mg/ml for 2–5 min). The success (IOP <21 mmHg) rate in infants who were less than 6 months old was 48%, and between 49 months and 84 months was 85%. The younger patients (<6 months) also needed more additional medications (40%) or surgery (60%), whereas above the age of 4 years, only 15% required additional treatment. The combined procedure was slightly more successful (57%) than trabeculectomy alone (39%) in infants less than 2 years old. Bleb-related complication rates were significantly higher in the older age groups. Dietlein et al. [12] found that trabeculotomy, trabeculectomy, and combined trabeculotomy-trabeculectomy seemed to be equally successful in primary congenital glaucoma. However, they noted that a patient age below 3 months and an axial length of 24 mm or more were two significant risk factors for surgical failure, regardless of the type of "ab externo" procedure chosen. Corneal diameter was not a significant factor in this particular study. On the other hand, Mandal et al. [23] in 2003 reported a 71.7 % 3-year survival rate for successful IOP control by combined trabeculotomy-trabeculectomy, in 47 eyes of infants who were less than 1 month old.

Nonpenetrating procedures are supposed to also be safe and effective in childhood glaucomas, but can be technically demanding in buphthalmic eyes, owing to the extreme thinness of the corneoscleral wall. Lüke et al. in 2002 [21] warned against a significant risk profile in eyes with refractory congenital glaucoma that underwent deep sclerectomy. In their review of ten eyes with a history of previous glaucoma surgery, they described a number of intraoperative difficulties and postoperative complications associated with deep sclerectomy. Difficulty in identifying Schlemm's canal, choroidal deroofing, and perforation of the "trabeculodescemetic membrane" were among the intraoperative problems. Spontaneously resolving hyphema occurred in 40% of the cases, and retinal detachment in one case.

Summary for the Clinician

- Goniotomy and trabeculotomy seem equally effective
- 360° Trabeculotomy with Prolene suture seems to achieve better IOP and vision
- Combination of trabeculotomy and trabeculectomy reported more effective than either procedure alone
- Nonpenetrating procedures technically demanding and may be risky in children

7.4.5
Glaucoma Drainage Implants

This type of surgery is reserved for cases of childhood glaucoma where conventional procedures fail. There are several types of glaucoma drainage implants (GDI). It is not the intention of this chapter to discuss which implant is better, nor to go into technical details. Let us just consider some aspects of GDI implantation that are specific to congenital glaucoma eyes. First of all, one is implanting an artificial device that is going to remain in the eye of an individual with a long life expectancy. What is going to become of this "foreign body," and what are its long-term effects on ocular tissues? It is difficult to prevent a child from rubbing his/her eye after surgery, which may predispose to corneal decompensation, if not erosion or extrusion of the implant. It has been my experience that the incidence of tube-cornea touch is high in buphthalmic eyes. I attribute that to the fact that the tube, which runs along a relatively flattened scleral surface (because of globe elongation), ends up with its tip pointing anteriorly and touching the cornea, no matter how much one tries to insert it away from the cornea, closer to the iris (Fig. 7.8). The same observation has been made by Djodeyre et al. [13], who describe an "elastic recoil that occurs when the intraocular pressure is normalized," causing the tube tip to rotate forward around the scleral spur. Therefore, one has to seriously consider the alternative procedures before choosing GDI surgery in very young children. We have reported on the use of the Molteno implant in childhood glaucoma, with a 68% success rate over a 3-year follow-up period [29]. Eid et al. [14] reported a limited success rate, high complication rate, and frequent surgical revisions of tube surgery in childhood glaucoma. The implants used in that review were all without valves. The valved implants that are available nowadays, the best example being the Ahmed implant, are supposed to be safer. The unidirectional valve mechanism opens at a specific pressure (around 8 mmHg), which minimizes the chances of hypotony and its sequelae [13]. Djodeyre et al. [13] reported a 64% cumulative probability of success by 2 years, in 35 eyes of patients younger than 15 years of age, treated with Ahmed valve implantation. About 25% of the cases had chamber shallowing, with or without choroidal detachment, and a similar number had malposition of the implant. Factors that seemed to influence the time to failure were diagnosis (of *congenital* glaucoma), number of previous glaucoma procedures, and surgeon's experience. In a report that has just been published (June 2003), Morad et al. [26] reviewed 60 eyes with pediatric glaucoma that had been treated with Ahmed valve implantation and followed for a mean of about 24 months. Pressure control (<21 mmHg) was achieved in 73% of the cases (but only 18.3% *without* medications), with a significant reduction in mean IOP and in the number of medications. Complications (mostly reversible) occurred in 50% of the cases, and four eyes ended up with severe visual loss. There was a significant association between tube exposure and uveitis. The probability of success (with or without medical treatment) decreased from 93% at 1 year to 45% at 4 years. Success did not seem to be influenced by age, specific diagnosis, or prior surgery.

In my own experience, it is not advisable (even in adult eyes) to insert the tube only under a scleral flap. This latter on its own is rarely sufficient to prevent tube erosion. Moreover, with only a thin scleral bed remaining, there will be greater chances of leakage around the entry site and of the tube tip moving forward closer to the cornea. My routine in all eyes is to pass the tube into the chamber through a relatively long tunnel, made with a 23-gauge hypodermic needle, and then to cover the tube with a patch graft of preserved donor sclera. This seems to greatly minimize tube erosion.

Summary for the Clinician

- Valved glaucoma drainage implants safer than non-valved
- Tube-cornea touch common due to globe elongation
- Patch graft of sclera (or equivalent) minimizes tube extrusion

7.4.6
Cyclodestructive Procedures

Cyclodestruction is probably the least desirable option in childhood glaucoma. Again, such procedures are resorted to only if all others fail. Cyclocryotherapy (CCT) has been the classical standard procedure. The main drawback of cyclodestruction, in general, is the difficulty of its titration, the inherent risk of loss of useful vision, and the risk of phthisis bulbi. It is highly advisable to localize the correct position of the ciliary body band by transillumination for more effective treatment, and to leave at least one quadrant untreated in order to reduce the risk of phthisis [16]. Wagle et al. [35] reported their experience with CCT in 64 eyes with refractory pediatric glaucoma. With a mean number of treatment sessions of four, success (IOP

<21 mmHg without additional surgery or complications) at 6 months was achieved in 66% of the cases, declining to 44% after about 5 years. Phthisis occurred in five eyes and retinal detachment in another five. The risk of phthisis was significantly higher in aniridic eyes.

With the advent of contact diode laser treatment, the morbidity of cyclodestruction seems to have decreased, although this technique is not as effective in young eyes [19]. Kirwan et al. [19] reported the results of diode laser cyclophotocoagulation (cyclodiode) in 77 eyes with refractory glaucoma in patients below 17 years of age. In all, 60% were aphakic, 35% had congenital glaucoma, and 64% had undergone previous surgery. Over half the eyes treated required more than one (up to eight) treatment sessions. With multiple sessions, 72% of the eyes were controlled (IOP reduction below 22 mmHg or by 30%) at 1 year, and 51% after 2 years. Aphakic eyes were found to achieve more sustained IOP reduction after the first treatment session. Also patients older than 5 years had a more sustained effect compared to the younger ones. Three of the aphakic eyes, two of which had undergone YAG laser cycloablation, developed retinal detachment and phthisis. A severe inflammatory reaction was seen in 6.2% of the treatment sessions. Autrata and Rehurek [4] in 2003 reported 41% success at 1 year with one session of transscleral cyclodiode treatment, and 79% with two sessions, in 69 eyes with refractory pediatric glaucoma. Complications (choroidal or retinal detachment) were low and occurred only in aphakic eyes.

Summary for the Clinician

- Cyclodestruction reserved for end-stage cases where other procedures fail repeatedly
- CCT still viable option but traumatic to the eye
- Aggressive treatment (more than 270° or multiple sessions) carries high risk of phthisis
- Diode laser seems more predictable and less destructive than cryo
- Young eyes respond less to laser than adults; repeated sessions may be required for IOP control

7.5
Postoperative Management

7.5.1
Periodic Clinical Examination

The first EUS is performed within the first 2 weeks after surgery. Thereafter, periodic examinations are scheduled in 4–6 weeks, then 3–4 months, and ultimately every 6 months to 1 year. Needless to say, much depends on how stable the clinical findings are. Recurrence of high IOP usually occurs within the first 6–12 months postoperatively [16]. Other than pressure measurement, the examiner must inspect the cornea for size and clarity, the optic nerve, with occasional photographic documentation if available, and monitor any changes in refraction. Periodic axial length measurements and B-scans in eyes with cloudy media may provide some additional useful information. It is helpful to tabulate all clinical findings for every examination using special forms. This has been illustrated very nicely by Jaafar [16].

Summary for the Clinician

- EUS 2 weeks postoperatively, then at 6 weeks, 3 months, and 6 months
- Recurrence of high IOP usually within 6–12 months
- IOP, corneal diameter, refraction, disc, and axial length are main parameters monitored during follow-up

7.5.2
Management of Amblyopia

Successful pressure control in congenital glaucoma is only half the job. Almost invariably all affected eyes require some form of visual rehabilitation, which involves addressing media opacities (usually corneal) and treating amblyopia. The latter can be deprivational and/or anisometropic, and a wide range of success rates of its treatment has been reported [6, 8, 9, 20, 27, 32]. It has long been recognized that a good proportion of eyes end up with poor vision despite adequate surgical IOP control and in the absence of optic nerve damage [32]. Over 35 years ago Richardson et al. [32] emphasized the role of anisometropia as a major cause of poor visual function in these eyes. Biglan and Hiles [6] reported success of occlusion therapy in six out of 12 eyes, observing that patients with five or more diopters of astigmatism "did not respond to optical and/or occlusion therapy". Only seven out of the total of 44 eyes studied had poor vision due to anatomical defects, and the rest due to large refractive errors or amblyopia. Kushner [20] reported successful amblyopia treatment in 10 out of 12 patients; the two failures were attributed to "extensive tears in Descemet's membrane." The axial myopia that results from globe elongation can be corrected using spectacles (or contact lenses where applicable), with aggressive treatment of amblyopia. Tears in Descemet's membrane may cause irregular astigmatism or corneal clouding, and deprivation amblyopia has been known to set in even after brief periods of corneal clouding [11]. Clothier et al. in 1979 [8] reported that corneal edema, anisometropia (especially with a difference of seven diopters or more), and strabismus, were the most important factors that contributed to the development of amblyopia. The authors also found that the end visual results were the same whether occlusion therapy was started in infancy or around the age of 2.5–3 years. Morin and Bryars in 1980 [27] reported that the main causes of visual loss in congenital glaucoma patients with controlled pressure were optic nerve damage, media opacities, and corneal opacities. "Anisometropic amblyopia was a relatively uncommon cause of poor vision" in their series (three out of the 76 bilateral cases, and three out of the 13 unilateral cases).

Media opacities are more difficult to handle. Irreversible corneal clouding (scarring) ideally requires penetrating keratoplasty (PKP). This procedure in children involves some serious obstacles, such as the difficulty of postoperative care of corneal grafts in children, the high rate of graft failure and rejection, and the presence of high astigmatism in the early postoperative period. This is not to mention the risk of recurrence of IOP elevation with repeated intraocu-

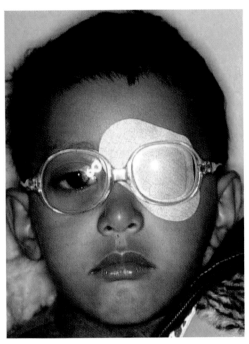

Fig. 7.8. The proper method of occlusion for treatment of amblyopia

lar surgery. Unfortunately, corneal grafting is not advisable before the age of 5 years, by which time deep amblyopia would have set in [16]. In 1994, Ariyasu et al. [3] reported that six out of nine corneal grafts (96%) performed in infants who were less than 2 years old remained clear over a mean follow-up period of 24 months. They were able to achieve ambulatory vision or better in 75% of the eyes with proper refraction and amblyopia treatment.

Despite the fact that cataract surgery in children nowadays has become much more refined than in the past, and even with the option of intraocular lens (IOL) implantation in some children, prevention of amblyopia in an aphakic or a pseudophakic infant is still quite a formidable task. The great significance of proper spectacle or contact lens correction and of occlusion therapy does not require re-emphasis (Fig. 7.8). As with all cases of amblyopia, successful treatment requires the utmost understanding and cooperation on the part of the parents.

7.5.3
Genetic Counseling

Finally, there is always an important role for genetic counseling [16, 18] and the field of congenital glaucoma genetics is an ever-expanding field; however, the scope of this chapter does not permit a more involved discussion of this aspect of childhood glaucomas.

Summary for the Clinician

- Amblyopia results from anisometropia, high astigmatism, and media opacities
- Refraction, occlusion therapy, and clearing of media opacities are important to restore and maintain vision after IOP control
- Corneal grafts are challenging in children because of difficult postoperative care, high astigmatism, and high rejection/failure rates
- Cataract surgery is equally challenging because of difficulty in visual rehabilitation (especially without IOL implants)
- Genetic counseling may help plan future pregnancies

7.6
Conclusions

Glaucoma in infants and children can present at birth or soon thereafter, or a little later in infancy or childhood. The underlying pathogenetic mechanism can range from isolated maldevelopment of the trabecular meshwork (*trabeculodysgenesis*), to involvement of iris tissue as well (*iridotrabeculodysgenesis*), to involvement of the cornea in addition to trabecular meshwork and iris (*irido-corneotrabeculodysgenesis*).

Childhood glaucoma may also be primary or secondary, depending on the absence or presence of associated ocular and/or systemic abnormalities. Cases that have the best surgical prognosis are those with primary trabeculodysgenesis that present *after* birth, at between 1 and 12 months of age and that do not have any undue corneal enlargement or globe stretching (buphthalmos).

Medical treatment in childhood glaucoma may be required in preparation for surgery or in cases where multiple surgical procedures fail to achieve adequate IOP control. Some glaucoma medications that are normally safe and effective in adult patients may not work very well for children, and may even cause very morbid systemic side effects. Miotics and adrenergic agents are not very effective and usually have annoying local and systemic side effects. Topical beta blockers have been associated with apnea in infants, and alpha-2 adrenergic agonists with severe central nervous system depression, coma, and even death. There is little justification for life-long treatment with systemic CAI, especially with the availability of topical preparations. Prostaglandin analogs may have some role, though their *very long-term* effects in young patients have yet to be established.

Goniotomy and trabeculotomy are still the standard surgical procedures in primary congenital glaucoma. The presence of a clear cornea is essential for performing goniotomy safely, whereas trabeculotomy can be done on any eye. Both procedures require special expertise, and must *not* be done by the general ophthalmologist who has limited experience in this type of glaucoma surgery. The results and success rates of the two procedures are very similar. The combination of trabeculotomy with trabeculectomy has been advocated by some. The latter procedure also requires special precautions in buphthalmic eyes, and the postoperative care in children following trabeculectomy may not be easy. Antimetabolites, especially MMC, do have a definite role in improving the success of filtration, but the rate of infection of the thin mitomycin blebs in young individuals has been unacceptably high. Nonpenetrating procedures may be safer than standard filtration in children, but with the thin corneoscleral layer, the procedure becomes technically very demanding. Glaucoma drainage devices also have a definite beneficial role in the refractory pediatric glaucomas. Valved implants are much safer and easier to manage in children than the non-valved ones, insofar as they reduce the chances of hypotony, chamber shallowing, or choroidal effusion/hemorrhage. Special problems related to valves implanted in stretched globes include tube-cornea touch and frequent malposition, migration or erosion of the implant. Cyclodestructive procedures are resorted to when repeated surgical procedures and medical treatment fail. The relatively recently introduced diode laser cyclophotocoagulation seems to have better results and less morbidity than the classical cyclocryotherapy, though it is not very effective in young eyes, and repeated treatment is often necessary. With any technique of cyclodestruction, there are always the risks of visual loss and of phthisis bulbi.

After achieving satisfactory IOP control, the ophthalmologist is still faced with the difficult task of treating or preventing amblyopia in the involved eye. Irregular astigmatism, anisometropia, strabismus, and media opacities, all contribute to the problem. Penetrating keratoplasty in infants and young children has its own difficulties and limitations, owing to the difficult postoperative care and the high rejection and failure rates in the young age groups. Even with the refined cataract surgical techniques practiced nowadays (oftentimes with IOL implantation), there is still the equally important task of postoperative visual rehabilitation and prevention of amblyopia. Amblyopia management requires a serious team effort from all parties involved: the glaucoma surgeon, the pediatric ophthalmologist, the orthoptist, and most importantly, the parents. The latter may also benefit from genetic counseling in planning future pregnancies.

Acknowledgments. I am deeply grateful to my colleagues Drs. Mohamad Jaafar, Baha' Noureddin, and Jamal Bleik for their help in preparing this chapter.

References

1. Al Hazmi A, Zwaan J, Awad A et al. (1998) Effectiveness and complications of mitomycin C use during pediatric glaucoma surgery. Ophthalmology 105:1915–1920
2. Anderson DR (1983) Trabeculotomy compared to goniotomy for glaucoma in children. Ophthalmology 90:805–806
3. Ariyasu RG, Silverman J, Irvine JA (1994) Penetrating keratoplasty in infants with congenital glaucoma. Cornea 13:521–526
4. Autrata R, Rehurek J (2003) Long-term results of transscleral cyclophotocoagulation in refractory pediatric glaucoma patients. Ophthalmologica 217:393–400
5. Azuara-Blanco A, Wilson RP, Spaeth GL et al. (1999) Filtration procedures supplemented with mitomycin C in the management of childhood glaucoma. Br J Ophthalmol 83:151–156
6. Biglan AW, Hiles DA (1979) The visual results following infantile glaucoma surgery. J Pediatr Ophthalmol Strabismus 16:377–381
7. Carlsen JO, Zabriskie NA, Kwon YH et al. (1999) Apparent central nervous system depression in infants after the use of topical brimonidine. Am J Ophthalmol 128:255–256
8. Clothier CM, Rice NS, Dobinson P et al. (1979) Amblyopia in congenital glaucoma. Trans Ophthalmol Soc UK 99:427–431
9. DeLuise VP, Anderson DR (1983) Primary infantile glaucoma (congenital glaucoma). Surv Ophthalmol 28:1–19
10. Dickens CJ, Hoskins HD (1996) Epidemiology and pathophysiology of congenital glaucoma. In: Ritch R, Shields MB, Krupin T (eds) The glaucomas, 2nd edn. Mosby, St. Louis, pp 729–738
11. Dickens CJ, Hoskins HD (1996) Diagnosis and treatment of congenital glaucoma. In: Ritch R, Shields MB, Krupin T (eds) The glaucomas, 2nd edn. Mosby, St. Louis, pp 739–749
12. Dietlein TS, Jacobi PC, Krieglstein GK (1999) Prognosis of primary ab externo surgery for primary congenital glaucoma. Br J Ophthalmol 83:317–322
13. Djodeyre MR, Peralta Calvo J, Abelairas Gomez J (2001) Clinical evaluation and risk factors of time to failure of Ahmed Glaucoma Valve implant in pediatric patients. Ophthalmology 108:614–620
14. Eid TE, Katz LJ, Spaeth GL et al. (1997) Long-term effects of tube-shunt procedures on management of refractory childhood glaucoma. Ophthalmology 104:1011–1016
15. Elder MJ (1994) Combined trabeculotomy-trabeculectomy compared with primary trabeculectomy for congenital glaucoma. Br J Ophthalmol 78:745–748
16. Jaafar MS (1988) Care of the infantile glaucoma patient. In: Reinecke RD (ed) Ophthalmology Annual 1988. Raven, New York, pp 15–28
17. Jaafar MS, Kazi GA (1993) Effect of chloral hydrate sedation on intraocular pressure measurement. J Pediatr Ophthalmol Strabismus 30:372–376
18. Kipp MA (2003) Childhood glaucoma. Pediatr Clin North Am 50:89–104
19. Kirwan JF, Shah P, Khaw PT (2002) Diode laser cyclophotocoagulation. Role in the management of refractory pediatric glaucomas. Ophthalmology 109:316–323

20. Kushner BJ (1988) Successful treatment of functional amblyopia associated with juvenile glaucoma. Graefes Arch Clin Exp Ophthalmol 226:150–153

21. Lüke C, Dietlein TS, Jacobi PC et al. (2002) Risk profile of deep sclerectomy for treatment of refractory congenital glaucomas. Ophthalmology 109:1066–1071

22. Luntz MH (1984) The advantages of trabeculotomy over goniotomy. J Pediatr Ophthalmol 21:150–153

23. Mandal AK, Gothwal VK, Bagga H et al. (2003) Outcome of surgery on infants younger than 1 month with congenital glaucoma. Ophthalmology 110:1909–1915

24. Mendicino ME, Lynch MG, Drack A et al. (2000) Long-term surgical and visual outcomes in primary congenital glaucoma: 360 degrees trabeculotomy versus goniotomy. JAAPOS 4:205–210

25. Meyer G, Schwenn O, Pfeiffer N et al. (2000) Trabeculotomy in congenital glaucoma. Graefes Arch Clin Exp Ophthalmol 238:207–213

26. Morad Y, Donaldson CE, Kim YM et al. (2003) The Ahmed drainage implant in the treatment of pediatric glaucoma. Am J Ophthalmol 135:821–829

27. Morin JD, Bryars JH (1980) Causes of loss of vision in congenital glaucoma. Arch Ophthalmol 98:1575–1576

28. Mullaney PB, Selleck C, Al-Awad A et al. (1999) Combined trabeculotomy and trabeculectomy as an initial procedure in uncomplicated congenital glaucoma. Arch Ophthalmol 117:457–460

29. Muñoz M, Tomey KF, Traverso C et al. (1991) Clinical experience with the Molteno implant in advanced infantile glaucoma. J Pediatr Ophthalmol Strabismus 28:68–72

30. Olson RJ, Bromberg BB, Zimmerman TJ (1979) Apneic spells associated with timolol therapy in a neonate. Am J Ophthalmol 88:120–122

31. Quigley HA (1982) Childhood glaucoma; results with trabeculotomy and study of reversible cupping. Ophthalmology 89:219–226

32. Richardson KT, Ferguson WJ Jr, Shaffer RN (1967) Long-term functional results in infantile glaucoma. Trans Am Acad Ophthalmol Otolaryngol 71:833–836

33. Senft SH, Tomey KF, Traverso CE (1989) Neodymium-YAG laser goniotomy vs surgical goniotomy. A preliminary study in paired eyes. Arch Ophthalmol 107:1773–1776

34. Sidoti PA, Belmonte SJ, Liebmann JM et al. (2000) Trabeculectomy with mitomycin-C in the treatment of pediatric glaucomas. Ophthalmology 107:422–429

35. Wagle NS, Freedman SF, Buckley EG et al. (1998) Long-term outcome of cyclocryotherapy for refractory pediatric glaucoma. Ophthalmology 105:1921–1926

What Have We Learned
from the Major Glaucoma Clinical Trials?

8

J.D. BRANDT, M.R. WILSON

Core Messages

- Clinical trials minimize bias but are often so rigidly controlled that they do not reflect common medical practice
- The AGIS study sought to answer the question "which is better when medical therapy fails, laser trabeculoplasty or trabeculectomy?" It showed that lower pressures were more effective at preventing glaucoma progression
- The CNTGS showed that lowering intraocular pressure decreased the rate of progression of normal tension glaucoma although not all patients progressed
- The CIGTS study demonstrated that both medical therapy and trabeculectomy were equally effective at lowering pressure and preventing progression of visual field loss although surgery had an increased rate of cataract formation
- The OHTS study showed that lowering IOP by at least 20% decreased the rate of progression of ocular hypertension to open angle glaucoma and that thin corneas, higher IOP, larger cups and older age were risk factors for open angle glaucoma
- The EMGT study demonstrated that lowering intraocular pressure was more likely to prevent progression of open angle glaucoma than not lowering the IOP and that each mmHg lowering was associated with a 10% decrease in risk
- Randomized clinical trials have provided some basic answers about management of glaucoma but have been expensive

8.1
Introduction

Arguably, the most important aspect of clinical research is the inference that a detected association between a variable and an outcome represents a cause-and-effect relationship. For example, elevated intraocular pressure is often associated with glaucoma; but does intraocular pressure cause glaucoma? A clinical trial is an experiment, i.e., variables may be manipulated to test its effect on outcome, and as such, it is the clinical study design that provides the strongest causal inference.

A well designed clinical trial minimizes the potential for bias in the conduct of the study. With strict adherence to standardized protocols, multiple sites may be used to conduct a trial. An advantage of using multiple sites is that large sample sizes can be achieved, thus increasing statistical strength. This is particularly advantageous when the outcome of interest is rare or takes a long time to detect, such as in the case of glaucoma, wherein the outcome of interest is typically loss of vision.

Despite these advantages, there are also disadvantages to clinical trials that have raised the question as to whether the conduct of clinical trials represents the most effective use of resources to answer important clinical questions. Because clinical trials attempt to control for the influence of potentially confounding factors, the application of the intervention is rigidly prescribed with little room for flexibility. The intervention protocol may thus not represent what actually occurs in practice. A related issue is that many clinical trials are of long duration, partic-

Table 8.1. Characteristics of recent clinical trials

Study name	Number clinical centers	Number of subjects or eyes analyzed	Recruitment completed (month/year)	Funding source
Advanced Glaucoma Intervention Study (AGIS)	11	789	November 1992	NEI
Collaborative Normal Tension Glaucoma Study	24	145	September 1998	GRF
Collaborative Initial Glaucoma Treatment Study (CIGTS)	14	607	April 1997	NEI
Ocular Hypertension Treatment Study (OHTS)	22	1636	October 1996	NEI
Early Manifest Glaucoma Trial (EMGT)	1	225	April 1997	NEI

NEI, National Eye Institute, National Institutes of Health, Bethesda, MD; GRF, Glaucoma Research Foundation, San Francisco, CA.

ularly when the primary outcome is rare or takes a long time to detect. The intervention protocol may thus not reflect changes in clinical practice and the results may be outdated by the time the study is completed. Additionally, clinical trials, particularly multicenter clinical trials, are typically very expensive. For example, the most recent National Eye Institute (NEI)-sponsored glaucoma clinical trials cost (through 2001) $16.7 million for the Advanced Glaucoma Intervention Study (AGIS), $19.4 million for the Collaborative Initial Glaucoma Treatment Study (CIGTS), $29.7 million thus far for the Ocular Hypertension Treatment Study (OHTS), and $7.6 million for the Early Manifest Glaucoma Treatment Study (EMGTS) (personal communication, John Whitaker, Office of Program Planning & Analysis, National Eye Institute, Bethesda, MD). This translates to an annual cost per enrolled subject averaging $3,600 per year for the OHTS and $5,600 per year for the CIGTS. Whether such costs represent a good investment ultimately depends on the extent to which these studies impact clinical practice.

The ophthalmologist who has stayed up to date with the glaucoma literature might regard the ultimate findings of the studies described below as fairly obvious and even pre-ordained, and therefore might question whether spending such large sums of money was an appropriate use of taxpayer dollars. It is important to note, however, that when these large trials were first conceived in the 1980s, a dispassionate review of many of the "big questions" in glaucoma – Does lowering pressure really work? Does it make sense to treat patients with ocular hypertension? Does treating early glaucoma make a difference? – revealed a remarkable lack of solid evidence to support contemporary clinical practice [26]. As a result, health economists and policy makers were challenging the assumptions our profession was making in screening and treating glaucoma patients [5].

The past two decades will likely be considered as the high point for ophthalmic clinical trials. The National Eye Institute has played a pivotal role in the promotion and performance of prospective, randomized multi-center clinical trials during these decades and its influence in the field of glaucoma is particularly noteworthy. As shown in Table 8.1, the majority of the major glaucoma clinical trials performed have been NEI sponsored. Historically, the NEI has spent approximately 10% of its extramural budget on clinical research, mostly on clinical trials. Glaucoma clinical trials have been well represented, and comprised 24% of the NEI glaucoma program budget in 2001. Major clinical trials reporting significant results in the past several years are described below.

8.2
Advanced Glaucoma Intervention Study (AGIS)

The Advanced Glaucoma Intervention Study [8, 28–38] was a long-term study of the clinical course and prognosis of glaucoma inadequately controlled by medications alone. All eligible eyes had intraocular pressure considered to be too high for the status of the visual field or optic disc, and surgery was considered to be an appropriate next treatment step. Between April 1988 and November 1992, 789 eyes of 591 subjects were enrolled and randomly assigned to one of two treatment sequences: (1) argon laser trabeculoplasty (ALT), followed by trabeculectomy should ALT fail (ATT sequence), followed by another trabeculectomy should the first trabeculectomy fail, or (2) trabeculectomy, followed by ALT should trabeculectomy fail, followed by a second trabeculectomy should ALT fail (TAT se-

quence). During the study, the protocol was modified to allow for the use of adjunctive 5-fluorouracil and mitomycin-C with trabeculectomy for eyes at high risk of surgical failure [29].

Supplemental medications were used as deemed necessary. The same criteria used to determine study eligibility were used to determine failure of an intervention. Because of an emphasis on visual field progression as an outcome measure, a visual field scoring algorithm using the 24–2 threshold program of the Humphrey Field Analyzer was used. The AGIS visual field defect score is based on the number and depth of clusters of adjacent depressed test sites in the upper and lower hemifields and in the nasal area of the total deviation printout of the STATPAC-2 analysis. The score ranges from 0 (no defect) to 20 (all test sites deeply depressed). Three outcome-related papers have been published as of November, 2003.

Because elevated intraocular pressure may lead to progressive visual field deterioration, it

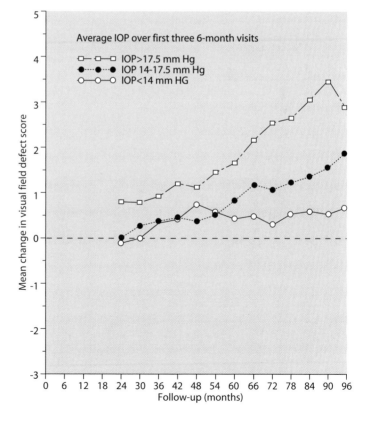

Fig. 8.1. Predictive analysis. Mean change from baseline in visual field defect score by intraocular pressure classified according to average value over the first three 6-month visits. (Reproduced from [37] with permission)

Average IOP over first three 6-month visits

□—□—□ IOP>17.5 mm Hg
●—●—● IOP 14-17.5 mm Hg
○—○—○ IOP<14 mm HG

had long been assumed that low intraocular pressure may have a protective role in visual field deterioration. A major contribution of AGIS has been the demonstration of an association of reduced progression of visual field defect with lower intraocular pressure [33]. In a predictive analysis based on IOPs during the first 18 months following randomization, eyes with average intraocular pressure greater than 17.5 mmHg had an estimated worsening during subsequent follow-up that was one unit of visual field defect score greater than eyes with average intraocular pressure less than 14 mmHg (Fig. 8.1). In an associative analysis of IOPs during *all* follow-up visits, eyes with 100 % of visits with intraocular pressure less than 18 mmHg over 6 years had mean changes from baseline in visual field defect score close to zero during follow-up, whereas eyes with less than 50 % of visits with intraocular pressure less than 18 mmHg had an estimated worsening over follow-up of

0.63 units of visual field score (Fig. 8.2). In both analyses, the difference in visual field worsening was greater at 7 years than at 2 years.

AGIS found that the efficacy of the two treatment sequences differed by race. Black patients experience less visual field loss whereas white patients experience more visual field loss with the ATT sequence. The results suggested that argon laser trabeculoplasty may be the preferred initial surgical treatment in black patients and trabeculectomy the preferred initial surgical treatment in white patients. No hypothesis for this race-specific treatment difference has been offered, and the clinical practice implication of this finding is, as yet, uncertain.

The AGIS participants represent some of the most closely studied patients undergoing either ALT or trabeculectomy. Analysis of pre- and peri-operative risk factors for failure of either procedure revealed that failure of either intervention was associated with younger age and

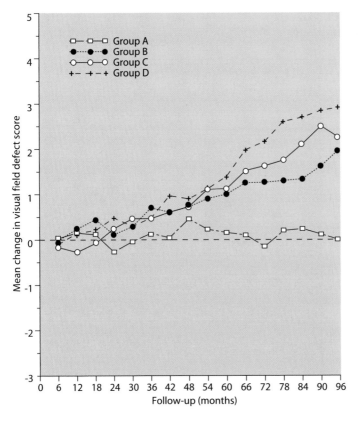

Fig. 8.2. Associative analysis. Mean change in visual field defect score by percent of visits over 6 years at which an eye presented with intraocular pressure less than 18 mmHg (group A is 100 %, group B is 75 % to less than 100 %, group C is 50 % to less than 75 %, and group D is 0 % to less than 50 %). (Reproduced from [37] with permission)

higher pre-intervention IOP; trabeculectomy failure was also associated with postoperative complications [37]. The results of 10-year follow-up are expected and will provide important information on the long-term clinical course and prognosis of advanced glaucoma. Additionally, AGIS should provide valuable information on the impact of surgical complications on vision outcomes and the effects of cataract surgery on the course of glaucoma.

Primary Study Question

- What is the best next step in a patient uncontrolled on medicines – laser trabeculoplasty or trabeculectomy?

Study Design

- Multi-center, prospective, randomized clinical trial.
- Patients randomly assigned to laser trabeculoplasty or trabeculectomy (without antimetabolite) as the first step in a prescribed sequence of interventions

Major Findings

- Efficacy of treatment effect varied by race (post-hoc analysis; see sidebar)
- Reduced progression of visual field defects associated with lower IOP

Use of Race and Ethnicity in Clinical Trials

Recent studies have reported differences in prevalence and cause of disease and in treatment response by racial and/or ethnic categories. However, racial and ethnic categorization is imprecise [39, 40]. There are no genetic alleles that define a unique population or race. On the other hand, the prevalence of certain alleles does vary among populations. There are estimated to be at least 15 million genetic polymorphisms. An undefined subgroup of these polymorphisms underlie variation in normal and disease traits and their frequency of occurrence may differ by racial and/or ethnic grouping. A lack of understanding of these can lead to substandard care in the affected racial or ethnic group. Yet, it is not possible for race, as we recognize it clinically, to provide both reasonable sensitivity and specificity for the presence of these genetic polymorphisms. Testing is the only way to be certain whether a patient has a particular polymorphism or not.

The use of single-nucleotide polymorphisms (SNP) creates an opportunity to scientifically determine the extent to which continental populations vary genetically. Though opinions differ, identifying these differences may have important implications for health. SNP is certainly more precise than race which is often left undefined in research studies. However, despite the advantages of its use, currently it is not practical for most clinical trials to collect SNP data.

At least for now, clinical trials will, and should, continue to collect race and ethnicity data. However, researchers must be clear about the choice and definition of terms and be careful about making inappropriate generalizations. In designing clinical trials, researchers should consider whether race is being collected as a proxy for genetic similarity (or diversity), or as a proxy for non-genetic factors such as socioeconomic status or both. It is important to collect data with as much precision as possible and to note how subjects were assigned to groups, such as on the basis of records, investigator-desig-nated, or self-assignment. To avoid post-hoc 'trolling' of databases, investigations that entail racial distinctions should begin with a plausible, clearly defined and testable hypothesis.

8.3 Collaborative Normal Tension Glaucoma Study (CNTGS)

The Collaborative Normal Tension Glaucoma Study [1, 4, 27] was designed to determine whether aggressive IOP lowering halts optic nerve damage or visual field loss in normal tension glaucoma and to assess the risks and side effects of aggressive treatment required to lower the IOP. Only one eye of each eligible patient was enrolled. All eyes had typical glaucoma-tous visual field and optic nerve changes and untreated IOPs were less than or equal to 24 mmHg with nine of ten readings being less than or equal to 21 mmHg.

One eye of each patient was randomized to either the untreated control arm or to the 30 %

intraocular pressure reduction arm of the study. Randomization occurred immediately if the eye had a visual field defect that threatened fixation or if recent progression was documented. Otherwise, the eligible eye was followed up until confirmed progression occurred; the eye was then randomized.

The study enrolled 230 subjects, but the analysis was based on 145 randomized eyes of 145 subjects. Three outcome-related papers have been published.

This study established that IOP is part of the pathogenic process of normal tension glaucoma. Lowering of IOP by at least 30 % from baseline slowed visual field loss and this IOP reduction was achieved by medication alone in more than half of the patients. There was a greater risk of cataract formation after surgery which obscured the protective effect of IOP reduction. When the influence of cataract on visual fields were censored, the favorable effects of IOP reduction were evident.

The CNTGS also showed that visual field progression rates in normal tension glaucoma vary considerably, and that the rate is slow in many eyes, even if left untreated. Only half of the untreated eyes experienced visual field progression by 5–7 years. Prognostic factors for progression included the occurrence of disc hemorrhage, history of migraine, and female gender.

Primary Study Question

- Is IOP lowering effective in preventing or delaying progressive visual field loss in patients with normal tension glaucoma?

Study Design

- Multi-center, prospective, randomized clinical trial
- Patients randomly assigned to close observation versus aggressive IOP reduction by 30 %

Major Findings

- IOP lowering by 30 % slowed visual field loss; effect was obscured by cataract development
- Aggressive IOP reduction often required trabeculectomy, resulting in frequent cataract development

8.4
Collaborative Initial Glaucoma Treatment Study (CIGTS)

The Collaborative Initial Glaucoma Treatment Study [6, 9, 14, 15, 22, 23] was designed to determine the long-term effect of treating newly diagnosed primary open-angle glaucoma (POAG) with trabeculectomy compared to treating with medication. Study outcome measures included visual function, which was evaluated by visual field and visual acuity testing, and health-related quality of life.

Eligibility was limited to patients with newly diagnosed open-angle glaucoma. Randomization was by patients (not eyes) with the two treatment arms being initial treatment with filtering surgery or initial treatment with medications. Patients were randomized in such a manner as to achieve balance between the two groups over five predetermined stratification variables: age, study center, gender, race, and diagnosis (primary, pigmentary, and pseudoexfoliation forms of open-angle glaucoma). If both eyes of a patient required treatment, the same treatment was used. Enrollment was competed in April, 1997 with 607 patients.

As of November 2003, two outcome-related papers reporting 5-year interim results have been published. In one publication, the primary outcome was visual field progression, whereas in the other, it was health-related quality of life. Visual field progression was minimal in both treatment arms and there was no statistically significant difference between the two (Fig. 8.3). Both treatment groups have shown a decline in symptom impact over time. The surgical group reported more symptom impact but the difference between groups was not statistically significant. The surgical group initially experienced more local eye symptoms than the medical group and this decrease was statistically significant, but the difference diminished with time.

The results of CIGTS suggest that treatment with trabeculectomy or with medication is equally effective for the first 5 years and do not support a major change in clinical practice. However, there has been relatively little visual field progression in both groups thus far on

Fig. 8.3. Percentage showing at least a 3-unit increase in Collaborative Initial Glaucoma Treatment Study visual field score by month of visit and treatment group. (Reproduced from [22] with permission)

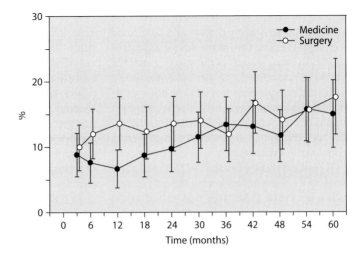

which to base definitive conclusions. Follow-up is ongoing with over 90% of the enrolled patients.

Primary Study Question

- What is the best initial step in a patient newly diagnosed with POAG – topical medication or trabeculectomy?

Study Design

- Multi-center, prospective, randomized clinical trial
- Patients randomly assigned to trabeculectomy (±5-FU at investigator's discretion) versus topical medication

Major Findings

- Medication and trabeculectomy equally effective in lowering IOP at 5-year time point
- No difference in visual field progression at 5 years
- Trabeculectomy was associated with more ocular symptoms than the medication group; this difference subsided after the first few years

8.5
Ocular Hypertension Treatment Study (OHTS)

The Ocular Hypertension Treatment Study [3, 7, 10, 11, 16–18, 24, 24] was designed to evaluate the efficacy of lowering IOP in preventing or delaying the development of clinical glaucoma in individuals with elevated IOP. Eligible subjects were randomized to either careful observation or a stepped medical regimen of all commercially-available topical IOP-lowering agents. The treatment goal was to lower IOP by at least 20% from baseline. Eligible patients were 40–80 years of age with best-corrected visual acuity in both eyes >20/40, had normal optic discs and normal visual fields, and had untreated intraocular pressure of 24–32 mmHg in at least one eye with the other eye having pressure of at least 21 mmHg.

Enrollment was completed in October 1996 with 1,636 subjects, 409 (25%) of whom were African Americans. The primary outcome of interest was the development of glaucoma as determined by confirmed visual field loss or optic disc change. Patients with co-morbidities that might result in endpoints unrelated to POAG (e.g., a history of demyelinating disease, optic disc drusen, diabetic retinopathy) were excluded from enrollment. Both the initial 'normal and reliable' status at study entry and the visual field and optic disc endpoints were determined by independent reading centers and confirmed with repeat testing. One of the unique aspects of the OHTS study design is the use of a masked 'endpoint committee' who attribute visual field or optic disc endpoints to POAG or other causes. In this manner, visual field loss from, for example, branch retinal vein occlusions or macular degeneration are differentiated from glaucomatous damage.

An early finding from the OHTS Visual Field Reading Center after reviewing the first 22,000 follow-up visual fields was that initial visual field defects are not reproduced on subsequent testing 85.9% of the time [18]. This finding highlights the significant variability of visual fields and the importance of confirming visual field defects or their progression before initiating or escalating potentially expensive and/or hazardous therapy.

A secondary goal of OHTS was to identify baseline demographic and clinical factors that predict which subjects will develop glaucoma. Some of the factors considered initially included age, gender, education, race, family history of glaucoma, baseline intraocular pressure, baseline visual field mean defect, pattern standard deviation and corrected pattern standard deviation, baseline cup-to-disc ratio and the presence of co-morbid conditions such as diabetes and hypertension. After the OHTS completed its enrollment, it became increasingly apparent from the literature that increased central corneal thickness (CCT) was more common among ocular hypertensive patients. Because altered CCT can influence the accuracy of Goldmann applanation tonometry, ultrasonic pachymetry was added to the testing of the OHTS patients approximately 2 years after enrollment was completed.

Confirming the observation of previous smaller studies, the OHTS found an increased average CCT among the ocular hypertensive participants of the OHTS compared to published normative data [3]. In fact, 25% of the OHTS subjects had CCTs greater than 600 μM. Several 'conversion factors' for correcting applanation readings with measured CCT to give a 'true' IOP have been published. Depending on which conversion algorithm is used, as many as 52% of the OHTS participants may have had 'true' IOPs below 21 mmHg upon entry into the study. This suggests that many patients diagnosed with ocular hypertension may have little more than thickened corneas that result in their mis-classification on the basis of Goldmann tonometry. The CCT data also demonstrated that the African-American OHTS subjects had thinner corneas than their Caucasian counterparts, more resembling the 'normal' population in terms of CCT than Caucasian ocular hypertensives.

In June, 2002, the OHTS reported on its 5 year results [11, 17, 24]. The two groups of 800+ patients were tightly comparable in all baseline parameters evaluated, and the treatment intervention (lowering IOP by 20% from baseline) was maintained throughout the study period. The onset of glaucoma was more common among the observation group than among the patients in the medication group (Fig. 8.4). Relatively modest lowering of IOP by 20% with commercially-available medications was found to reduce the onset of glaucoma by almost 60%. "All cause" endpoints (combining POAG and other causes of visual field loss or optic disc damage) were also reduced in the medication group. The safety of topical medication was also confirmed; there were no significant differences in a wide variety of safety measures between the medication and observation groups.

The predictive factor analysis of the OHTS provided confirmation in a multivariate model that increased IOP, increased age, and increased cup-to-disc ratio are all independent predictive factors for the development of POAG among ocular hypertensives. An unexpected finding of the OHTS was that CCT proved to be a most potent predictive factor for the development of POAG – patients with CCTs only 40 μM thinner than the OHTS average had a 71% increased incidence of POAG endpoints. This risk relationship was independent of IOP (Fig. 8.5) or baseline cup to disc ratio. Most strikingly, in the multivariate model the increased incidence of POAG among African-American OHTS subjects was explained by thinner CCT and increased cup-to-disc ratio at baseline.

The OHTS demonstrated the importance of pachymetry in assessing risk among ocular hy-

Fig. 8.4. Kaplan Meier plot of the cumulative probability of developing primary open-angle glaucoma (POAG) by randomization group. The number of participants at risk are those who had not developed POAG at the beginning of each 6-month period. The number of participants classified as developing POAG is given for each interval. Participants who did not develop POAG and withdrew before the end of the study or who died are censored from the interval of their last completed visit. (Reproduced from [23])

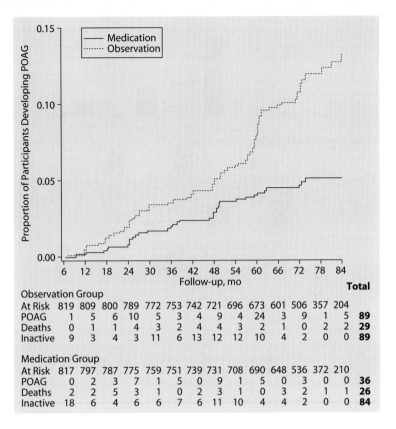

Observation Group														Total
At Risk	819	809	800	789	772	753	742	721	696	673	601	506	357	204
POAG	1	5	6	10	5	3	4	9	4	24	3	9	1	5	89
Deaths	0	1	1	4	3	2	4	4	3	2	1	0	2	2	29
Inactive	9	3	4	3	11	6	13	12	12	10	4	2	0	0	89

Medication Group														Total
At Risk	817	797	787	775	759	751	739	731	708	690	648	536	372	210
POAG	0	2	3	7	1	5	0	9	1	5	0	3	0	0	36
Deaths	2	2	5	3	1	0	2	3	1	0	3	2	1	1	26
Inactive	18	6	4	6	6	7	6	11	10	4	4	2	0	0	84

pertensive and glaucoma suspect patients and recommended its general use. For example, when applying the OHTS risk model to a 60-year-old patient presenting with IOPs of 24 mmHg and minimal cupping, the 5-year risk of developing POAG can vary from as little as 1% if the CCT is 600 µM to 20% if the CCT is 490 µM. An older patient with somewhat larger cup-to-disc ratios and thin corneas can have a 5-year risk of POAG approaching 40%.

The OHTS was the first large clinical trial designed from the outset to prove that lowering IOP is protective against the onset of POAG. Although the study demonstrated the efficacy and safety of IOP-lowering therapy in ocular hypertensive patients, it is wrong to conclude that all patients with elevated IOP should be treated. The risk model analysis demonstrated that there are large numbers of ocular hypertensive patients (e.g., those with thick corneas and small cup-to-disc ratios) who have a negligible likeli-

hood of developing glaucoma and for whom therapy is not indicated. Others (e.g., older patients with thin corneas and larger cup-to-disc ratios) are far more likely to develop glaucoma and therapy in these patients is strongly indicated. The OHTS provides clinicians with the 'proof of concept' justifying the therapy of ocular hypertensives, as well as the tools to identify those who will benefit the most from treatment.

Additional ancillary studies have been performed on subsets of the OHTS patients. These include prospective studies of short-wavelength automated perimetry (SWAP) and confocal scanning laser ophthalmoscopy (CSLO; HRT, Heidelberg Engineering GmbH, Germany) testing performed since the beginning of the study. Baseline data from these two ancillary studies are currently in press [41, 42]. The reading centers for these ancillary studies were masked to the overall OHTS results until the 5-year reports were released. In 2004–5, we should begin to

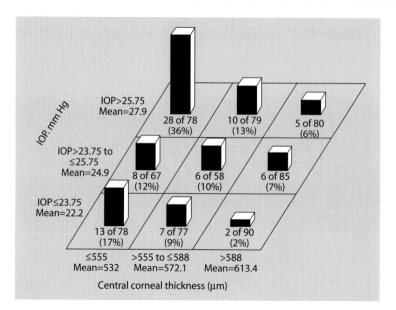

Fig. 8.5. The percentage of participants in the observation group who developed primary open-angle glaucoma (median follow-up, 72 months) grouped by baseline intraocular pressure (IOP) of ≤23.75 mmHg, >23.75 mmHg to ≤25.75 mmHg, and >25.75 mmHg and by central corneal thickness measurements of ≤555 μm, >555 μm to ≤588 μm, and >588 μm. These percentages are not adjusted for length of follow-up. The means are not identical to those given in the text, which includes all participants in the Ocular Hypertension Treatment Study rather than just the observation group. (From [22] with permission)

learn whether these new technologies were successful in predicting which patients would develop glaucoma and whether they can accurately follow progression of disease.

The OHTS will continue for several more years, with patients in the observation group encouraged to begin treatment with IOP-lowering medications. It is hoped that continued careful follow-up of the OHTS patients will provide better characterization of the risk model and the natural history of early glaucoma and determine whether a delay in treatment alters the long-term outcome of the disease.

Primary Study Question

- Is lowering IOP in patients with ocular hypertension safe and effective in delaying or preventing the development of primary open-angle glaucoma?

Study Design

- Multi-center, prospective, randomized clinical trial.
- Patients randomly assigned to close observation versus treatment with topical medications to lower IOP 20 % from baseline.

Major Findings

- Lowering IOP by 20 % reduced the incidence of glaucomatous endpoints (confirmed visual field defects or optic nerve changes)
- Baseline characteristics predictive of increased risk of glaucoma included IOP, age, and central corneal thickness (CCT)
- The study recommended that CCT be measured in patients with ocular hypertension to better assess risk

8.6
Early Manifest Glaucoma Trial (EMGT)

The Early Manifest Glaucoma Trial [12, 13, 19, 20, 21] was designed to determine the efficacy of glaucoma treatment in subjects with documented glaucomatous damage. Initiated with local support in Sweden, the NEI has provided additional support to fund a statistical coordinating center in the United States. The EMGT randomized patients with primary open-angle glaucoma, normal-tension glaucoma, and pseudoexfoliation glaucoma to either treatment with topical betaxolol, a β_1 selective adrenergic antagonist, combined with argon laser trabeculoplasty, or to observation. As a safety measure for eyes with sustained IOP elevation $\geq$35 mmHg, delayed treatment was permitted for the observation group, as was the addition of latanoprost, a topical prostaglandin analog, after it became commercially available in 1996.

Eligible subjects were from 50 to 80 years of age, with newly diagnosed, previously untreated chronic open-angle glaucoma. The diagnosis of glaucoma required repeatable visual field defects in at least one eye and included primary open-angle glaucoma, normal-tension glaucoma, and pseudoexfoliation glaucoma. The study outcome was glaucoma progression as measured by quantitative visual field criteria and optic disc changes as determined by a disc reading center. The identification of subjects took place in Malmö and Helsingborg, Sweden. A total of 255 patients were enrolled with randomization concluded in April 1997.

The primary outcome result, with median follow-up of 6 years, was published in October 2002 [12]. The treatment group maintained a mean IOP reduction from baseline of 25%, whereas the observation group maintained its baseline IOP through the course of follow-up. Progression was less frequent in the treatment group (45%) compared to the observation group (62%) and occurred later. The median time to progression was 66 months in the treatment and 48 months in the observation groups. The EMGT provided unequivocal evidence that reducing the IOP makes a difference in slowing glaucomatous damage. It thus corroborates the

major conclusion of OHTS, but at a more advanced stage of the disease process, and it reaffirms the primary role of IOP in the pathogenesis of glaucomatous damage.

Few adverse systemic and ocular events were identified, but both occurred more commonly in the treatment group. An unexpected increased incidence of nuclear opacities was found in the treatment group. This finding is consistent with the increased frequency of cataract surgery in the treatment group of OHTS, and further research to investigate the possible association between glaucoma treatment and lens opacities is warranted [2].

Factors related to glaucoma progression were reported in a subsequent publication [20]. The magnitude of initial IOP reduction was a major factor influencing outcome. The importance of IOP as a prognostic factor was reinforced in that each mmHg of IOP lowering on follow-up was associated with an approximate 10% decrease in risk of progression. Other factors associated with progression were higher baseline IOP, exfoliation, bilateral disease, worse mean deviation, and older age, as well as frequent disc hemorrhages during follow-up. In contrast to the OHTS, the EMGT did not find a strong predictive relationship between CCT and glaucoma progression.

To understand this disparity, it is important to recognize that the OHTS used IOP (as measured by Goldmann tonometry) as its primary entry criterion, with normality of VFs and nerves confirmed afterwards. If CCT's influence as a predictive factor results primarily from its effect as an artifact influencing the accuracy of Goldmann tonometry, then the entry criteria for OHTS and the study design were perfectly set up to show that CCT causes a mis-classification of IOP-related risk. Consider two otherwise identical OHTS participants with the same baseline IOPs but with very different CCTs – these two individuals likely had very different 'true' IOPs at the beginning of the OHTS, and the only baseline measurement able to reveal this difference would be CCT. In such a scenario, a thinner central cornea would 'predict' an increased risk of glaucoma.

In contrast, in the EMGT, patients were recruited based on the presence of damage, regardless of IOP and without the recruitment bias an IOP cutoff might cause; in fact, a large portion of the patients were those whom many would consider classifying as having normal tension glaucoma. Thus at the outset, the EMGT started with patients who had demonstrated the propensity to sustain damage at *whatever* their 'true' IOP might be – errors in IOP measurement become less important in such a situation.

This explanation for the disparity between the EMGT and the OHTS results assumes that the CCT story is primarily one of a measurement artifact. It is entirely plausible (but at this point purely speculative) that CCT is also a surrogate for other structural factors in the eye, such as the thickness of the lamina cribrosa. These and other hypotheses are likely to be the focus of both laboratory and clinical investigation in coming years.

Primary Study Question

- Is IOP-lowering treatment effective in preventing or delaying progression of glaucoma in patients newly-diagnosed with mild to moderate disease?

Study Design

- Multi-center, prospective, randomized clinical trial
- Patients randomly assigned to close observation versus betaxolol and laser trabeculoplasty

Major Findings

- Progression less frequent (and occurred later) in the treated group
- Each mmHg of IOP associated with 10 % increased progression
- Increased incidence of nuclear cataract in treated group

8.7 Conclusions

Through the proper use of randomized clinical trials over the last 5–10 years, we now have the evidence necessary to answer the questions that loomed so large in the 1980s and early 1990s. As in all good science, however, new questions arise as old ones are put to rest: Do patients pay a price for a delay in treatment? What are the economic costs of treating early glaucoma? How do we reliably measure disease progression? Does neuroprotection work? These are just some of the questions that loom large at the beginning of the 21st century.

We can hope that in the next 5–10 years ongoing and future randomized clinical trials will provide more answers (and more questions) for our profession's next generation.

Acknowledgment. Portions of this chapter have been reprinted with permission from Focal Points: Clinical Modules for Ophthalmologists, "Update on Glaucoma Clinical Trials," San Francisco: American Academy of Ophthalmology, 2003.

References

1. Anderson DR, Drance SM, Schulzer M (2001) Natural history of normal-tension glaucoma. Ophthalmology 108:247–253
2. Brandt JD (2003) Does benzalkonium chloride cause cataract. Arch Ophthalmol 121:892–893
3. Brandt JD, Beiser JA, Kass MA, Gordon MO (2001) Central corneal thickness in the Ocular Hypertension Treatment Study (OHTS). Ophthalmology 108:1779–1788
4. Drance S, Anderson DR, Schulzer M (2001) Risk factors for progression of visual field abnormalities in normal-tension glaucoma. Am J Ophthalmol 131:699–708
5. Eddy DM, Billings J (1988) The quality of medical evidence: implications for quality of care. Health Aff (Millwood) 7:19–32
6. Feiner L, Piltz-Seymour JR (2003) Collaborative Initial Glaucoma Treatment Study: a summary of results to date. Curr Opin Ophthalmol 14:106–111

7. Feuer WJ, Parrish RK, Schiffman JC, Anderson DR, Budenz DL, Wells MC, Hess DJ, Kass MA, Gordon MO (2002) The Ocular Hypertension Treatment Study: reproducibility of cup/disk ratio measurements over time at an optic disc reading center. Am J Ophthalmol 133:19–28

8. Gaasterland DE, Blackwell B, Dally LG, Caprioli J, Katz LJ, Ederer F (2001) The Advanced Glaucoma Intervention Study (AGIS): 10. Variability among Academic Glaucoma Subspecialists in Assessing Optic Disc Notching. Trans Am Ophthalmol Soc 99:177–184; discussion 184–175

9. Gillespie BW, Musch DC, Guire KE, Mills RP, Lichter PR, Janz NK, Wren PA (2003) The collaborative initial glaucoma treatment study: baseline visual field and test-retest variability. Invest Ophthalmol Vis Sci 44:2613–2620

10. Gordon MO, Kass MA (1999) The Ocular Hypertension Treatment Study: design and baseline description of the participants. Arch Ophthalmol 117:573–583

11. Gordon MO, Beiser JA, Brandt JD, Heuer DK, Higginbotham EJ, Johnson CA, Keltner JL, Miller JP, Parrish RK, Wilson MR, Kass MA (2002) The Ocular Hypertension Treatment Study: baseline factors that predict the onset of primary open-angle glaucoma. Arch Ophthalmol 120:714-20; discussion 829-30

12. Heijl A, Leske MC, Bengtsson B, Hyman L, Bengtsson B, Hussein M (2002) Reduction of intraocular pressure and glaucoma progression: results from the Early Manifest Glaucoma Trial. Arch Ophthalmol 120:1268–1279

13. Heijl A, Leske MC, Bengtsson B, Bengtsson B, Hussein M (2003) Measuring visual field progression in the Early Manifest Glaucoma Trial. Acta Ophthalmol Scand 81:286–293

14. Janz NK, Wren PA, Lichter PR, Musch DC, Gillespie BW, Guire KE, Mills RP (2001) The Collaborative Initial Glaucoma Treatment Study: interim quality of life findings after initial medical or surgical treatment of glaucoma. Ophthalmology 108:1954–1965

15. Janz NK, Wren PA, Lichter PR, Musch DC, Gillespie BW, Guire KE, Mills RP (2001) The Collaborative Initial Glaucoma Treatment Study: interim quality of life findings after initial medical or surgical treatment of glaucoma. Ophthalmology 108:1954–1965

16. Johnson CA, Keltner JL, Cello KE, Edwards M, Kass MA, Gordon MO, Budenz DL, Gaasterland DE, Werner E (2002) Baseline visual field characteristics in the ocular hypertension treatment study. Ophthalmology 109:432–437

17. Kass MA, Heuer DK, Higginbotham EJ, Johnson CA, Keltner JL, Miller JP, Parrish RK, Wilson MR, Gordon MO (2002) The Ocular Hypertension Treatment Study: a randomized trial determines that topical ocular hypotensive medication delays or prevents the onset of primary open-angle glaucoma. Arch Ophthalmol 120:701-13; discussion 829-30

18. Keltner JL, Johnson CA, Quigg JM, Cello KE, Kass MA, Gordon MO (2000) Confirmation of visual field abnormalities in the Ocular Hypertension Treatment Study. Ocular Hypertension Treatment Study Group. Arch Ophthalmol 118:1187–1194

19. Leske MC, Heijl A, Hyman L, Bengtsson B (1999) Early Manifest Glaucoma Trial: design and baseline data. Ophthalmology 106:2144–2153

20. Leske MC, Heijl A, Hussein M, Bengtsson B, Hyman L, Komaroff E (2003) Factors for glaucoma progression and the effect of treatment: the early manifest glaucoma trial. Arch Ophthalmol 121: 48–56

21. Lichter PR (2002) Expectations from clinical trials: results of the Early Manifest Glaucoma Trial. Arch Ophthalmol 120:1371–1372

22. Lichter PR, Musch DC, Gillespie BW, Guire KE, Janz NK, Wren PA, Mills RP (2001) Interim clinical outcomes in the Collaborative Initial Glaucoma Treatment Study comparing initial treatment randomized to medications or surgery. Ophthalmology 108:1943–1953

23. Mills RP, Janz NK, Wren PA, Guire KE (2001) Correlation of visual field with quality-of-life measures at diagnosis in the Collaborative Initial Glaucoma Treatment Study (CIGTS). J Glaucoma 10:192–198

24. Palmberg P (2002) Answers from the ocular hypertension treatment study. Arch Ophthalmol 120:829–830

25. Piltz J, Gross R, Shin DH, Beiser JA, Dorr DA, Kass MA, Gordon MO (2000) Contralateral effect of topical beta-adrenergic antagonists in initial one-eyed trials in the ocular hypertension treatment study. Am J Ophthalmol 130:441–453

26. Rossetti L, Marchetti I, Orzalesi N, Scorpiglione N, Torri V, Liberati A (1993) Randomized clinical trials on medical treatment of glaucoma. Are they appropriate to guide clinical practice?. Arch Ophthalmol 111:96–103

27. Schulzer M (1992) Intraocular pressure reduction in normal-tension glaucoma patients. The Normal Tension Glaucoma Study Group. Ophthalmology 99:1468–1470

28. Schwartz AL, Van Veldhuisen PC, Gaasterland DE, Ederer F, Sullivan EK, Cyrlin MN (1999) The Advanced Glaucoma Intervention Study (AGIS): 5. Encapsulated bleb after initial trabeculectomy. Am J Ophthalmol 127:8–19

29. The AGIS Investigators (1994) The Advanced Glaucoma Intervention Study (AGIS): 1. Study design and methods and baseline characteristics of study patients. Control Clin Trials 15:299–325

30. The AGIS Investigators (1994) The Advanced Glaucoma Intervention Study (AGIS): 2. Visual field test scoring and reliability. Ophthalmology 101:1445–1455

31. The AGIS Investigators (1998) The Advanced Glaucoma Intervention Study (AGIS): 3. Baseline characteristics of black and white patients. Ophthalmology 105:1137–1145

32. The AGIS Investigators (1998) The Advanced Glaucoma Intervention Study (AGIS): 4. Comparison of treatment outcomes within race. Seven-year results. Ophthalmology 105:1146–1164

33. The AGIS Investigators (2000) The Advanced Glaucoma Intervention Study (AGIS): 7. The relationship between control of intraocular pressure and visual field deterioration. Am J Ophthalmol 130:429–440

34. The AGIS Investigators (2000) The advanced glaucoma intervention study. 6. Effect of cataract on visual field and visual acuity. Arch Ophthalmol 118:1639–1652

35. The AGIS Investigators (2001) The Advanced Glaucoma Intervention Study (AGIS): 8. Risk of cataract formation after trabeculectomy. Arch Ophthalmol 119:1771–1779

36. The AGIS Investigators (2001) The Advanced Glaucoma Intervention Study (AGIS): 9. Comparison of glaucoma outcomes in black and white patients within treatment groups. Am J Ophthalmol 132:311–320

37. The AGIS Investigators (2002) The Advanced Glaucoma Intervention Study (AGIS): 11. Risk factors for failure of trabeculectomy and argon laser trabeculoplasty. Am J Ophthalmol 134:481–498

38. The AGIS Investigators (2002) The Advanced Glaucoma Intervention Study (AGIS): 12. Baseline risk factors for sustained loss of visual field and visual acuity in patients with advanced glaucoma. Am J Ophthalmol 134:499–512

39. Wilson MR (2003) The use of "race" for classification in medicine: is it valid? J Glaucoma 12:293–294

40. Wilson MR (2003) What is race? Int Ophthalmol Clin 43:1–8

41. Zangwill LM, Weinreb RN, Berry CC, Smith AR, Dirkes KA, Coleman AL, Piltz-Seymour JR, Liebmann JM, Cioffi GA, Trick G, Brandt JD, Gordon MO, Kass MA, and the Ocular Hypertension Treatment Study Group (2004) Racial Differences of Optic Disc Topography in Ocular Hypertensive Eyes: Results from the Confocal Scanning Laser Ophthalmoscopy Ancillary Study to the Ocular Hypertension Treatment Study. Archives of Ophthalmology 122(1):22–28

42. Zangwill LM, Weinreb RN, Berry CC, Smith AR, Dirkes KA, Liebmann JM, Brandt JD, Trick G, Cioffi GA, Coleman AL, Piltz-Seymour JR, Gordon MO, Kass MA, and the Ocular Hypertension Treatment Study Group (2004) The Confocal Scanning Laser Ophthalmoscopy Ancillary Study to the Ocular Hypertension Treatment Study. Study Design and Baseline Factors. American Journal of Ophthalmology 137(2):219–227

C. MIGDAL

Core Messages

- Approximately 90%–55% of progressive glaucoma damage is pressure dependent
- In normal tension glaucoma, 30% IOP reduction slowed visual field progression significantly
- Fluctuations of IOP are a significant risk factor for progression
- Starting IOP, degree of pre-existing glaucoma damage, life expectancy, and other risk factors such as myopia, family history, and microvascular disease are to be considered for estimation of target IOP
- Target IOP defines the upper limit of an IOP range at which it is supposed glaucoma damage will not progress
- OHTS, CIGTS, CNTG, AGIS, and EMGT studies provide evidence of the importance of target IOP in glaucoma treatment

9.1
Introduction

The ophthalmologist managing glaucoma is faced with a complex task. After initially assessing the glaucoma damage already present, the likely rate of development of the disease and the pressure at which damage occurred, other factors will need to be taken into account, including age, race, life expectancy, family history of glaucoma, other individual circumstances and preferences of the patient, before an individualized treatment plan can be initiated. The patient is monitored at regular intervals, and necessary changes in treatment introduced where indicated. The ultimate goal of glaucoma treatment is to preserve visual function throughout life at minimal costs of time, money and side effects of therapy.

Information that has emerged about the long-term outcomes of glaucoma therapy necessitates a reassessment of our glaucoma management strategy in order to direct more aggressive treatment to those patients who have aggressive disease. While most patients do well in the short term, so that patient encounters would seem to suggest that our treatment strategies are adequate, long-term outcomes indicate that this is not necessarily the case. For example, although population statistics suggest that only 2% of glaucoma patients are legally blind, a recent study from the Mayo Clinic [10] indicates that after 20 years of follow-up, 22% of glaucoma patients in the local county were bilaterally blind, and 54% blind in one eye. About 12% were blind at 12 years of follow-up, which has been estimated to be the life expectancy of the average glaucoma patient. It is reasonable to presume that even higher percentages of patients may have suffered functional visual impairment. Other studies have suggested a lesser amount of blindness from glaucoma. A study in Denmark reported an estimated glaucoma prevalence of 45 per 100,000 among the Danish population 50 years or older [8]. Results from the Baltimore Eye Survey indicated that blindness due to open-angle glaucoma increased with age among whites and blacks, began 10 years earlier among blacks, and was the leading cause of non-remediable blindness among blacks [20, 21]. However, the number of cases of blindness was small.

These results indicate that having primary open-angle glaucoma and being treated conventionally, carries a fairly high risk of blindness, with about the same lifetime risk of visual loss as having insulin-dependent diabetes.

9.2
The Relationship Between IOP and the Risk of Visual Field Progression

There is published evidence of long-term outcomes of intraocular pressure (IOP)-lowering. Odberg [17] documented the long-term efficacy of medical and/or surgical therapy on patients with advanced glaucoma. A dose–response relationship was noted between the IOP during follow-up and the risk of field progression. The greatest therapeutic benefit was noted in those achieving pressures in the low normal range. Palmberg reviewed the outcomes of patients undergoing filtering surgery with either 5-fluorouracil or mitomycin C carried out at the Bascom Palmer Eye Institute [18, 19] and showed that those patients with the lower pressures had better preservation of visual field. These studies indicate that, in eyes sufficiently damaged to warrant surgery, the dose–response relationship between IOP and risk of field progression takes place within the normal range (i.e. IOP less than 21 mmHg). It would thus appear that 90%–95% of progressive glaucoma damage is pressure-dependent. It is important to remember that risk is given for group mean IOPs and not for individuals at that pressure.

Patients with progressive normal tension glaucoma and/or split fixation and randomised to an untreated control group, had a 60% risk of visual field progression, compared with those in whom the IOP had been reduced by 30%, in whom 20% progressed (mean IOP was 16 vs 11 mmHg). This limited dose–response relationship is parallel to and shifted to the left from that of primary open-angle glaucoma (POAG) [6].

Summary for the Clinician

- In glaucoma, the therapeutic benefit is not obtained simply by reaching the upper normal limit of IOP

- A dose response–curve has been noted with regard to IOP during follow-up and the risk of progression in long-term follow-up studies

9.3
Target Pressures in Glaucoma Management

In glaucoma, the therapeutic benefit is not obtained by simply approaching the upper normal limit of the treated factor (i.e. IOP). This differs from other chronic diseases such as systemic hypertension or insulin-dependent diabetes. Factors other than pressure may also be important, for example blood supply, such that upper normal IOP may further impede an already compromised blood supply to the optic nerve. Lowering of the IOP to the low-normal range allows improved perfusion. Mechanical factors may also be important with lower pressures reducing the strain on the lamina cribrosa. Whatever the damage mechanism, the considerable variation in the individual range of susceptibility to pressure complicates the setting of a therapeutic goal or 'target pressure'.

9.4
Target Pressure

Target IOP is defined as an estimate of the mean IOP obtained with treatment that would be expected to prevent further glaucomatous damage [7]. This level is obviously chosen from clinical experience and uses the outcomes of clinical trials for guidance. The level chosen should be the highest IOP in a given eye at which IOP does not contribute to further glaucomatous optic nerve head damage. This is selected after individual patient assessment (Fig. 9.1), and may need to be adjusted during the course of follow-up, depending on whether visual function is maintained, or continues to deteriorate [1, 2].

There are, however, limitations to the target IOP concept. The effect of IOP is continuous, but IOP is infrequently measured in clinical practice. Individual IOPs may vary considerably, either in the course of a day (diurnal variation), or over different days. In addition, there

Fig. 9.1. Target IOP: a guideline for target IOP estimation, noting patient factors such as IOP at which damage occurred, degree of glaucomatous damage and life expectancy of the patient. (From [7] with permission)

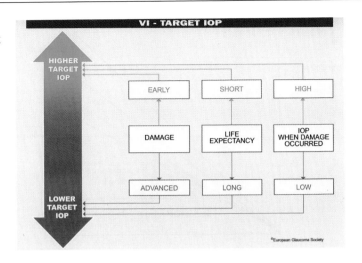

is no way to directly assess at which level of IOP damage occurred. Should the target pressure selected be the peak IOP value, the mean value, or the mean value over different days, for example? Other points to consider are that pressures may differ diurnally, at night in the supine position, that the relationship of IOP with blood pressure may be important (perfusion pressure), measurements may differ due to corneal thickness, and certain postures or pastimes may cause sudden and extreme alterations in IOP, e.g. yoga, head stands, etc.

Clinical assessment of the glaucoma patient does need to consider both mean IOP and peak IOP (this emphasizes the importance of the diurnal pressure curve measurements in order to assess the effects of a topical hypotensive drop more accurately). In addition, untreated glaucoma patients show an exaggerated variation in diurnal pressures. Thus IOPs recorded during office hours may not be a true reflection of overall IOP control. These large fluctuations are a significant risk factor [3].

IOP is the most important risk factor in glaucoma, and accumulating evidence supports the benefits of lowering IOP in slowing or halting loss of visual function. This evidence comes from both retrospective studies [15, 17] as well as prospective clinical trials [6, 13, 23, 25].

It is not possible to assess accurately and in advance the exact level of IOP that will prevent further damage as this varies in the individual patient and indeed the individual eye, nor is there a single IOP level that is safe for every patient. The goal should be the least amount of medication (and least amount of side effects) necessary to achieve this therapeutic response. If medications are unable to achieve the desired effects, then laser or surgery could be considered.

There is no single level of IOP that could be considered an ideal target for all patients. The target pressure selected will depend on a number of factors, including the starting IOP, the degree of pre-existing glaucoma damage, and the life expectancy of the patient, as discussed in more detail in the following:

1. Starting IOP (IOP level before treatment)
   Reduction of IOP can be considered in terms of millimetres of IOP reduction, and percentage IOP reduction (Fig. 9.2). Thus, a patient with a high starting IOP (e.g. 40 mmHg), reduced to 20 mmHg may have a 20 mmHg reduction or 50% reduction, compared with an NTG patient with starting IOP 18 mmHg reduced to 12 mmHg (i.e. 6 mmHg or 33% reduction). Some of the randomized controlled trials have aimed at a particular percentage reduction in IOP [6].

2. Degree of pre-existing glaucoma damage
   The greater the pre-existing damage, the lower the target IOP should be. Results of the Advanced Glaucoma Intervention Study

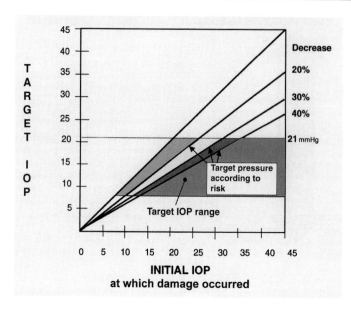

Fig. 9.2. Target IOP according to risk: evaluation of the desired therapeutic outcome in the form of IOP lowering. The target IOP should be situated in the *shaded area*. Obviously, the lower the initial IOP, the lower the target IOP will be and vice versa. The percentage of IOP reduction targeted (i.e. 20%, 30%, 40%, respectively) depends mainly on the degree of visual field damage at diagnosis and on the rate of progression. (From [7] with permission)

(AGIS) have shown that patients whose IOPs were in the lower range and maintained at this level had better protection of visual field [23]. Thus, mean IOPs less than 14.0 mmHg during the first 3 months of the study predicted a better later outcome than pressures between 14.0 and 17.5 mmHg, or greater than 17.5 mmHg. In addition, patients with IOPs measuring less than or equal to 18 mmHg at all visits showed better field preservation than patients who had IOPs maintained within this level at only a certain percentage of follow-up visits [23].

3. Life expectancy of the patient
   The natural course of the disease needs to be considered when selecting and then attempting to achieve a desired target IOP. Glaucoma damage is a chronic long-term process, and, if functional vision is not threatened, side effects of treatment and quality of life of the individual also need to be taken into account.

4. Other risk factors
   Other than IOP, there may be additional risk factors present, e.g. family history of glaucoma, myopia, microvascular disease, etc. These patients may therefore require even lower target IOPs.

The concept of target pressure should encourage the ophthalmologist initiating glaucoma therapy to consider the features of the individual case in the light of the above, and select a pressure for that patient that they feel is low enough to prevent progressive damage. This target IOP may, of course, need adjustment during the course of the disease. When a patient is seen subsequently for follow-up, a pressure above the goal should trigger a consideration of additional pressure readings, or additional therapeutic options of low risk, e.g. medication or laser trabeculoplasty. If the target is not attained by these measures, and there is a high risk of progressive damage, then surgery could be considered, taking into account the relative risks.

The adequacy of the level of target IOP chosen needs to be validated by periodic visual field tests and optic disc assessment. The value may need to be lowered if further damage is seen, or may even be raised if no damage occurs during follow-up.

Attempts have been made to select more complex target pressure values, such as in the Collaborative Initial Glaucoma Treatment Study where there is a 'goal' target pressure that triggers low-risk additions of therapy, and a 'mandatory' target pressure that initiates major interventions [16].

As a general rule, it has been suggested that, in cases with minimal damage, the target pressure should be set at approximately 20% below the baseline pressure before therapy has been initiated. In cases with moderate damage (with no paracentral field points involved), perhaps a 30% reduction is indicated, while in advanced cases, a reduction to 15 mmHg or less and a minimal 30% reduction is probably indicated.

There is no accurate method of precisely preselecting the ideal target IOP in any individual patient. Thus a target pressure sufficiently low to avoid axon death and preserve visual function must be arrived at indirectly using visual field deterioration or increasing optic disc damage for guidance. This process is relatively imprecise: visual fields may vary and optic nerve damage may already be impaired by the time that visual field damage has been detected. Little or no safety margin may be present in patients with advanced damage, and treatment must be relatively aggressive from the outset.

Summary for the Clinician

- There are limitations to the concept of target IOP, both mean and peak IOPs need to be considered
- It is not possible to assess accurately and in advance the exact level of IOP that will prevent further damage; this varies from patient to patient and in the individual eye
- There is no single target IOP that might be considered ideal for all patients
- In setting the target IOP, factors to be considered include: starting IOP, degree of preexisting glaucoma damage, life expectancy of the patient, as well as other risk factors
- The target IOP may have to be adjusted during follow-up

9.5 Randomized Controlled Trials and Target IOPs

Several randomized controlled prospective clinical trials have recently been published, the results of which may prove relevant and modify clinical decision making in the individual glaucoma patient. Patients included in these trials comprised different clinical subgroups of glaucoma, and outcomes deal solely with the patient groups included. Moreover, group outcomes may not exactly mimic those of the individual patient. For purposes of this chapter, details of the trials will not be included, and only comments relevant to clinical management of IOP addressed.

1. OHTS [4, 9, 25]: Mean IOP reduction was 22.5% (SD 9.9) in the treated group and 4.0% (SD 11.9) in the controls. The cumulative proportion developing POAG at 5 years was 4.4% in treated eyes, compared with 9% in controls ($p<0.0001$): a 50% reduction of risk. The difference between the treated and controls appears to increase with time. Risk of progression decreased 10% with each mmHg IOP reduction from baseline to the first follow-up visit. Central corneal thickness was important in estimating the need to treat [4]. Factors that were good predictors for conversion to POAG included age, CD ratio of the optic disk, PSD (pattern standard deviation) of the visual field, and IOP [9]. Not all patients with OHT require treatment: a large percentage of untreated patients (>90%) did not convert to POAG over time. Estimates of the individual risk factors are therefore important. Another point of note is that aiming for an IOP reduction of only 20% may be insufficient (in this study 4.4% of the treated eyes still progressed).

2. CIGTS [14, 16]: In this study, a target IOP algorithm was used to guide the IOP-lowering treatment. Patients were treated aggressively, as needed, in an effort to reduce IOP to a level at or below a predetermined target pressure specific for each individual eye. Visual

field loss did not differ significantly between initial treatment groups (despite a lower average IOP with surgery (average 14–15 mmHg) compared to medications (average 17–18 mmHg).

3. CNTG [5, 6]: Goal of treatment was a 30% reduction from average baseline IOPs. Progression occurred in 12% of treated eyes and 35% of controls. No correlation with absolute IOP level maintained during follow-up was found in either group. The 2:1 difference in progression between the control and treated groups may be because the progression was IOP-related in a proportion of patients. Treated patients that progressed may be explained by their progression not being related to IOP, or that their IOP was not at target.

4. AGIS [22–24]: This trial investigated further interventional treatments in advanced glaucoma patients not controlled on maximal tolerated medical therapy alone. In the Predictive Analysis of this trial, eyes with average IOP greater than 17.5 mmHg over the first three 6-month visits showed a significantly greater visual field deterioration compared with eyes that had mean IOPs less than 14 mmHg over the same period. The amount of deterioration increased over the period of follow-up. In the Associative Analysis of the same trial, eyes with less than 18 mmHg at 100% of the visits over the 6-year follow-up period did not show any increase in their initial visual field defect, whereas eyes that had IOPs of less than this level at only 75%–100%, 50%–75%, or less than 50% of visits all showed a significant increase in their visual field deterioration. These results indicate that low IOP levels and low IOP fluctuation are associated with reduced progression of the field defect in advanced glaucoma. It must be noted that both these analyses were post-hoc.

5. EMGTS [11–13]: In this trial which evaluated the effectiveness of treatment by IOP reduction versus no treatment in cases with early

glaucoma, a 25% decrease of IOP from baseline and a maximum absolute level of IOP of 25 mmHg reduced the risk of disease progression (usually determined by loss of visual field) by 50%. This risk of progression decreased 10% with every mmHg IOP reduction from baseline to the first follow-up visit. It should also be noted that some patients did not show any disease progression even after several years without treatment.

Although these trials show that IOP reduction is beneficial in OHT and POAG of various stages and that lower IOP provides better protection against loss of visual function, lowering the IOP is inevitably not always beneficial for all. It is essential to evaluate each individual patient for specific risk factors, lifestyle, degree of existing damage, etc. The aim of treatment need not be no progression at all, but rather a reduction of the rate of progression to such a level that functional vision is not endangered during the patient's lifetime.

The target IOP concept is now generally accepted as a useful guideline on which to base the active management of the glaucoma patient. As with all guidelines, individual factors need to be taken into account that will modify treatment choice and indeed, choice of the target IOP itself. Glaucoma is a chronic long-term disease, and target pressures need to be reviewed and adjusted during the course of the disease, depending on individual patient circumstances and behaviour of the disease.

Summary for the Clinician

- The results of certain recently published random controlled glaucoma clinical trials may modify clinical decision-making
- Remember that outcomes deal solely with the groups included in the trials, and that group outcomes may not mimic those in the individual patient
- The aim of treatment may not be no progression at all, but rather a reduction in the rate of progression to such a level that functional vision is not endangered during the patient's lifetime

References

1. American Academy of Ophthalmology (1989) Preferred practice pattern for primary open angle glaucoma. American Academy of Ophthalmology, San Francisco

2. American Academy of Ophthalmology (1996) Preferred practice pattern for primary open angle glaucoma. American Academy of Ophthalmology, San Francisco

3. Asrani S, Zeimer R, Wilensky J, Gieser D, Vitale S, Lindenmuth K (2000) Large diurnal fluctuations in intraocular pressure are an independent risk factor in patients with glaucoma. J Glaucoma 9:134–142

4. Brandt JD, Beiser JA, Kass MA, Gordon MO (2001) Central corneal thickness in the Ocular Hypertension Treatment Study (OHTS). Ophthalmology 108:1779–1788

5. Collaborative Normal-Tension Glaucoma Study Group (1998) Comparison of glaucomatous progression between untreated patients with normal-tension glaucoma and patients with therapeutically reduced intraocular pressures. Am J Ophthalmol 126:487–497

6. Collaborative Normal-Tension Glaucoma Study Group (1998) The effectiveness of intraocular pressure reduction in the treatment of normal-tension glaucoma. Am J Ophthalmol 126:498–505

7. European Glaucoma Society (2003) European Glaucoma Society Guidelines, 2nd edn. DOGMA, Savona

8. Fuchs J, Nissen KR, Goldschmidt E (1992) Glaucoma blindness in Denmark. Acta Ophthalmol (Copenh) 70:73–78

9. Gordon MO, Beiser JA, Brandt JD, Heuer DK et al (2002) The Ocular Hypertension Treatment Study. Baseline factors that predict the onset of primary open-angle glaucoma. Arch Ophthalmol 120:714–720

10. Hattenhauer MG, Johnson DM, Img HH et al (1998) The problem of blindness from open angle glaucoma. Ophthalmology 105:2099–2104

11. Heijl A, Leske MC, Bengtsson B, Hyman L, Bengtsson B, Hussein M (2002) Reduction of intraocular pressure and glaucoma progression: results from the Early Manifest Glaucoma Trial. Arch Ophthalmol 120:1268–1279

12. Leske MC, Heijl A, Hyman L, Bengtsson B (1999) Early Manifest Glaucoma Trial: design and baseline data. Ophthalmology 106:2144–2153

13. Leske MC, Heijl A, Hussein M, Bengtsson B, Hyman L, Konaroff E (2003) The Early Manifest Glaucoma Trial. Factors for glaucoma progression and the effect of treatment. Arch Ophthalmol 121:48–56

14. Lichter PR, Musch DC, Gillespie BW, Guire KE, Janz NK, Wren PA, Mills RP (2001) Interim clinical outcomes in the Collaborative Initial Glaucoma Treatment Study comparing initial treatment randomized to medications or surgery. Ophthalmology 108:1943–1953

15. Mao LK, Stewart WC, Shields MB (1991) Correlation between intraocular pressure control and progressive glaucomatous damage in primary open-angle glaucoma. Am J Ophthalmol 111:51–55

16. Musch DC, Lichter PR, Guire KE, Standardi CL (1999) The CITGS Study Group. The Collaborative Initial Glaucoma Treatment Study. Study design, methods and baseline characteristics of enrolled patients. Ophthalmology 106:653–662

17. Odberg T (1987) Visual field prognosis in advanced glaucoma. Acta Ophthalmol Scan 65[suppl 182]: 27–29

18. Palmberg P (1998) Clinical controversies: target pressures – what are they? In: Leader B, Calkwood JC (eds) Peril in the nerve – glaucoma and clinical neuro-ophthalmology. Proceedings of the New Orleans Academy of Ophthalmology, 1996. Kugler, The Hague, pp87–95

19. Palmberg P (1998) Filtering surgery with antimetabolites. In: Leader B, Calkwood JC (eds) Peril in the nerve – glaucoma and clinical neuro-ophthalmology. Proceedings of the New Orleans Academy of Ophthalmology, 1996. Kugler, The Hague, pp171–177

20. Sommer A, Tielsch JM, Katz J, Quigley HA, Gottsch JD, Javitt JC, Martone JF, Royall RM, Witt KA, Ezrine S (1991) Racial differences in the cause-specific prevalence of blindness in east Baltimore. N Engl J Med 325:1412–1417

21. Sommer A, Tielsch JM, Katz J, Quigley HA, Gottsch JD, Javitt J, Singh K (1991) Relationship between intraocular pressure and primary open angle glaucoma among white and black Americans. The Baltimore Eye Survey. Arch Ophthalmol 109:1090–1095

22. The AGIS Investigators (1998) The Advanced Glaucoma Intervention Study (AGIS): 4. Comparison of treatment outcomes within race. Ophthalmology 105:1146–1164

23. The AGIS Investigators (2000) The Advanced Glaucoma Intervention Study (AGIS): 7. The relationship between control of intraocular pressure and visual field deterioration. Am J Ophthalmol 130:429–440

24. The AGIS Investigators (2001) The Advanced Glaucoma Intervention Study (AGIS): 9. Comparison of glaucoma outcomes in black and white patients within treatment groups. Am J Ophthalmol 132:311–320

25. Kass MA, Heuer DK, Higginbotham EJ et al (2002) The Ocular Hypertension Treatment Study. A randomized trial determines that topical ocular hypotensive medication delays or prevents the onset of primary open angle glaucoma. Arch Ophthalmol 120:701–703

A Practical Approach to the Management of Normal Tension Glaucoma

R. A. HITCHINGS

Core Messages

- Normal tension glaucoma is a variety of primary open angle glaucoma where the intra ocular pressure lies within the normal range
- In Caucasian societies it is relatively common and may in rare instances be familial
- The condition usually progresses quite slowly, but in 10% of cases progression may be detected within a short period of follow-up
- A significant reduction in intraocular pressure has been shown to benefit the course of the disease in about 60% of cases
- Other forms of neuroprotection have not been demonstrated to be of benefit but could be considered should intraocular pressure reduction fail to be of use

10.1
Introduction

The management of normal tension glaucoma (NTG) has been a therapeutic challenge for the writer over the past 20 years. For this period of time he has had responsibility for managing a clinic comprising entirely of patients with (possible) NTG. His views on management are based on this practical experience.

10.1.1
Background

10.1.1.1
Diagnosis and Definition

NTG forms a subset of primary open-angle glaucomas (POAG). Phenotypically they differ little from other 'types' of POAG other than the fact that they have a (mean) intraocular pressure (IOP) consistently within the statistically normal range. This glaucoma shares a number of characteristics with high pressure glaucoma (HPG). They tend to have recurrent optic disc haemorrhages [14], peripapillary atrophy is common, as is focal notching of the optic nerve [9, 10], and they appear to progress slowly [5]. Different optic disc phenotypes have been described as myopic, senile sclerotic and focal [9, 10]. Additionally the left eye appears to be affected before the right [25], and they are more likely to have a history of migraine and vasospasm [7]. However, none of these are absolute identifiers for NTG.

Genotypically, however, there may be differences. MYOC mutations are seen in high pressure POAG but less commonly in NTG [1]. The position is reversed with OPTN mutations [27]. While both are commonly seen in families with dominantly inherited open-angle glaucoma, MYOC comprises 3%–5% of its respective population. OPTN mutations with the E 50 K variant were found in 1.5% sporadic NTG, while the M98 K variant was found in 10.6% compared with 4.4% HPG and 3.2% controls (Table 10.1) [2]. To date there is no data for phenotypic separation between NPG patients with and without OPTN mutations.

Table 10.1. Prevalence of E50 K and M98 K by subgroup. (From [2] with permission)

	E50K	χ2 Test Odds ratio (95% CI)	M98K	χ2 Test Odds ratio (95% CI)
HTG (n=183)	0 (0%) (0–2.0)	χ2=2.8, p=0.18, RR=1.02 (0.99–1.04) (1.9–8.4)	8 (4.4%) (1.1–6.4)	χ2=4.6, p=0.03, CR=2.6
NTG (n=132)	2 (1.5%) (0.2–5.4)	χ2=1.5, p=0.51, RR=1.02 (0.99–1.04)	14 (10.6%) (5.9–17.2)	χ2=4.4, p=0.04, CR=3.6 (1.02–13.0)
Controls (n=95)	0 (0%) (0–3.8)		3 (3.2%) (0.7–9.0)	

10.1.1.2
Natural History

Management of patients with NTG has been greatly facilitated by knowledge of the natural history of the condition. This has been obtained in two ways. Firstly, for many years it was the practice of the Moorfields NTG clinic to follow patients without treatment until or unless progression was identified on 'White on White' perimetry. Secondly, the untreated arm of the collaborative NTG (CNTG) study also provided a subset of patients without threat to fixation for which the natural history was available [4, 5]. (A significant but as yet unrealized proportion of the untreated arm of the Early Manifest Glaucoma Study [13] will also have had NTG). The time to progression was very similar in both the Moorfields patients and the CNTG. Both centres noted that progression could be identified in about 10% within 12 months [21], and that no progression could be identified in approximately 30% within 5 years. Threat to fixation was not found in the Moorfields Clinic to result in a greater risk of progression, but if it did occur it was more likely to be noticed by the patient (Fig. 10.1) [21].

As the Moorfields patients were also followed with point-wise linear progression (PROGRESSOR) the rate for individual retinal locations could be established [6]. This was found to exceed 5 dB/year in a few cases, but in the majority to be difficult to distinguish from normal age-related change. Importantly, a change in rate could be established using PROGRESSOR following surgery [3].

Knowledge of this rate of change would be important when deciding on what, if any treatment should be prescribed in this condition.

Long term follow-up of the untreated patient has shown that only a small proportion develop an increase in IOP over time [8]. Should this occur prophylactic IOP reduction ought to be undertaken before further progression of visual field damage be given for the minority whose IOP rises with time.

Summary for the Clinician

- Information is available from white-on-white perimetry from different patient groups confirming that rapid progression occurs in 10%, and no detectable progression within 5 years occurs in 30%

10.1.2
Differential Diagnosis

The differential diagnosis of NTG would include the following:
- Other glaucoma
- Other optic nerve disease
- Retinal disease
- Unreliable visual fields

Fig. 10.1. KM curve indicating time to the detection of W-on-W field loss. Moorfields Data. Values in parentheses refer to the number of eyes. (From [10] with permission)

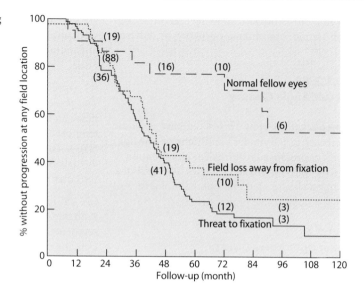

Fig. 10.2. Changes in IOP during sleeping and waking periods. Data from a sleep laboratory demonstrating IOP change with sleep and posture change. Two groups (*open* and *filled* symbols) were measured in the sitting (*circles*) and supine (triangles) positions at daytime and in the supine position (*triangles*) during night. (From [19] with permission)

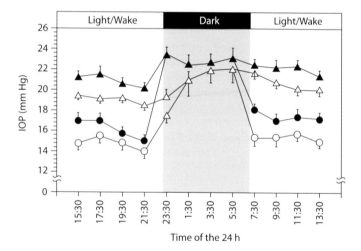

10.1.2.1
Other Glaucoma

10.1.2.1.1
'High Pressure' Glaucoma (HPG)

Increased trabecular resistance results in greater diurnal variation in HPG. This can result in levels that exceed the normal range only occasionally in the 24 h, or with adoption of supine posture [19] (Fig. 10.2).

10.1.2.1.2
Secondary Glaucoma

Steroid-induced increase in outflow resistance can disappear following steroid withdrawal. However, by the time this occurs there may be optic disc cupping and visual field loss. A history of previous topical medication, and/or coincidental eye disease such as vernal conjunctivitis typically treated with topical steroids should alert the ophthalmologist to this possibility – both from the point of view of making the correct diagnosis, but also knowing that future topical steroid use should normally be advised against.

10.1.2.1.3
Occult Angle Closure

Patients with narrow angles can have episodic increases in IOP under conditions of low light levels or prolonged reading. The combination of narrow anterior chamber angles, PAS and disc changes should alert the ophthalmologist and suggest appropriate provocative tests.

10.1.2.2
Other Optic Nerve Disease

10.1.2.2.1
Acquired Optic Nerve Disease: Anterior Ischaemic Optic Neuropathy (AION)

Glaucomatous cupping produces rim thinning without overt pallor. Non-arteritic anterior ischaemic optic neuropathy will usually produce pallor without focal rim thinning. Both will produce retinotopic visual field defects. Non-arteritic AION will often depress colour recognition and reduce foveal sensitivity. Examples of this condition that show progression are rare.

10.1.2.2.2
Developmental Optic Nerve Disease

(a) Large discs
Congenitally large discs will have large C/D ratios. They are usually symmetric between eyes. Often they are seen with coincidental myopia. It would appear that some ethnic groups such as South Indian, and Afro-Caribbean have a disproportionate number of people with large discs. Scanning laser ophthalmoscopy or planimetry that gives quantitative optic disc measurements will allow recognition of this harmless anomaly.

(b) Coloboma
Failure of the foetal fissure to fully close in utero gives rise to large misshapen discs. These may be associated with choroidal and iris colobomata and can on occasion be misdiagnosed as

glaucoma. However the overall disc shape, inequalities in cup depth and an abnormally high number of opticociliary vessels assist diagnosis.

(c) Optic disc pit
The presence of a focal area of laminar weakness can be congenital (when it is usually sited temporally) or polar (when it is acquired in NTG). The former is seen with central visual disturbances from a central serous retinopathy, the latter with focal arcuate visual field defects.

(d) Optic disc drusen
Both buried and exposed drusen can give rise to segmental field defects, mimicking NTG. However, the combination of small disc size plus visualization of the drusen is usually sufficient for the diagnosis. It is important to remember that sudden loss of visual field can occur from drusen due to peripapillary haemorrhage and from an associated AION.

10.1.2.3
Retinal Disease

Visual field defects mimicking glaucoma can be associated with retinal dialyses and retinoschisis. They give rise to atypical visual field defects and may be slowly progressive.

Retinal vascular occlusions can also create sector visual field defects. These will not be associated with concomitant signs of glaucomatous cupping, but will have retinal signs to indicate the correct diagnosis.

10.1.2.4
Visual Pathways Disease

(a) Pre-chiasmal
Optic nerve disease arising from orbital lesions can produce anomalous visual field defects together with optic atrophy but rarely optic nerve head cupping. An exception is the extensive cupping that follows acute intraorbital haemorrhage (typically from orbital roof fractures), resulting in retro laminar infarcts of the optic nerve. The appearance is similar to arteritic AION. In both instances the history and other physical signs should allow the correct diagnosis.

(b) Post-chiasmal
Bilateral visual field defects with or without optic atrophy occur with lesions at varying sites along the visual pathway. Glaucomatous cupping is rarely a feature. However, atrophy in an eye with a pre-existing large C/D ratio can mimic glaucoma. Eyes with visual field defects that do not respect the horizontal meridian, and that have atrophy exceeding manifest cupping should always be referred for a neurological consultation. Routine skull X-rays are insufficient and often misleading, and play little part in the ophthalmological workup. In an elderly population coincidental lesions such as an 'empty sella' can be associated without being causative pathology.

> **Summary for the Clinician**
>
> • Careful examination of the optic nerve and visual field defect should allow differentiation between glaucoma as the cause of visual loss and visual pathway disease as a cause of visual loss

10.1.3
Investigation

10.1.3.1
For the Purpose of Making the Diagnosis

(a) Is the IOP normal?
Day-time diurnal curves may reveal abnormal ranges of IOPs suggesting concomitant reduction in outflow facility. If the mean IOP rises above normal it is reasonable to reclassify the patient.

Recent evidence for nocturnal increases in IOP (especially when associated with falls in systemic blood pressure) suggests another cause for a reduction in perfusion pressure [19]. A surrogate for this rise is to measure the IOP 20 min after the patient has adopted a supine posture. Dramatic increases are worth correcting (see below).

(b) Has the IOP been raised in the past?
A history of previously elevated IOP, or a suggestion of angle closure should be requested.

(c) Does the optic disc have glaucomatous cupping?
The optic nerve should be checked for alternatives to glaucomatous optic neuropathy (GON) with indirect funduscopy using a condensing lens viewing through the dilated pupil. Visibility or otherwise of the RNFL, and the presence of optic atrophy should be checked for.

(d) Is there a developmental cause for a large C/D ratio?
Quantitative measurements of the optic disc size will reveal the presence of 'megadiscs' that would account for a large C/D ratio.

(e) Is there visual field loss?
White-on-white perimetry is not the most sensitive measure of visual function. Repeated perimetry is often needed to confirm the presence of early 'W-on-W' visual field defects.

(f) Is the field loss retinotopic?
The visual field defect needs to follow the pathway of the retinal nerve fibres, and correspond with changes visible at the optic nerve head.

(g) Does the visual loss respect the vertical and not the horizontal meridian?
The visual field defect needs to respect the horizontal and not the vertical meridian.

10.1.3.2
For the Purposes of Identifying Precipitating and Risk Factors

(a) Systemic blood pressure
Incidence data from the Barbados study has shown increased risk of developing GON with reduced systolic and diastolic perfusion pressure [18]. This is likely to be a factor in a proportion of cases of NTG, and is, therefore, worth investigating.

(b) Episodes of massive blood loss
In theory sudden and uncontrolled blood loss could precipitate GON. However, sudden blood loss seems, at best, to be a rare contributor to the pathogenesis of GON.

(c) Nocturnal 'dips'
Severe falls in blood pressure during sleep ('big dips') are associated with progressive visual field loss, and are worth looking for [12]. If asso-

ciated with treatment for essential hypertension the 'dips' can be corrected by a review of the patient's hypotensive medication. If not, mineralocorticoids have been recommended by one centre, but, as yet, there is no prospective evidence for a beneficial effect following their use. An increase in daily exercise is, however, worth recommending.

(d) Reversible changes in vessel diameter – 'vasospasm'

Many (female) patients have a history of 'migraine' either on diagnosis or in the past. The relevance of this to their glaucoma is difficult to ascertain. Peripheral vasospasm, shown as cold hands and feet, and elicited (often from the partner) with the question 'are your hands/feet cold in bed' may also be associated with 'central vasospasm' affecting the vessel calibre in the optic nerve [7]. Peripheral vasospasm can be studied by measuring nail-fold capillary blood flow, and vasospasm identified by the response of these capillaries to stress (such as cold water immersion) [22]. Such changes are probably due to high levels of endothelin release [16].

(e) Rheological changes

Hyperviscosity has been found in a proportion of patients with NTG, and may be a contributory factor in a few cases [14].

(f) Other systemic diseases – diabetes, dysthyroid eye disease

Any associated systemic disease that can affect the integrity of small blood vessels could in theory contribute, but in most instances are not needed for NTG to develop.

(g) Other ocular abnormality – myopia

High myopia is associated with optic atrophy, and may contribute to the development of GON.

> **Summary for the Clinician**
>
> - The investigation of a patient with normal pressure glaucoma should be first to confirm the diagnosis, secondly to monitor to see whether progression is present or is likely to occur, thirdly to assess the presence of any systemic risk factor

10.1.4
Investigation for the Purpose of Management

10.1.4.1
IOP Phasing

It is important to establish a baseline level of IOP. Normally the IOP range does not exceed 3–4 mmHg, so the mean can be taken as the baseline IOP. IOP reduction would aim to achieve a specific fall from this baseline.

Supine levels of IOP can reflect nocturnal levels and if significantly raised above the mean suggest that additional IOP reduction therapy is needed during sleep [12].

10.1.4.2
Optic Nerve and RNFL

Baseline assessment is required, preferably by one of the commercially available imaging devices. Planimetry or stereo photography are both useful, but lack the capability for reliable detection of change (progression). Quantitative methods of optic disc and retinal nerve fibre layer assessment are beginning to demonstrate practical usefulness in detecting change. In one study optic disc change was detected before 'W-on-W' disc change in ocular hypertensives [17]. A second study documented sequential changes in the retinal nerve fibre layer shown with the GDx [26].

10.1.4.3
Visual Function

White-on-white perimetry remains the standard. It is important to take the average sensitivity for each retinal point from the most reliable two of the first three fields. Sequential perimetry is necessary to detect change. Visual fields should be performed every 3–4 months at least for the first 2 years to facilitate the identification of change [30]. Patients who have been followed with stable fields for 5 years can have perimetry every 6 months.

Alternatives to 'W-on-W' perimetry such as 'blue-on-yellow', have been demonstrated to be effective in identifying change in visual function before 'W-on-W' perimetry [15].

10.1.4.4
Optic Nerve Head Perfusion

Perfusion pressure can be estimated from IOP and systemic blood pressure [18]. The range of systemic blood pressure can be found from ambulatory blood pressure monitoring, and should be undertaken in all cases of NTG.

The pulsatile component of total ocular blood flow can be estimated, but as it mainly reflects choroidal rather than optic nerve blood flow changes in pulsatile ocular blood flow (POBF) may bear little correlation to ONH changes.

10.1.4.5
Neurological Consultation

The help of a neurologist should always be sought when there are doubts about the type of visual field loss or whether the optic nerve head change fits the visual loss.

10.1.5
Management

10.1.5.1
Observation

From the remarks above concerning the natural history of NTG and because there is no marker to distinguish between those eyes with rapidly progressing disease, and those without, it is reasonable to choose 'watch without treatment' as the initial approach. Indications for treatment *before* documented progression would include:

(a) An inability to obtain reliable visual fields with the necessary frequency and/or an inability to quantify progressive optic-RNFL changes

(b) Cases with a family history of NTG that suggest rapid progression

(c) Eyes with threat to fixation – where any progression will lead to visual symptoms

(d) Recurrent optic disc haemorrhages – eyes that will progress rapidly

(e) Youth – where any progression is likely to affect quality of life over the patients expected lifetime

10.1.5.2
IOP Reduction

The EMGT [13] and CNTG studies [4], as well as the MEH audit [21], showed that 25%–30% reduction in IOP from baseline is needed to slow if not stabilize the disease.

Initial therapy is best with a prostaglandin-prostamide analogue. If this fails to achieve the required percentage fall then the choice lies between adding a beta blocker, and carbonic anhydrase inhibitors (CAI) inhibitor or an alpha agonist. The topical beta-blocker should only be given in the morning because of possible effects of the beta blocker on systemic blood pressure without simultaneously lowering IOP, thus reducing perfusion pressure [11]. The effects of three different drug combinations on supine and nocturnal IOPs have been studied in a short-term crossover trials, demonstrating rather better IOP stabilization with Latanoprost than a fixed beta blocker CAI inhibitor, than Brimonidine [23] (Fig. 10.3).

A trial of therapy to one eye for a few weeks is the simplest way of assessing IOP fall, and as the amount may be small objective measurements (such as by finding the end point without looking at the tonometer dial) are required.

Fistulizing surgery has been shown to achieve the 30% fall and has been used as treatment for progressing glaucoma [4, 20] (Fig. 10.4).

One study highlighted the complications that can follow the use of peri-operative mitomycin [20].

IOP reduction in this way has been shown to slow the rate of progression in individual cases as well as improve the prognosis for groups. However, even with a 30% reduction a significant proportion will still progress (40% at 4 years; see Fig. 10.4); therefore, alternative approaches that do not affect IOP are needed.

Fig. 10.3. Cross over trial of three drug combinations in eyes with elevated IOP looking at the effect of different topically applied drugs on diurnal IOP curves. (From Orzalezi et al ref 23)

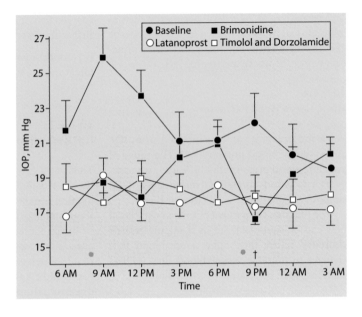

Fig. 10.4. Survival curves showing the effect of IOP falls exceeding 30 % fall from baseline in eyes that had undergone glaucoma surgery. Visual field survival defined as lack of visual field progression following surgery in two groups separated by difference in IOP fall postoperatively. Numbers indicate eyes remaining. (From [20] with permission)

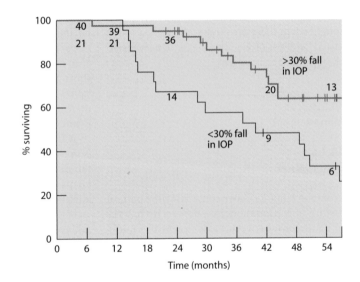

10.1.5.3
Optic Nerve Head Perfusion

As has been identified above, perfusion pressure can be improved by attending to both IOP and systemic blood pressure over the 24 h [12].

Calcium channel blockers and magnesium can counter reversible constriction arteriolar constriction [24, 29]. There is some evidence from Japanese studies that these have been of benefit [28]. However, as some calcium channel blockers will also lower systemic blood pressure their use might be counterproductive! The help of an internist should be sought when considering this approach.

10.1.5.4
Neurorescue

Neurorescue is a recently introduced term in ophthalmology that addresses the concept of continuing neuronal loss from agents released by neurones damaged from the disease itself [31]. The evidence comes from studies that have looked at experimental animal models of glaucoma. Alpha agonists, NMDA antagonists as well as calcium channel blockers have all been suggested as possible agents for this purpose. Randomized controlled trials of alpha agonists and NMDA antagonists for the management of NTG are currently underway. To date there is no evidence that they are beneficial in the long term.

Summary for the Clinician

- Initial treatment is justified if progression is occurring. Management should therefore take the form of intensive perimetry, possibly augmented by sequential optic nerve head imaging; treatment is justified for progression and may not be justified in the absence of progression

Therapeutic Approach

- Unless otherwise indicated an initial "wait and see" approach is justified.
- Initial treatment is by IOP reduction, by an initial trial of therapy and if necessary by combination therapy or surgery
- Failure of a 30% reduction to eliminate progression justifies the use of other neuroprotectant approaches

References

1. Alward L, Fingert JH, Cooke M A, Johnson AT, Lerner SF, Junquez D et al. (1998) Clinical features associated with mutations in the chromosome 1 open angle glaucoma gene. N Engl J Med 338: 1022–1027
2. Aung T, Ebenezer ND, Brice G, Child A, Prescott O, Lehmann OJ et al. (2003) Prevalance of optoneurin sequence variants in adult primary open angle glaucoma, implications for diagnostic testing. J Med Genet 40:e101
3. Bhandari A, Crabb DP, Poinoosawmy D, Fitzke FW, Hitchings RA, Noureddin BN (1997) Effect of surgery on visual field progression in normal-tension glaucoma. Ophthalmology 104:1131–1137
4. Collaborative normal tension glaucoma study group (1998) The effectiveness of intraocular pressure reduction in the treatment of normal-tension glaucoma. Am J Ophthal 126:498–505
5. Drance S, Anderson DR, Schulzer M, Collaborative Normal-Tension Glaucoma Study Group (2001) Risk factors for progression of visual field abnormalities in normal-tension glaucoma. Am J Ophthalmol 131:699–708
6. Fitzke FW, Hitchings.R A, Poinoosawmy D, McNaught AI (1996) Analysis of visual field progression in glaucoma. Br J Ophthalmol 80:40–48
7. Flammer J, Pache M, Resink T (2001) Vasospasm, its role in the pathogenesis of diseases with particular reference to the eye. Prog Retin Eye Res 20:319–349
8. Fontana L, Poinoosawmy D, Wu J, Hitchings RA (1996) The natural history of the intraocular pressure in untreated normal tension glaucoma: a long-term follow up study. Invest Ophthalmol Vis Sci 37:S927
9. Geijssen HC, Greve EL (1987) The spectrum of primary open angle glaucoma. I: Senile sclerotic glaucoma versus high tension glaucoma. Ophthalmic Surg 18:207–213
10. Geijssen HC, Greve EL (1990) Focal ischaemic normal pressure glaucoma versus high pressure glaucoma. Doc Ophthalmol 75:291–301
11. Greve EL, Rulo AH, Drance SM, Crichton AC, Mills RP, Hoyng PF (1997) Reduced intraocular pressure and increased ocular perfusion pressure in normal tension glaucoma: a review of short-term studies with three dose regimens of latanoprost treatment. Surv Ophthalmol 41[Suppl 2]:S89–S92
12. Hayreh SS, Zimmerman MB, Podhajsky P, Alward WL (1994) Nocturnal arterial hypotension and its role in optic nerve head and ocular ischemic disorders. Am J Ophthalmol 117:603–624

13. Heijl A, Leske MC, Bengtsson B, Bengtsson B, Hussein M (2002) EMGT group. Reduction of intraocular pressure and glaucoma progression: results from the Early Manifest Glaucoma Trial. Arch Ophthalmol 120:1268–1279
14. Hoyng PF, de Jong N, Oosting H, Stilma J (1992) Platelet aggregation, disc haemorrhage and progressive loss of visual fields in glaucoma. A seven year follow-up study on glaucoma. Int Ophthalmol 16:65–73
15. Johnson CA, Sample PA, Cioffi GA, Liebmann JR, Weinreb RN (2002) Structure and function evaluation (SAFE): I. criteria for glaucomatous visual field loss using standard automated perimetry (SAP) and short wavelength automated perimetry (SWAP). Am J Ophthalmol 134:177–185
16. Kaiser HJ, Flammer J, Wenk M, Luscher T (1995) Endothelin-1 plasma levels in normal-tension glaucoma: abnormal response to postural changes. Graefes Arch Clin Exp Ophthalmol 233:484–488
17. Kamal DS, Viswanathan AC, Garway-Heath DF, Hitchings RA, Poinoosawmy D, Bunce C (1999) Detection of optic disc change with the Heidelberg retina tomograph before confirmed visual field change in ocular hypertensives converting to early glaucoma. Br J Ophthalmol 83:290–294
18. Leske MC, Wu SY, Nemesure B, Hennis A (2002) Incident open-angle glaucoma and blood pressure. Arch Ophthalmol 120:954–959
19. Liu JH, Kripke DF, Twa MD, Hoffman RE, Mansberger SL, Rex KM et al. (1999) Twenty-four-hour pattern of intraocular pressure in the aging population. Invest Ophthalmol Vis Sci 40:2912–2917
20. Membrey WL, Bunce C, Poinoosawmy DP, Fitzke FW, Hitchings RA (2001) Glaucoma surgery with or without adjunctive antiproliferatives in normal tension glaucoma: 2. Visual field progression. Br J Ophthalmol 85:696–701
21. Membrey WL, Poinoosawmy DP, Bunce C, Fitzke FW, Hitchings RA (2000) Comparison of visual field progression in patients with normal pressure glaucoma between eyes with and without visual field loss that threatens fixation. Br J Ophthalmol 84:1154–1158
22. Orgul S, Kaiser HJ, Flammer J, Gasser P (1995) Systemic blood pressure and capillary blood-cell velocity in glaucoma patients: a preliminary study. Eur J Ophthalmol 5:88–91
23. Orzalesi N, Rossetti L, Bottoli A, Fumagalli E, Forgagnola P (2003) The effect of Latanoprost, Brimonidine or a fixed combination of Timolol and Dorzolamide on circadian intraocular pressure in patients with glaucoma or ocular hypertension. Arch Ophthalmol 121:453–457
24. Piltz JR, Bose S, Lanchoney D (1998) The effect of nimodipine, a centrally active calcium antagonist, on visual function and mascular blood flow in patients with normal-tension glaucoma and control subjects [see comments]. J Glaucoma 7:336–342
25. Poinoosawmy D, Fontana L, Wu J, Bunce C, Hitchings RA (1998) Frequency of asymmetric visual field defects in normal-tension and high tension glaucoma. Ophthalmolgy 105:988–991
26. Poinoosawmy D, Tan JC, Bunce C, Membrey LW, Hitchings RA (2000) Longitudinal nerve fibre layer thickness change in normal-pressure glaucoma. Graefes Arch Clin Exp Ophthalmol 238:965–969
27. Rezai T, Child A, Hitchings RA, Brice G, Miller L, Coca-Prados M et al. (2002) Adult onset primary open angle glaucoma caused by mutations in optineurin. Science 295:1077–1079
28. Sawada A, Kitazawa Y, Yamamoto T, Okabe I, Ichien K (1996) Prevention of visual field defect progression with brovincamine in eyes with normal-tension glaucoma. Ophthalmology 103:283–288
29. Strenn K, Matulla B, Wolzt M, Findl O, Bekes MC, Lamsfuss U et al. (1998) Reversal of endothelin-1-induced ocular hemodynamic effects by low-dose nifedipine in humans. Clin Pharmacol Ther 63:54–63
30. Viswanathan AC, Hitchings RA, Fitzke FW (1997) How often do patients need visual field tests? Graefes Arch Clin Exp Ophthalmol 235:563–568
31. Weinreb RN, Levin LA (1999) Is neuroprotection a viable therapy for glaucoma? Arch Ophthalmol 117:1540–1544

Pseudoexfoliation Glaucoma

Ursula Schlötzer-Schrehardt, Gottfried O.H. Naumann

11

Core Messages

- PEX syndrome has been characterized a generalized disorder of the extracellular matrix, an elastic microfibrillopathy, which is associated with excessive production and progressive accumulation of an abnormal extracellular fibrillar material in intra- and extraocular tissues
- Diagnostic criteria of PEX syndrome comprise the observation of PEX material deposits after pupillary dilation, dispersion and deposition of pigment on anterior segment structures, peripupillary atrophy, and poor mydriasis; early stages can be diagnosed by the presence of a diffuse-matte film on the surface of the anterior lens capsule
- The probability of PEX eyes to develop glaucoma is up to 40% within 10 years. Clinical characteristics of this PEX-associated secondary open-angle glaucoma include high intraocular pressure levels, marked diurnal pressure fluctuations and spikes, increased chamber angle pigmentation, small optic disks, rapid progression of glaucomatous damage, and often poor response to medications
- The primary cause of chronic pressure elevation is an increased outflow resistance in the trabecular meshwork caused by blockage of the outflow channels by locally produced PEX material in the juxtacanalicular tissue followed by degenerative changes of Schlemm's canal wall
- Clinical management of patients with PEX glaucoma should consider diurnal pressure monitoring, vigorous reduction and stabilization of intraocular pressure, close follow-up examinations, and expectation of a higher complication rate during and after surgery

11.1
Background

Pseudoexfoliation (PEX) syndrome is a common age-related, though often overlooked disorder which predisposes to a number of ocular complications, most notably glaucoma [32]. It is presently acknowledged as the most common identifiable cause of open-angle glaucoma, accounting for the majority of glaucoma in some countries and for about 25% of all open-angle glaucomas worldwide [42]. PEX-associated open-angle glaucoma (PEX glaucoma, exfolia-tion glaucoma, capsular glaucoma) develops in about half of patients with PEX syndrome over time [44]. It has been estimated that the number of people with PEX syndrome in the world varies between 60 and 100 million [43], and thus, the socioeconomic importance of the associated glaucoma has increased considerably in recent years. With an increasing mean age in western populations, PEX is increasing in prevalence, although it is not an integral part of aging but represents a distinct clinical entity. Despite its clinical significance and many new insights in recent years, the PEX-associated glaucoma still is amazingly underestimated, often not exactly diagnosed and not clearly differentiated from primary open-angle glaucoma (POAG) leading to unexpected problems in clinical management and surgery.

Despite extensive research, the etiology of PEX remains unclear; however, it has been characterized as a disorder of the extracellular matrix associated with the multifocal production of an abnormal extracellular matrix product [32]. This results in the gradual accumulation of a specific fibrillar substance (PEX material) in virtually all tissues of the anterior segment of the eye, diagnostically most important on the lens and pupillary margin. There is active involvement of the lens, the iris, the ciliary body, the zonular apparatus, the trabecular meshwork, and the cornea. These changes in turn predispose to a spectrum of intraocular complications including chronic open-angle glaucoma, angle-closure glaucoma, lens subluxation or dislocation, pigment dispersion, insufficient mydriasis, posterior synechiae, blood-aqueous barrier defects and anterior chamber hypoxia, early corneal endothelial decompensation, and a significantly higher rate of intra- and postoperative complications in cataract surgery (Table 11.1) [32, 43].

Recent evidence indicates that the ocular features of PEX syndrome are actually only one facet of a broader systemic process, since PEX deposits have been found in the skin and in connective tissue portions of various visceral organs, such as lungs, liver and heart [47, 53]. Although the clinical consequences of these systemic deposits are not yet fully clear, there is increasing evidence for an association of PEX with cerebrovascular and cardiovascular disease. Preliminary reports suggest a relationship with transient ischemic attacks, aneurysms of the abdominal aorta, and a history of angina, hypertension, myocardial infarction, or stroke [31, 51]. Hyperhomocystinemia has been suggested as one possible cause for an increased vascular risk in PEX patients [59]. However, the mortality rate appears to be not increased in PEX patients. Other investigators reported on an association of PEX syndrome and hearing loss or Alzheimer's disease [43].

Table 11.1. Clinical complications of PEX syndrome

1. Involvement of lens, ciliary body, zonules
   Cataract
   Phacodonesis
   Lens subluxation
   Angle-closure glaucoma
   Complications in cataract surgery
      (e.g., zonular rupture, vitreous loss,
      IOL decentration)

2. Involvement of the iris
   Pigment dispersion
   Poor mydriasis
   Capillary hemorrhages
   Blood–aqueous barrier defects and increased
      aqueous flare
   Anterior chamber hypoxia
   Posterior synechiae

3. Involvement of the trabecular meshwork
   Intraocular hypertension
   Open-angle glaucoma
   Retinal vein occlusion

4. Involvement of the cornea
   Corneal endothelial decompensation
   Corneal endothelial proliferation/migration

11.2
Pathobiology of PEX Syndrome

11.2.1
Pathogenesis

The exact pathogenesis of PEX syndrome is still not known. However, the pathologic process is characterized by the progressive accumulation of an abnormal fibrillar matrix product, which is either the result of an excessive production or an insufficient breakdown and is regarded as pathognomonic for the disease based on its unique ultrastructural criteria (Fig. 11.1 A,B) [32, 43]. The characteristic fibrils, which are composed of microfibrillar subunits resembling elastic microfibrils (Fig. 11.1 C), contain predominantly epitopes of elastic fibers, such as elastin, tropoelastin, amyloid P, vitronectin, and components of elastic microfibrils, such as fibrillin-1, microfibril-associated glycoprotein MAGP-1, and the latent TGF-β binding proteins LTBP-1 and LTBP-2 by immunohistochemistry (Fig. 11.1 D). Antibodies to such elastic mi-

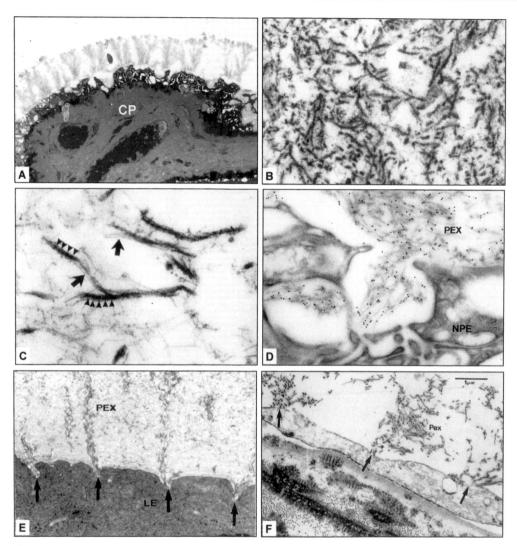

Fig. 11.1 A–F. Light and transmission electron micrographs showing structure and origin of PEX material. **A** Bush-like, feathery PEX deposits on ciliary process (*CP*) by light microscopy (toluidine blue; ×400). **B** Ultrastructure of PEX fibrils. **C** Aggregation of microfibrils (*arrows*) into mature PEX fibrils showing cross-bands at 50 nm (*arrowheads*). **D** Immuno-gold labeling using antibodies against fibrillin-1 showing clear association of the gold marker with PEX fibrils emerging from a nonpigmented ciliary epithelial cell (*NPE*). **E** Intracapsular PEX fibrils emerging from pits (*arrows*) in the preequatorial lens epithelium (*LE*). **F** Apparent production of PEX fibrils (*arrows*) by a trabecular endothelial cell

crofibril components, particularly LTBP-1, have been proven useful as markers for PEX deposits in intra- and extraocular tissues. These immunohistochemical and recent molecular biologic data confirming an overexpression of fibrillin-1 and LTBP mRNA in most cell types involved [49] give strong support to the elastic microfibril theory first proposed by Streeten [52], which explains PEX syndrome as a type of elastosis particularly affecting elastic microfibrils.

These PEX fibrils appear to be multifocally produced by various intra- and extraocular cell types, including the preequatorial lens epithelium (Fig. 11.1 E), non-pigmented ciliary epithelium, trabecular endothelium (Fig. 11.1 F), corneal endothelium, vascular endothelial cells, and virtually all cell types in the iris, by active fibrillogenesis [32, 43]. This fibrillogenesis is accompanied by a destruction of the normal extracellular matrix of the cells, normally represented by their basement membrane, and is followed by a degeneration of the cells involved due to a disturbed cell–matrix interaction (degenerative fibrillopathy).

11.2.2
Pathogenetic Factors

Excessive matrix accumulation may be due either to increased de novo synthesis or decreased turnover of matrix components or both and may be influenced by growth factors, proteolytic enzymes and their inhibitors, and free radicals.

Biochemical analyses showed significantly increased concentrations of the transforming growth factor TGF-β1, both in its latent and active form, in the aqueous humor of PEX patients with and without glaucoma compared to age-matched controls with cataract or POAG [49]. This growth factor has been known as a powerful modulator of matrix formation in many fibrotic diseases. Evidence has been also provided for an enhanced mRNA expression and local synthesis of TGF-β1 by anterior segment tissues, suggesting a central role for TGF-β1 in the promotion of this fibrotic process [49].

Aqueous humor from PEX patients also had higher levels of matrix metalloproteinases MMP-2 and MMP-3, as well as their inhibitors TIMP-1 and TIMP-2, as compared to controls [50]. However, levels of endogenously active MMP-2, which is the major MMP in human aqueous humor, were significantly decreased as was the ratio of MMP-2 to TIMP-2. These findings suggest that an excess of TIMP-2 over MMP-2 and a reduced MMP-2 activity in the aqueous humor of PEX eyes may promote the abnormal matrix accumulation due to impaired matrix turnover. TIMPs also bind to PEX material creating so-called cold spots for proteolysis.

Significantly reduced levels of ascorbic acid, an important free radical scavenger in the eye,

and concomitantly increased levels of 8-Isoprostaglandin-F2α, a marker of oxidative stress, have further been reported in the aqueous humor of PEX patients [16], suggesting a faulty antioxidative defense system and increased oxidative stress in the pathogenesis of PEX syndrome.

11.2.3
Pathogenetic Concept

The currently acknowledged pathogenetic concept describes PEX syndrome as a specific type of a stress-induced elastosis, an elastic microfibrillopathy, associated with the excessive production of elastic microfibrils and their aggregation into typical PEX fibrils by a variety of potentially elastogenic cells (Fig. 11.2) [43, 44]. Growth factors, particularly TGF-β1, increased cellular and oxidative stress, but also the stable aggregation of misfolded stressed proteins in the sense of a conformational disease, appear to be involved in this fibrotic process. Due to an imbalance of MMPs and TIMPs and extensive cross-linking processes involved in PEX fiber formation, the newly formed material is not properly degraded but progressively accumulates within the tissues over time with potentially deleterious effects, e.g. in the trabecular meshwork. In this scenario, TGF-β1 and TIMP-1/2 may be key molecules, which represent potential target molecules for specific therapeutic approaches in PEX patients.

11.2.4
Etiology

The role of genetic and environmental factors in the pathogenesis of PEX syndrome is not known, although a genetic predisposition is very likely. Lines of evidence that support a genetic basis for PEX include familial aggregation, transmission in two-generation families, higher concordance rates in monozygous twins, an increased risk of PEX in relatives of affected patients, loss of heterozygosity, HLA studies, and geographic clustering [3, 35]. Preliminary linkage analyses identified two putative gene loci,

Fig. 11.2. Pathogenetic concept of PEX syndrome

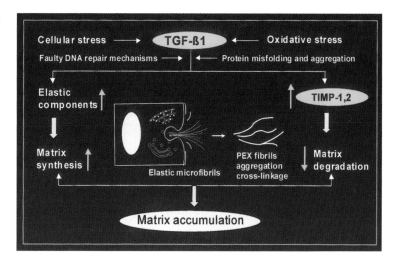

2p16 and 2q35–36, in association with PEX syndrome. PEX syndrome appears to be inherited as an autosomal dominant trait whose late onset and incomplete penetrance pose considerable problems to genetic analyses [35].

However, a number of nongenetic environmental factors have also been implicated in pathogenesis. These include ultraviolet light, dietary factors, autoimmunity, infectious agents, and trauma. Therefore, it appears that a combination of genetic and nongenetic factors may be involved in the etiopathogenesis of PEX.

Summary for the Clinician

- PEX syndrome is a generalized disorder of the extracellular matrix associated with the excessive production and progressive accumulation of an abnormal fibrillar material in intra- and extraocular tissues
- The pathologic matrix product appears to be multifocally produced by various intra- and extraocular cell types involving all tissues of the anterior segment
- Recent research data suggest a special form of an elastosis, an elastic microfibrillopathy
- The fibrogenic growth factor TGF-β1, the tissue inhibitors of matrixmetalloproteinases TIMP-1/2, and oxidative stress appear to be causally involved in pathogenesis
- There is evidence for a genetic basis of PEX syndrome

11.3
Clinical Diagnosis

11.3.1
Manifest PEX Syndrome

The most important diagnostic criteria of PEX syndrome are the whitish flake-like deposits of PEX material on anterior segment structures, particularly on the anterior lens surface and the pupillary margin (Fig. 11.3 A–C), occasionally also on the posterior surface of the cornea (Fig. 11.3 D), on the anterior surface of intraocular lens implants, and on the anterior vitreous face in aphakic eyes [43]. However, the majority of intraocular PEX deposits cannot be observed by direct biomicroscopy, and the accumulations on zonules, ciliary processes (Fig. 11.3 E), and trabecular meshwork may be only detected on gonioscopy or cycloscopy or may be visualized by high resolution ultrasound biomicroscopy [12].

The characteristic target-shaped pattern on the lens, consisting of a rather homogenous central disc, an intermediate clear zone, and a peripheral granular zone, can be only seen after pupillary dilation. In routine examinations without pupillary dilation, the diagnosis may be easily missed, because the central disc may be very subtle or even absent in 20 %–50 % of cases. The central disc, corresponding to the size of the pupil, appears to result from diffuse sedi-

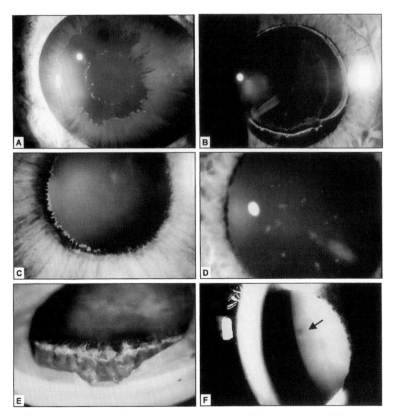

Fig. 11.3 A–F. Clinical signs of PEX syndrome. **A** Classic target-shaped pattern on the lens with the central disc and peripheral zone separated by a clear zone. **B** The central disc may be absent and the peripheral zone may show curled edges as illustrated here. **C** PEX deposits on the pupillary border. **D** Retro-corneal PEX deposits. **E** PEX deposits on ciliary processes and zonules as observed through an iris defect. **F** Appearance of an early stage with a rub-off defect (*arrow*) in the homogenous precapsular layer of the supranasal area of the lens

mentation of PEX material from the aqueous, whereas the peripheral granular zone builds up by undisturbed accumulation of nodular PEX aggregates produced by the iris pigment epithelium; the intermediate clear zone is created by abrasive movements of the peripupillary iris during pupillary movement [32]. Variations of this general pattern include, e.g., the lack of a central disc (Fig. 11.3 B), bridges of PEX material crossing the intermediate clear zone, and a layered or striated peripheral granular zone with or without curled edges (Fig 3B). In the clinically invisible preequatorial region of the lens, PEX aggregates appear to be locally produced by the metabolically active preequatorial lens epithelium, to penetrate the lens capsule and loosen the

attachment of the zonular fibers to the anterior lens capsule, giving rise to a pronounced zonular weakness in PEX eyes [32].

In addition to deposits of PEX material, several other clinical signs aid in the diagnosis (Table 11.2) [32, 43]. Pigment loss from the peripupillary iris pigment epithelium and its deposition on anterior chamber structures is a hallmark of PEX syndrome. Pigment dispersion is caused by rubbing of the peripupillary iris against the rough anterior lens surface during pupillary movement and rupture of the degenerative iris pigment epithelial cells with liberation of melanin granules (Fig. 11.4 A). This manifests clinically in a peripupillary atrophy producing a characteristic "moth-eaten" transil-

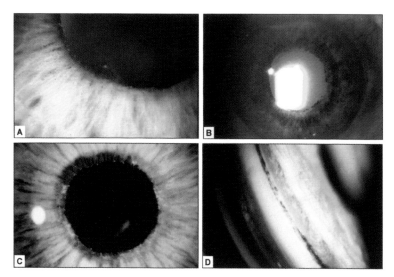

Fig. 11.4 A–D. Additional clinical signs in PEX eyes. **A** Pigment loss from the peripupillary iris pigment epithelium. **B** Peripupillary atrophy producing a characteristic "moth-eaten" transillumination pattern. **C** Pupillary ruff defects. **D** Uneven trabecular meshwork pigmentation

lumination pattern (Fig. 11.4 B), pupillary ruff defects (Fig. 11.4 C), pigment dispersion after pupillary dilation, and deposition of melanin granules on the iris surface, the corneal endothelium, and the trabecular meshwork (Fig. 11.4 D). Increased trabecular meshwork pigmentation, particularly in the inferior half, is a prominent sign of PEX syndrome. Unlike pigment dispersion syndrome, the distribution of the pigment tends to be uneven or patchy and less well defined. Pigment is also characteristically deposited on or anterior to Schwalbe's line (Sampaolesi's line).

Further PEX-associated clinical signs that alert the clinician to the presence of PEX include phacodonesis, iris stroma atrophy, iris hemorrhages after pupillary dilation, increased aqueous flare values, elevated intraocular pressure, and insufficient pupillary dilation, particularly if asymmetrically present.

Table 11.2. Clinical signs of PEX syndrome

1. Diagnostic signs
   PEX material on anterior segment structures
2. Pigment-related signs
   Pigment dispersion in anterior chamber after pupillary dilation
   Peripupillary atrophy, transillumination defects, loss of pupillary ruff
   Pigment deposition on anterior segment structures (iris, cornea, trabecular meshwork)
3. Other signs (asymmetry!)
   Insufficient mydriasis, unequal pupil sizes and pupil responses
   Iris stroma atrophy
   Iris hemorrhages after pupillary dilation
   Increased aqueous flare values
   Elevated intraocular pressure
   Phacodonesis

11.3.2
Masked PEX Syndrome

Posing a diagnostic challenge, the deposits on the lens may be obscured by posterior synechiae. In cases of circular posterior synechiae, which frequently form in PEX eyes, particularly under miotic therapy, the evaluation of the anterior lens surface may be hindered and PEX deposits may be masked by the synechiae ("masked PEX syndrome") [29]. In these cases, high resolution ultrasound biomicroscopy may be useful to reveal PEX deposits on the lens or zonules [12, 32].

11.3.3
Early Stages of PEX Syndrome

The classical picture of lens deposits represents, however, a very late stage of the disease, which is preceded by a long, chronic, preclinical course. By thorough biomicroscopic examination, a diffuse-matte homogenous film on the surface of the anterior lens capsule can be observed prior to the formation of typical PEX deposits [32, 55]. To visualize these early changes at the slit-lamp, it has been suggested to place the slit beam at 45° to the axis of observation, reducing the light source, and focus temporally from the center of the lens to highlight the subtle deposits on the lens surface [43]. Electron microscopy shows this surface film to consist of a layer of microfibrils, a precursor of PEX fibrils, diffusely deposited on the entire surface of the anterior lens capsule from the aqueous humor. As the precapsular layer becomes thicker, focal defects begin to form in this precapsular layer by abrasive movements of the iris, often in the upper nasal quadrant, which further enlarge and become confluent to form the classical picture of manifest PEX syndrome (Fig. 11.3 F).

Additional clinical signs, which help alert the ophthalmologist to the presence of these early stages, comprise pupillary atrophy of the iris pigment epithelium, melanin dispersion associated with pupillary dilation, an increased trabecular pigmentation, and poor mydriasis [36]. As PEX often is an asymmetric condition, comparison with the fellow eye is diagnostically helpful in highlighting these early changes.

11.3.4
Asymmetry of Involvement

For unknown reasons, patients can present with either unilateral or bilateral involvement, which can be markedly asymmetric. Unilateral involvement is often regarded as a precursor to bilateral involvement. PEX syndrome manifests unilaterally in about 50 %–70 % of patients and the conversion rates from clinically unilateral to bilateral disease were found to vary from 15 % to 40 % within 5 years [43].

Clinically, the involved eye often has a poorer visual acuity, more advanced lens opacity, higher intraocular pressure, a smaller pupil, and a more pronounced trabecular pigmentation than the noninvolved fellow eye. Histopathologically however, both eyes are involved, with PEX material being almost invariably present on electron microscopy in the conjunctiva [36] and in the iris of the clinically uninvolved fellow eye [10, 15]. These early changes noted in fellow eyes, particularly subtle PEX deposits in the dilator muscle and blood vessel walls of the iris, may account for the clinical signs characteristic of early stages, such as pigment dispersion, peripupillary atrophy, insufficient mydriasis, and blood–aqueous barrier defects leading to increased aqueous flare values. They further support the concept of PEX syndrome as a generalized, basically bilateral disorder with a clinically marked asymmetric presentation. Whether subtle differences in ocular blood flow, aqueous humor dynamics, or blood–aqueous barrier function might be responsible for this asymmetric manifestation, remains to be determined.

11.3.5
Differential Diagnosis

The differential diagnosis of PEX syndrome has to consider the rare true exfoliation of the lens, fibrin and amyloid deposits on the anterior lens capsule, and disorders associated with melanin dispersion in the anterior segment, e.g., pigment dispersion syndrome or pigmentary glaucoma, Fuchs' heterochromic iridocyclitis, uveitis, diabetes mellitus, etc. Retrocorneal PEX accumulations may be misdiagnosed as inflammatory precipitates.

True exfoliation of the lens capsule is a rare clinical entity, which typically results from exposure to extremely high temperatures, but idiopathic cases have also been described. In contrast to PEX syndrome, where a newly formed material is deposited on the surface of the intact lens capsule, true lens exfoliation is characterized by a splitting and delamination of the anterior lens capsule.

In pigment dispersion syndrome or glaucoma, the trabecular pigmentation is dense and even compared to the irregular patchy pigmentation in PEX syndrome/glaucoma. The iris transillumination defects of pigment dispersion syndrome/glaucoma appear as midperipheral radial spokes, whereas those in PEX appear as moth-eaten patches around the pupil. However, PEX syndrome may subsequently develop after long-standing pigmentary glaucoma and may lead to an uncontrolled pressure rise in those patients [54].

Although pigment dispersion after mydriasis or surgery can be so pronounced that heterochromia iridium is produced in PEX patients, Fuchs' heterochromic iridocyclitis, uveitis, diabetes, and other conditions associated with pigment changes can usually be readily distinguished.

Summary for the Clinician

- Pupillary dilation is essential for an accurate clinical diagnosis
- Pigment-related signs, e.g., pigment dispersion and peripupillary atrophy, and other signs, e.g., poor mydriasis and iris hemorrhages, aid in the diagnosis in addition to PEX material depositions
- Circular posterior synechiae may impede the diagnosis (masked PEX syndrome)
- Early stages of PEX syndrome can be diagnosed by presence of a diffuse-matte film on the surface of the anterior lens capsule accompanied by pigment-related signs
- Ultrastructural alterations of the iris of all fellow eyes in clinically unilateral cases suggest PEX syndrome to be a bilateral disorder with asymmetric manifestation

11.4
Open-Angle Glaucoma in PEX Syndrome

11.4.1
Epidemiology

PEX syndrome occurs in all geographic regions worldwide with reported prevalence rates varying between 5% and 40% of the general population over the age of 60 [4, 43]. All studies report on a significant increase of PEX syndrome with age, with its incidence doubling every decade after the age of 50. Only exceptionally, PEX can be diagnosed in younger patients under the age of 40, mostly as a consequence of prior intraocular surgery or trauma to the anterior segment, particularly to the iris, which may serve as a trigger for the premature development of PEX in a predisposed individual or point to the possibility of an infectious etiology.

Among glaucoma patients, the frequency of PEX syndrome is usually high and has been reported to range from 10% to 30% in the United States, from 50% to 60% in Northern Europe, and up to 87% of glaucoma patients requiring trabeculectomy in Greece. At our department, about 40% of all glaucoma patients undergoing filtering surgery have PEX syndrome.

Elevated intraocular pressure with or without glaucomatous damage occurs in 15%–50% of PEX patients, or about 6–10 times the rate in eyes without PEX syndrome. The probability of PEX eyes to develop glaucoma has been reported to vary from 5% to 35% within 5 years and from 15% to 40% within 10 years; the progression from unilateral to bilateral glaucoma was found to be 48% of patients with bilateral PEX syndrome within 15 years. In a recent study involving patients with clinically unilateral PEX syndrome, conversion to PEX glaucoma was 32% in the initially involved eyes and 38% in the initially noninvolved fellow eyes within 10 years, suggesting that glaucoma may develop before there are any clinical signs of PEX material [38]. The relative risk of conversion to glaucoma was found to be dependent on initial intraocular pressure, degree of pupillary dilation, and difference in pressure between the fellow eyes.

11.4.2
Clinical Features

Compared to POAG, PEX glaucoma has a more serious clinical course and worse prognosis. It is typically associated with higher mean intraocular pressure levels, greater diurnal pressure fluctuations, marked pressure spikes, a higher fre-

Table 11.3. Clinical features of PEX glaucoma

High intraocular pressure (>35 mmHg) at the time of diagnosis
Significant fluctuations in the diurnal curve of intraocular pressure
Marked spiking and pressure peaks
Acute intraocular pressure rises following mydriasis
More often asymmetric (2/3 unilateral)
Significant amount of pigment dispersion and trabecular pigmentation
Rapid progression of optic nerve damage and loss of visual field
Often poor response to medical therapy
Frequent and early need for surgical intervention

quency and severity of optic nerve damage, more rapid visual field loss, poorer response to medications, and more frequent necessity for surgical intervention (Table 11.3) [19, 20].

PEX glaucoma further differs from POAG by a more frequent asymmetry of manifestation, more pronounced chamber angle pigmentation, and acute pressure rises after mydriasis. In contrast to patients with POAG, patients with PEX glaucoma behave like normal persons after steroid application, i.e., only one third responds with a distinct pressure rise.

The percentage area of optic disk pallor was shown to be significantly greater in PEX eyes than in control eyes and the mean disk area has been reported to be significantly smaller in eyes with PEX, with or without glaucoma, than in POAG eyes and normal control eyes [14]. There were, however, no significant differences in neuroretinal rim area, area of peripapillary atrophy, rim:disk ratio, cup area and cup volume between PEX eyes and control or POAG eyes [14, 39], but cupping and neuroretinal rim defects tended to be more diffuse in PEX glaucoma compared to POAG [57]. The occurrence of a relatively small optic disk in eyes with PEX glaucoma is diagnostically important, because a small optic cup indicating glaucomatous optic nerve damage in small disks may erroneously be considered normal.

A significant correlation between the intraocular pressure level at the time of diagnosis and the mean visual field defect could be only established in PEX glaucoma but not in POAG patients [56], suggesting intraocular pressure as the main risk factor for glaucomatous damage in this type of glaucoma. Correspondingly, decrease in intraocular pressure fluctuations and lowering of mean intraocular pressure level has been shown to improve visual field prognosis much more in PEX glaucoma than in POAG [1]. These findings suggest that glaucomatous damage in patients with PEX glaucoma may be more directly related to intraocular pressure than in POAG patients, where the situation may be more complex. The rapid progression of PEX glaucoma probably reflects the cumulative effects of the daily trauma of intraocular pressure spikes on the optic nerve.

11.4.3
Pathomechanisms of Glaucoma Development

11.4.3.1
PEX Material Deposition

The cause of chronic pressure elevation in PEX eyes is an increased outflow resistance in the trabecular meshwork [5], most probably caused by a blockage of the outflow channels by PEX material. Although there may be deposits of PEX material throughout the trabecular meshwork, the focus of PEX material accumulation and pathologic alterations is the juxtacanalicular tissue beneath the inner wall of Schlemm's canal, the site of greatest resistance to aqueous outflow, which becomes thickened through gradual deposition of PEX material (Fig. 11.5 A,B), often associated with degenerative changes of Schlemm's canal including narrowing, fragmentation, and obstruction in advanced cases (Fig. 11.5 C) [8, 46]. Ultrastructural indications suggest that the PEX fibrils are locally produced by the endothelial cells lining Schlemm's canal leading to a progressive accumulation of the pathologic matrix product in the subendothelial area, thus limiting access of aqueous humor to Schlemm's canal (Fig.

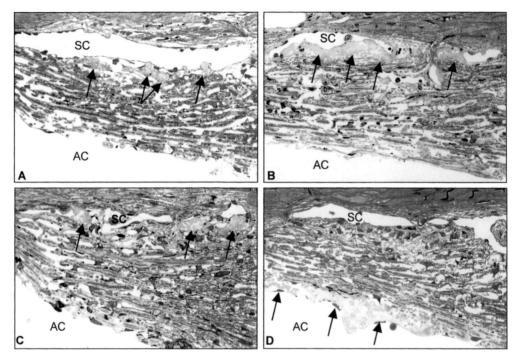

Fig. 11.5 A–D. Light micrographs showing involvement of the trabecular meshwork in PEX syndrome (semithin sections, toluidine blue; ×250; *AC*, anterior chamber; *SC*, Schlemm's canal). **A** Accumulation of small deposits of PEX material (*arrows*) in the juxtacanalicular meshwork. **B** Accumulation of large masses of PEX material (*arrows*) in the juxtacanalicular tissue. **C** Disorganization of Schlemm's canal area by PEX material accumulation (*arrows*) in the juxtacanalicular tissue. **D** Pretrabecular sheet of PEX material covered by proliferating/migrating corneal endothelial cells (*arrows*)

11.6 A,B) [46]. From these changes it can be appreciated that therapeutic efforts to improve outflow need to address the changes in this area to obtain lasting intraocular pressure reduction. PEX material accumulations can be also found along the outer wall of Schlemm's canal and in the periphery of collector channels and scleral aqueous veins, occasionally leading to collapse of aqueous veins.

The amount of PEX material within the juxtacanalicular region correlated with the presence of glaucoma, the average thickness of the juxtacanalicular tissue, and the mean cross-sectional area of Schlemm's canal in one study [46] and also with the intraocular pressure level and the axon count in the optic nerve in another [8]. These findings indicate a direct causative relationship between the buildup of PEX material in the meshwork and glaucoma development and progression.

Histopathological analyses indicated fundamental differences in the nature of PEX glaucoma and POAG, which might help to explain the differences in clinical course and management: Whereas POAG is characterized by increased juxtacanalicular plaque material and decreased trabecular meshwork cellularity (Fig. 11.6 C), both plaque material and cellularity are unchanged in PEX glaucoma compared to normal eyes, but there is production and deposition of the characteristic fibrillar PEX material instead [46].

Thus, the primary cause of chronic pressure elevation in PEX eyes appears to be the active participation of the trabecular endothelial cells, particularly Schlemm's canal endothelial cells, in the generalized abnormal matrix process, leading to local production and accumulation of PEX material in the juxtacanalicular region of the meshwork and subsequent degenerative al-

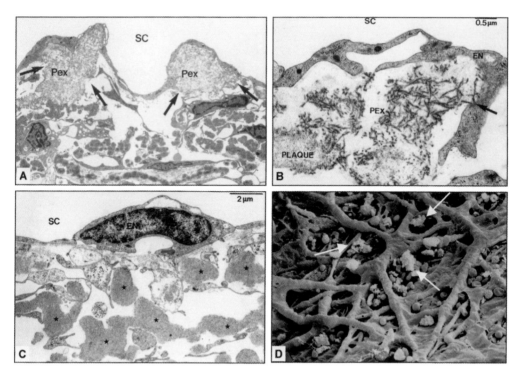

Fig. 11.6 A–D. Electron micrographs showing involvement of the trabecular meshwork in PEX syndrome and POAG. **A** Accumulation of PEX material (*arrows*) in the subendothelial juxtacanalicular tissue along the inner wall of Schlemm's canal (*SC*). **B** Apparent production of PEX fibrils (*arrow*) by the inner wall endothelium (*EN*) lining Schlemm's canal (*SC*). **C** Accumulation of plaque material (*asterisks*) in the juxtacanalicular tissue in POAG. **D** Scanning electron micrograph of the inner surface of the trabecular meshwork showing PEX deposits (*arrows*) in the uveal pores

terations of Schlemm's canal wall. Partly, PEX clumps may be also passively washed in with the aqueous flow after abrasion from the lens and pupillary margin and may become trapped in the uveal pores of the meshwork (Fig. 11.6 D).

Even though it is most widely held that obstruction of the trabecular pores by PEX material, either locally produced or passively deposited, is the major mechanism of chronic pressure elevation, contributions due to pigment dispersion and increased aqueous protein concentrations have also been proposed (Table 11.4) [48]. Another interesting observation has been the proliferation of corneal endothelial cells beyond Schwalbe's line resulting in a pretrabecular layer of extracellular material including PEX fibrils produced by migrating/proliferating endothelial cells (Fig. 11.5 D) [46, 48]. This may be a consequence of anterior chamber hypoxia in PEX eyes, stimulating corneal endothelial cell proliferation. Such observations may partially explain why there is a variable response to medical therapy with some patients seeming to respond so poorly.

Although PEX glaucoma is characteristically a high-pressure disease, pressure-independent risk factors, such as an impaired ocular and retrobulbar perfusion and abnormalities of elastic tissue of the lamina cribrosa, may be present and further increase the risk for glaucomatous damage [33, 62]. In a prospective study, Puska et al. [39] found that in patients with clinically unilateral involvement, in whom intraocular pressure was equal throughout the follow-up period, disk changes took place only in the involved eye, suggesting that the PEX process itself may be a risk factor for optic disk changes.

Table 11.4. Pathomechanisms of intraocular pressure elevation and glaucoma development

1. Pathomechanisms of intraocular pressure elevation

   Accumulation of locally produced PEX material in the juxtacanalicular tissue and subsequent degenerative changes in Schlemm's canal wall

   Passively deposited PEX material in the uveal meshwork washed in with aqueous flow

   Pigment dispersion and accumulation in the trabecular meshwork

   Increased protein concentration and viscosity of aqueous humor

   Proliferation/migration of corneal endothelial cells over the chamber angle

2. Pathomechanisms of glaucoma development
   High intraocular pressure levels and pressure spikes

   Vascular factors (impaired ocular and retrobulbar perfusion)

   Structural factors (elastosis of the lamina cribrosa)

However the question remains as to why some eyes with PEX appear to never develop glaucoma. This may be explained simply by the individual amount of PEX material present in the outflow structures, by interindividual differences in managing the metabolic disturbance, by additionally required predisposing or genetic factors, or by interindividual differences in the susceptibility to optic nerve damage, mediated by vascular or structural factors. An underlying defect in aqueous humor dynamics or involvement of a glaucoma susceptibility gene may also be considered as a requirement for glaucoma development in PEX eyes, because patients with unilateral PEX syndrome may also have glaucoma in the fellow eye [38]. Degeneration of the ciliary epithelium is part of the disease, and reduced aqueous secretion may explain why some eyes with PEX syndrome do not develop glaucoma.

11.4.3.2
Pigment Dispersion

A characteristic clinical feature and early diagnostic sign of PEX syndrome is an increased pigmentation of the trabecular meshwork. The degree of trabecular pigmentation is always more pronounced in the involved eye and appears to correlate in some [37, 61], but not in all studies, with the intraocular pressure level and the severity of glaucomatous damage.

Therefore, the role of melanin dispersion in chronic pressure elevation and glaucoma development still remains controversial. Unlike that in primary pigment dispersion syndrome, the distribution of the pigment tends to be less dense and rather uneven or patchy. Histomorphometric analyses confirmed a high circumferential variation of melanin concentration in the trabecular meshwork and failed to show a direct relationship between the melanin density and glaucoma status [46]. By electron microscopy, pigment granules are invariably present within trabecular endothelial cells, preferably in the innermost uveal portions of the meshwork [45].

It therefore has been suggested that pigment dispersion and accumulation do not appear to play a significant role in chronic pressure elevation in PEX eyes, but may exert an additional stress on the metabolically damaged cells and may lead to acute and transient pressure rises, when sudden melanin showers are provoked by diagnostic mydriasis.

11.4.3.3
Vascular Factors

Although the mechanical component of optic nerve damage certainly predominates in this hypertensive glaucoma type, the risk of glaucomatous damage may be further increased by vascular factors and PEX-associated alterations of blood vessels. In fact, many studies have reported on a general disturbance of ocular and retrobulbar perfusion in PEX patients with and without glaucoma, including the demonstration of a pronounced vasculopathy of the iris with hypoperfusion and anterior chamber hypoxia, a reduction of pulsatile ocular blood flow, and significantly diminished blood flow velocities and increased resistivity indices in the ophthalmic artery, the central retinal artery, and short posterior ciliary arteries [62]. The blood flow in the lamina cribrosa and the neuroretinal rim area was found to decrease with progressing glaucomatous damage [11]. Moreover, higher rates of disk hemorrhages and central retinal vein occlusions have been reported in PEX glaucoma patients [7].

Morphological correlates of these pathophysiologic findings are perivascular accumulations of PEX material and elastotic alterations of vessel walls, as they have been demonstrated by electron microscopy in the walls of iris vessels, aqueous veins, ciliary arteries, and the central retinal artery [32, 44, 47].

11.4.3.4
Structural Factors

The lamina cribrosa of the optic disk appears to undergo elastosis, although PEX material has not been identified in this region. Netland et al. [33] demonstrated a marked and site-specific elastosis of the lamina cribrosa, which is more pronounced in eyes with PEX glaucoma than in POAG eyes, suggesting an abnormal regulation of elastin synthesis and/or degradation. These alterations of the connective tissue at the level of the lamina cribrosa may increase the susceptibility of optic nerve fibers towards mechanical and ischemic damage.

11.4.4
Acute Open-Angle Glaucoma

Dispersion of melanin granules and PEX material in the anterior chamber is common after diagnostic pupillary dilation and may lead to marked rises in intraocular pressure, sometimes causing, together with an early corneal endothelial decompensation and diffuse corneal edema, the clinical picture of an acute glaucoma [32]. Such pressure peaks can even mimic an acute pupillary block with a red eye, corneal edema, and pressure rises over 50 mmHg, in spite of an open angle [6]. Krause et al. [24] noted a positive correlation between the degree of pressure rise and the amount of pigment liberation, which both reach a maximum after 2 h following mydriasis and may go back to normal levels after 10–24 h. Post-dilation intraocular pressure should be, therefore, checked in all patients receiving mydriatics.

In rare cases, the spontaneous luxation of the lens into the vitreous or of lens fragments in complicated cataract surgery may induce the development of an acute phacolytic glaucoma [28].

Summary for the Clinician

- The probability of PEX eyes to develop glaucoma is up to 40% within 10 years; risk factors for conversion are initial intraocular pressure level and degree of pupillary dilation
- Eyes with PEX glaucoma are characterized by marked chamber angle pigmentation, small optic disks, high intraocular pressure levels, marked diurnal pressure fluctuations and spikes, rapid progression of glaucomatous damage, and often poor response to medication; intraocular pressure appears to be the main risk factor for glaucomatous damage
- The primary cause of chronic pressure elevation is an increased outflow resistance in the trabecular meshwork caused by blockage of the outflow channels by locally produced PEX material in the juxtacanalicular region of the meshwork followed by degenerative changes of Schlemm's canal wall
- Pressure-independent risk factors, such as an impaired ocular and retrobulbar perfusion and abnormalities of elastic tissues of the lamina cribrosa, may further increase the risk for glaucomatous damage
- Dispersion and trabecular accumulation of pigment granules and PEX flakes may lead to acute and transient pressure rises following mydriasis

11.5
Angle-Closure Glaucoma in PEX Syndrome

Glaucoma in PEX syndrome usually occurs in the presence of an open chamber angle, but an association between PEX and angle-closure glaucoma is also not rare (Table 11.5) [9]. Ritch [41] found signs of PEX in 28% of consecutive patients with angle-closure glaucoma. Because

Table 11.5. PEX-associated types of glaucoma

Secondary chronic open-angle glaucoma

Secondary angle-closure glaucoma
(pupillary/ciliary block); predisposing factors:
weak zonules, posterior synechiae, rigid iris,
protein-rich aqueous humor

Secondary angle-closure glaucoma with rubeosis
iridis following retinal vein occlusion
(neovascular glaucoma)

"Acute open-angle glaucoma"
(caused by dispersion of pigment and PEX
material after mydriasis)

eyes with PEX syndrome often have narrowed chamber angles and smaller anterior chamber volumes [5, 9, 61] in the presence of a weak zonular apparatus, a minimal anterior subluxation of the lens predisposes to the development of angle-closure glaucoma via a pupillary block mechanism. The decrease in anterior chamber depth between the supine and prone position was shown to be greater in eyes with PEX than in fellow eyes [27].

Characteristic features of PEX eyes that may predispose to the development of pupillary block angle-closure glaucoma include the formation of posterior synechiae, an increased iris rigidity and decreased iris motility, an impairment of the blood–aqueous barrier and increased protein concentrations of aqueous humor, and anterior movement of the lens secondary to zonular weakness [32]. In extreme and rather rare cases with marked zonular laxity, anterior displacement of the lens may be so pronounced that a ciliary block angle-closure glaucoma ("malignant glaucoma") is induced by contraction of the ciliary muscle [60]. Miotics may aggravate both pupillary block and forward movement of the lens-iris diaphragm. A narrow angle associated with PEX syndrome may, therefore, represent an additional argument for prophylactic iridotomy.

Secondary angle-closure glaucoma following central retinal vein occlusion with rubeosis iridis (neovascular glaucoma) may also occur in PEX eyes, because retinal vein occlusion appears to be more common in patients with PEX syndrome/glaucoma, perhaps due to high intraocular pressure values [7].

Summary for the Clinician

- Development of angle-closure glaucoma in PEX eyes is predisposed by weak zonules, decreased iris motility, posterior synechiae, and small anterior chamber volumes
- Miotics may aggravate pupillary block in eyes with marked zonular instability

11.6 Management

In the past, little emphasis has been put on making an accurate diagnosis of PEX syndrome and on differentiating it from POAG, since the treatment modalities of both glaucoma types are classically identical. However, distinguishing PEX glaucoma from POAG has direct clinical importance, because intraocular pressure is generally more difficult to control and refractory to medical therapy than in POAG [2] and because reduction and stabilization of intraocular pressure may be more important than in POAG [1]. In practice, patients with PEX syndrome should be examined at regular intervals, always including careful examination of the optic discs. Intraocular pressure measurements have to take into account that the central corneal thickness is significantly higher in PEX eyes than in control eyes, which may reflect decompensation of the barrier function of the corneal endothelial cells [40]. Konstas et al. [18] found that the peak level of intraocular pressure occurs more frequently outside office hours, indicating that a single intraocular pressure measurement during office hours is not reliable. Glaucoma, once diagnosed, requires standard medical treatment, often requiring combination therapy, along with examinations at shorter intervals and diurnal pressure monitoring. Despite treatment with more antiglaucoma medications, the mean intraocular pressure was still significantly higher in PEX glaucoma compared with that in POAG patients in another study by Konstas and coworkers [20].

11.6.1
Medical Therapy

Unfortunately, to date there are few comparative studies with respect to the efficacy of medications in controlling the intraocular pressure in PEX glaucoma patients. Konstas et al. [21] showed that, as primary therapy, timolol maleate solution twice daily controlled intraocular pressure similarly to timolol maleate gel once daily. Despite a greater initial pressure reduction in patients with PEX glaucoma by timolol, significant fluctuations in the diurnal curve were still present in contrast to POAG patients [17]. Apraclonidine added to timolol further reduced intraocular pressure by 17% in PEX glaucoma eyes [21]. Latanoprost is also effective in lowering intraocular pressure in eyes with PEX glaucoma, but no significant differences between the effects of latanoprost and a fixed combination of timolol and dorzolamide have been reported [23]. Latanoprost and pilocarpine had a similar diurnal efficacy when added to timolol and dorzolamide as a third-line therapy in PEX glaucoma [22].

Despite good pressure lowering effects and several potential benefits of miotic agents, e.g., reduction of pupillary movement [43], there are some hazards of miotic use in PEX patients. Aggravation of blood–aqueous barrier breakdown, reduced pupillary movement promoting the formation of posterior synechiae, aggravation of lens opacities, and induction of pupillary or ciliary block glaucoma in eyes with marked zonular instability, may complicate management.

11.6.2
Laser Trabeculoplasty

Argon laser trabeculoplasty often has an immediate pressure lowering effect, with reported initial success rates of up to 80%, perhaps by easier heat absorption due to increased trabecular pigmentation. Although the initial response to laser treatment is greater in PEX glaucoma patients than in POAG patients, the long-term outcome is similar for both groups. The success rates decrease with time, and by 3 years there is a substantial failure rate averaging 50% in both POAG and PEX eyes [58]. Postlaser complications are, however, more common in PEX eyes and comprise inflammatory reactions and intraocular pressure spikes, requiring careful follow-up together with anti-inflammatory therapy and pressure control in the early postoperative phase.

11.6.3
Filtration Surgery

Because long-term effects of medical therapy and laser treatment are often unsatisfactory, surgical intervention may be necessary earlier and more frequently than in other forms of glaucoma. Whereas routine filtration surgery is most often applied, a relatively new surgical approach to improve chamber angle facility by aspiration of debris and PEX material on the surface of the meshwork, trabecular aspiration, has been specifically developed for treatment of PEX glaucoma [13]. Although efficacious in decreasing intraocular pressure in the early course, there seems to be a slight regression in effect over time, but further studies are needed to assess the long-term results of this new technique.

Although results of glaucoma filtering surgery in PEX eyes are usually comparable to those in eyes with POAG, peri- and postoperative surgical complications, such as inflammatory responses, fibrin reactions, formation of synechiae, and intraocular pressure fluctuations, are more common in PEX eyes. These postoperative complications can be directly attributed to the characteristic chronic defects in blood–aqueous barrier [26], which are exaggerated in the early postoperative phase with a more prolonged return to basal levels compared to controls [34]. After surgery, frequent and thorough follow-up examinations are important for detection and treatment of complications in the early period. Pre-operative treatment with corticosteroids may, therefore, be beneficial along with more intensive and prolonged topical post-operative corticosteroid therapy.

In cases of coexisting cataract, an early combined cataract and glaucoma surgery has to be considered. Simultaneous cataract extraction has been reported to reduce, though not eliminate, the frequency and magnitude of post-operative pressure elevation [25]. Cataract extraction alone may also improve intraocular pressure control in patients with PEX syndrome and may be more effective than in POAG and cataract patients [30].

Summary for the Clinician

- Emphasis should be put on reduction and stabilization of intraocular pressure, on diurnal pressure monitoring considering the greater corneal thickness in PEX patients, and on optic disk examinations at regular intervals
- Post-laser and post-surgery complications should be expected and met by careful follow-up and anti-inflammatory therapy

11.7
Summary and Perspectives

The awareness of the importance of PEX syndrome has increased considerably in recent years. We have realized that it is a common disorder affecting a considerable proportion of our cataract and glaucoma patients, we have improved the diagnosis of early stages, we are beginning to understand the underlying pathophysiology, and we have learned that it is a systemic condition, which may be associated with an increased risk for cardiovascular disease. It may not only cause severe chronic open-angle glaucoma, but also a spectrum of other ocular complications including lens subluxation, blood–aqueous barrier impairment, posterior synechiae, corneal endothelial decompensation, and serious complications in cataract surgery.

Secondary chronic open-angle glaucoma associated with PEX syndrome accounts for approximately 25% of all glaucomas and represents the most common identifiable cause of glaucomas overall. Due to high intraocular pressure levels and diurnal pressure fluctuations, PEX-associated open-angle glaucoma represents a relatively severe and progressive type of glaucoma. The underlying disorder, PEX syndrome, is a generalized process of the extracellular matrix characterized by production and progressive accumulation of an abnormal extracellular material in intra- and extraocular tissues. Recent data support the pathogenetic concept of PEX syndrome as a type of elastosis affecting particularly elastic microfibrils. Active involvement of the trabecular meshwork cells in this characteristic matrix process may lead to glaucoma development in about half of patients. The primary cause of chronic pressure elevation is an increased outflow resistance in the trabecular meshwork caused by blockage of the outflow channels by locally produced PEX material in the juxtacanalicular region of the meshwork followed by degenerative changes of Schlemm's canal wall. Additional pathogenetic factors contributing to pressure rise and glaucoma development include marked pigment dispersion, increased aqueous humor protein concentrations, vascular factors, and connective tissue alterations of the lamina cribrosa. Other types of glaucoma, such as acute open-angle glaucoma due to sudden pigment liberation after diagnostic mydriasis, or secondary angle-closure glaucoma due to pupillary or ciliary block mechanisms in the presence of an unstable zonular apparatus, are also common in PEX patients.

In relation to the clinical management of these patients, the importance of early recognition and accurate diagnosis of the pathologic features, reduction and stabilization of intraocular pressure, diurnal pressure monitoring, expectations of a higher complication rate during surgery, and close attention to post-operative follow-up, has to be emphasized. The diagnosis of the condition by careful biomicroscopy should alert the clinician to the potential for glaucoma and for systemic cardiovascular disease.

In spite of completely different pathomechanisms, treatment of PEX glaucoma still is identical to that of POAG. Future therapeutic options should, however, be guided by the specific underlying pathophysiology. Pathogenetic factors, which appear to be causally involved in this fibrotic matrix process, are the growth factor

TGF-β1 and the inhibitors of matrix metalloproteinases TIMP-1 and TIMP-2, stimulating abnormal matrix formation and inhibiting its degradation. Both TGF-β1 and TIMP-1/2, therefore, represent potential target molecules for a specific rational therapeutic approach in PEX patients, and neutralization of one of these key molecules may be one possibility to interfere with this matrix process before glaucomatous damage has occurred.

References

1. Bergea B, Bodin L, Svedbergh B (1999) Impact of intraocular pressure regulation on visual fields in open-angle glaucoma. Ophthalmology 106:997–1004
2. Brinchmann-Hansen O, Albrektsen T, Anmarkrud N (1993) Pilocarpine drops do not reduce intraocular pressure sufficiently in pseudoexfoliation glaucoma. Eye 7:511–516
3. Damji KF, Bains HS, Stefansson E, Loftsdottir M, Sverrison T, Thorgeirsson E, Jonasson F, Gottfredsdottir M, Allingham R (1998) Is pseudoexfoliation syndrome inherited? A review of genetic and nongenetic factors and a new observation. Ophthalmic Genetics 19:175–85
4. Forsius H (1988) Exfoliation syndrome in various ethnic populations. Acta Ophthalmol 184[Suppl]: 71–85
5. Gharagozloo NZ, Baker RH, Brubaker RF (1992) Aqueous dynamics in exfoliation syndrome. Am J Ophthalmol 114:473–78
6. Gillies WE, Brooks AM (1988) The presentation of acute glaucoma in pseudoexfoliation of the lens capsule. Aust NZ J Ophthalmol 16:101–106
7. Gillies WE, Brooks AMV (2002) Central retinal vein occlusion in pseudoexfoliation of the lens capsule. Clin Exp Ophthalmol 30:176–178
8. Gottanka J, Flügel-Koch C, Martus P, Johnson DH, Lütjen-Drecoll E (1997) Correlation of pseudoexfoliative material and optic nerve damage in pseudoexfoliation syndrome. Invest Ophthalmol Vis Sci 38:2435–46
9. Gross FJ, Tingey D, Epstein DL (1994) Increased prevalence of occludable angles and angle-closure glaucoma in patients with pseudoexfoliation. Am J Ophthalmol 117:333–336
10. Hammer Th, Schlötzer-Schrehardt U, Naumann GOH (2001) Unilateral or asymmetric pseudoexfoliation syndrome? An ultrastructural study. Arch Ophthalmol 119:1023–31
11. Harju M, Vesti E (2001) Blood flow of the optic nerve head and peripapillary retina in exfoliation syndrome with unilateral glaucoma or ocular hypertension. Graefes Arch Clin Exp Ophthalmol 239:271–77
12. Inazumi K, Takahashi D, Taniguchi T, Yamamoto T (2002) Ultrasound biomicroscopic classification of zonules in exfoliation syndrome. Jpn J Ophthalmol 46:502–509
13. Jacobi PC, Krieglstein GK (1995) Trabecular aspiration. A new mode to treat pseudoexfoliation glaucoma. Invest Ophthalmol Vis Sci 36:2270–76
14. Jonas JB, Papastathopoulos KI (1997) Optic disk appearance in pseudoexfoliation syndrome. Am J Ophthalmol 123:174–80
15. Kivelä T, Hietanen J, Uusitalo M (1997) Autopsy analysis of clinically unilateral exfoliation syndrome. Invest Ophthalmol Vis Sci 38:2008–2015
16. Koliakos GG, Konstas AGP, Schlötzer-Schrehardt U, Hollo G, Katsimbris IE, Georgiadis N, Ritch R (2003) 8-isoprostaglandin F_{2A} and ascorbic acid concentration in the aqueous humour of patients with exfoliation syndrome. Br J Ophthalmol 87: 353–56
17. Konstas AGP, Mantziris DA, Cate EA, Stewart WC (1997) Effect of timolol on the diurnal intraocular pressure in exfoliation and primary open-angle glaucoma. Arch Ophthalmol 115:975–979
18. Konstas AGP, Mantziris DA, Stewart WC (1997) Diurnal intraocular pressure in untreated exfoliation and primary open-angle glaucoma. Arch Ophthalmol 115:182–85
19. Konstas AGP, Stewart WC, Stromann GA (1997) Clinical presentation and initial treatment patterns in patients with exfoliation glaucoma versus primary open-angle glaucoma. Ophth Surg Lasers 28:111–17
20. Konstas AGP, Tsatsos I, Kardasopoulos A (1998) Preoperative features of patients with exfoliation glaucoma and primary open-angle glaucoma. The AHEPA study. Acta Ophthalmol Scand 76:208–12
21. Konstas AGP, Maltezos A, Mantziris DA, Sine CS, Stewart WC (1999) The comparative ocular hypotensive effect of apraclonidine with timolol maleate in exfoliation versus primary open-angle glaucoma patients. Eye 13:314–318
22. Konstas AGP, Lake S, Maltezos AC, Holmes KT, Stewart WC (2001) Twenty-four hour intraocular pressure reduction with latanoprost compared with pilocarpine as third-line therapy in exfoliation glaucoma. Eye 15:59–62
23. Konstas AGP, Kozobolis VP, Tersis I, Leech J, Stewart WC (2003) The efficacy and safety of the timolol/dorzolamide fixed combination vs latanoprost in exfoliation glaucoma. Eye 17:41–46

24. Krause U, Helve J, Forsius H (1973) Pseudoexfoliation of the lens capsule and liberation of iris pigment. Acta Ophthalmol 51:39–46

25. Krupin T, Feitl ME, Bishop KI (1989) Postoperative intraocular pressure rise in open-angle glaucoma patients after cataract or combined cataract-filtration surgery. Ophthalmology 96: 579–584

26. Küchle M, Nguyen N, Hannappel E, Naumann GOH (1995) The blood-aqueous barrier in eyes with pseudoexfoliation syndrome. Ophthalmic Res 27(Suppl1):136–42

27. Lanzl IM, Merté RL, Graham AD (2000) Does head positioning influence anterior chamber depth in pseudoexfoliation syndrome? J Glaucoma 9:214–218

28. Lim MC, Doe EA, Vroman DT, Rosa RH, Parrish RK (2001) Late onset lens particle glaucoma as a consequence of spontaneous dislocation of an intraocular lens in pseudoexfoliation syndrome. Am J Ophthalmol 132:261–63

29. Mardin CY, Schlötzer-Schrehardt U, Naumann GOH (2001) "Masked" pseudoexfoliation syndrome in unoperated eyes with circular posterior synechiae. Arch Ophthalmol 119: 1500–04

30. Merkur A, Damji KF, Mintsioulis G, Hodge WG (2001) Intraocular pressure decrease after phacoemulsification in patients with pseudoexfoliation syndrome. J Cataract Refract Surg 27:528–32

31. Mitchell P, Wang JJ, Smith W (1997) Association of pseudoexfoliation syndrome with increased vascular risk. Am J Ophthalmol 124:685–87

32. Naumann GOH, Schlötzer-Schrehardt U, Küchle M (1998) Pseudoexfoliation syndrome for the comprehensive ophthalmologist. Intraocular and systemic manifestations. Ophthalmology 105:951–68

33. Netland PA, Ye H, Streeten BW, Hernandez MR (1995) Elastosis of the lamina cribrosa in pseudoexfoliation syndrome with glaucoma. Ophthalmology 102:878–86

34. Nguyen NX, Küchle M, Martus P, Naumann GOH (1999) Quantification of blood-aqueous barrier breakdown after trabeculectomy: pseudoexfoliation versus primary open-angle glaucoma. J Glaucoma 8:18–23

35. Orr AC, Robitaille JM, Price PA, Hamilton JR, Falvey DM, De Saint-Sardos AG, Pasternak S, Guernsey DL (2001) Exfoliation syndrome: clinical and genetic features. Ophthalmic Genetics 22:171–185

36. Prince AM, Streeten BW, Ritch R, Dark AJ, Sperling M (1987) Preclinical diagnosis of pseudoexfoliation syndrome. Arch Ophthalmol 105:1076–82

37. Puska P (1995) The amount of lens exfoliation and chamber-angle pigmentation in exfoliation syndrome with or without glaucoma. Acta Ophthalmol Scand 73:226–32

38. Puska PM (2002) Unilateral exfoliation syndrome: conversion to bilateral exfoliation and to glaucoma: a prospective 10-year follow-up study. J Glaucoma 11:517–524

39. Puska P, Vesti E, Tomita G, Ishida K, Raitta C (1999) Optic disc changes in normotensive persons with unilateral exfoliation syndrome: a 3-year follow-up study. Graefe's Arch Clin Exp Ophthalmol 237:457–462

40. Puska P, Vasara K, Harju M, Setälä K (2000) Corneal thickness and corneal endothelium in normotensive subjects with unilateral exfoliation syndrome. Graefe's Arch Clin Exp Ophthalmol 238:659–663

41. Ritch R (1994) Exfoliation syndrome and occludable angles. Trans Am Ophthalmol Soc 92:845–944

42. Ritch R (1996) Exfoliation syndrome – the most common identifiable cause of open-angle glaucoma. J Glaucoma 3:176–78

43. Ritch R, Schlötzer-Schrehardt U (2001) Exfoliation syndrome. Surv Ophthalmol 45:265–315

44. Ritch R, Schlötzer-Schrehardt U, Konstas AGP (2003) Why is glaucoma associated with exfoliation syndrome? Progr Ret Eye Res 22:253–275

45. Sampaolesi R, Zarate J, Croxato O (1988) The chamber angle in exfoliation syndrome. Clinical and pathological findings. Acta Ophthalmol 184[Suppl]:48–53

46. Schlötzer-Schrehardt U, Naumann GOH (1995) Trabecular meshwork in pseudoexfoliation syndrome with and without open-angle glaucoma. Invest Ophthalmol Vis Sci 36:1750–64

47. Schlötzer-Schrehardt U, Koca M, Naumann GOH, Volkholz H (1992) Pseudoexfoliation syndrome: ocular manifestation of a systemic disorder? Arch Ophthalmol 110:1752–56

48. Schlötzer-Schrehardt U, Küchle M, Naumann GOH (1999) Mechanisms of glaucoma development in pseudoexfoliation syndrome. In: Gramer E, Grehn F (eds) Pathogenesis and risk factors of glaucoma. Springer, Berlin Heidelberg New York, Springer, pp 34–49.

49. Schlötzer-Schrehardt U, Zenkel M, Küchle M, Sakai LY, Naumann GOH (2001) Role of transforming growth factor-β1 and its latent form binding protein in pseudoexfoliation syndrome. Exp Eye Res 73:765–80

50. Schlötzer-Schrehardt U, Lommatzsch J, Küchle M, Konstas AGP, Naumann GOH (2003) Matrix metalloproteinases and their inhibitors in aqueous humor of patients with pseudoexfoliation syndrome, pseudoexfoliation glaucoma, and primary open-angle glaucoma. Invest Ophthalmol Vis Sci 44:1117–25

51. Schumacher S, Schlötzer-Schrehardt U, Martus P, Lang W, Naumann GOH (2001) Pseudoexfoliation syndrome and aneurysms of the abdominal aorta. The Lancet 357:359–60

52. Streeten BW (1993) Aberrant synthesis and aggregation of elastic tissue components in pseudoexfoliative fibrillopathy: a unifying concept. New Trends Ophthalmol 8:187–196

53. Streeten BW, Li ZY, Wallace RN, Eagle RCJ, Keshgegian AA (1992) Pseudoexfoliative fibrillopathy in visceral organs of a patient with pseudoexfoliation syndrome. Arch Ophthalmol 110:1757–1762

54. Tarkkanen A, Kivelä T (1999) Unilateral capsular glaucoma after long-standing bilateral pigmentary glaucoma. Eye 13:212–214

55. Tetsumoto K, Schlötzer-Schrehardt U, Küchle M, Dörfler S, Naumann GOH (1992) Precapsular layer of the anterior lens capsule in early pseudoexfoliation syndrome. Graefe's Arch Clin Exp Ophthalmol 230, 252–57

56. Teus MA, Castejón MA, Calvo MA, Pérez-Salaíces P, Marcos A (1998) Intraocular pressure as a risk factor for visual field loss in pseudoexfoliative and in primary open-angle glaucoma. Ophthalmology 105:2225–30

57. Tezel G, Tezel TH (1993) The comparative analysis of optic disc damage in exfoliative glaucoma. Acta Ophthalmol 71:744–750

58. Threlkeld AB, Hertzmark E, Sturm RT, Epstein DL, Allingham RR (1996) Comparative study of the efficacy of argon laser trabeculoplasty for exfoliation and primary open-angle glaucoma. J Glaucoma 5:311–316

59. Vessani RM, Ritch R, Liebmann JM, Jofe M (2003) Plasma homocysteine is elevated in patients with exfoliation syndrome. Am J Ophthalmol 136:41–46

60. Von der Lippe I, Küchle M, Naumann GOH (1993) Pseudoexfoliation syndrome as a risk factor for acute ciliary block angle closure glaucoma. Acta Ophthalmol 71:277–79

61. Wishart PK, Spaeth GL, Poryzees EM (1985) Anterior chamber angle in the exfoliation syndrome. Br J Ophthalmol 69:103–107

62. Yüksel N, Karabas L, Arslan A, Demirci A, Caglar Y (2001) Ocular hemodynamics in pseudoexfoliation syndrome and pseudoexfoliation glaucoma. Ophthalmology 108:1043–49

Robert Ritch

Core Messages

- Pigment dispersion syndrome is more common than previously realized
- PDS is associated with a high rate of retinal detachment
- Posterior bowing of the iris and thus iridozonular contact may be facilitated by a larger and more posteriorly inserted iris
- Blinking allows aqueous humor to flow from the posterior chamber to the anterior chamber. The inability of aqueous to equilibrate between the two chambers due to greater than normal iridolenticular contact produces reverse pupillary block
- PDS goes through active and regressive phases
- The probability of PDS converting to glaucoma is about 10 % in 5 years and 15 % in 15 years
- Laser iridotomy has not shown a clear benefit in this condition but medical therapy and laser trabeculoplasty have been effective

12.1
Introduction

Pigment dispersion syndrome (PDS) is a unique and fascinating entity. It is far more prevalent, actually by an order of magnitude, than previously suspected, comprising 2.45 % of the screened Caucasian population in one study [76]. PDS and pigmentary glaucoma (PG) are characterized by disruption of the iris pigment epithelium (IPE) and deposition of the dispersed pigment granules throughout the anterior segment. The classic diagnostic triad consists of corneal pigmentation (Krukenberg spindle), slit-like, radial, mid-peripheral iris transillumination defects, and dense trabecular pigmentation. The iris insertion is typically posterior and the peripheral iris tends to bow posteriorly. The basic abnormality in this hereditary disorder remains unknown.

12.2
Clinical Findings

12.2.1
Anterior Segment

Loss of iris pigment appears clinically as a mid-peripheral, radial, slit-like pattern of transillumination defects seen most commonly inferonasally and more easily in blue eyes than in brown ones (Fig. 12.1). Although the defects can sometimes be seen by retroillumination, they are more easily detected by a dark adapted examiner using a fiberoptic transilluminator in a darkened room. Infrared videography provides the most sensitive method of detection [3]. Pigment particles deposited on the iris surface tend to aggregate in the furrows. Rarely, this pigment can be dense enough to darken the iris or to cause heterochromia when involvement is asymmetric. Anisocoria may occur with asymmetric involvement, the larger pupil corresponding to the eye with greater pigment loss from the iris [1]. The pupil may be distorted in the direction of maximal iris transillumination.

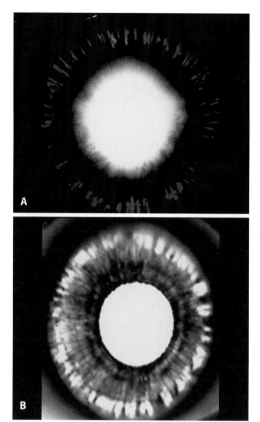

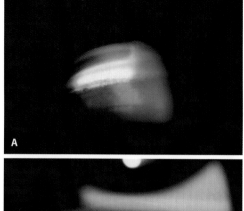

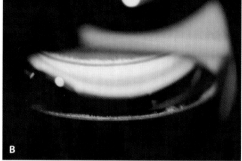

Fig. 12.3 A,B. Pigment reversal sign in a 48-year-old man. **A** Inferior angle. **B** Superior angle. The pigment is denser in the superior angle. Note that the pigment band has sharp anterior and posterior margins and appears smooth, indicating that this pigment was deposited in the past and is now localized to the region of the filtering portion of the trabecular meshwork. The iris is inserted posteriorly

Fig. 12.1 A,B. Mid-peripheral, slit-like, radial iris transillumination defects. **A** Slit-lamp appearance. **B** Infrared pupillography

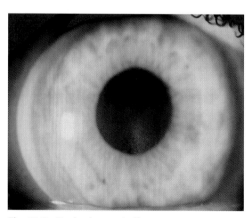

Fig. 12.2. Krukenberg spindle

Corneal endothelial pigment generally appears as a central, vertical, brown band (Krukenberg spindle; Fig. 12.2), the shape being attributed to aqueous convection currents. The pigment is phagocytosed by trabecular cells. Coincident PDS and megalocornea has been reported.

The anterior chamber is deeper both centrally and peripherally and the anterior chamber volume significantly greater in PDS patients compared to controls [22]. In patients with unilateral PDS, the anterior chamber was deeper and the lens flatter in the involved eyes [92]. Patients with PDS have flatter corneas than myopic age- and refraction-matched controls, but no difference in axial length [53].

The angle is characteristically wide open, with a homogeneous, dense hyperpigmented band on the trabecular meshwork (Fig. 12.3). Pigment may also be deposited on Schwalbe's line and on the corneal shelf anterior to it. The iris insertion is posterior and the peripheral iris approach is often concave. The iris is most concave in the mid-periphery. In younger patients, the scleral spur may be poorly demarcated, blending with the ciliary face due to pigment deposition on these structures. Pigment may be deposited on the zonules, on the posterior capsule of the lens, where it is apposed to the anterior hyaloid face at the insertion of the posterior zonular fibers (Zentmayer ring) and on the posterior lens central to Weigert's ligament.

12.2.2
Posterior Segment

PDS is associated with a high incidence of retinal detachment [84]. Most detachments occur in phakic men who are not highly myopic. Miotics have been incriminated in precipitating these. It is significant that the incidence of retinal detachment in PDS is 6%–8% independent of miotic treatment, and when detachment is associated temporally with miotics, a preexisting lesion was most likely present. Lattice degeneration is commonly found in myopes and may be hereditary. Its incidence appears to be higher for all degrees of myopia in patients with PDS than in the general population [97]. Despite the fact that comparable prevalences of lattice degeneration in blacks and whites have been demonstrated at autopsy, PDS and retinal detachment are both uncommon in blacks. Eyes with PG are similar to those with primary open-angle glaucoma in size and shape of the optic disc, configuration of the neuroretinal rim, depth of the optic cup, area of the alpha zone of parapapillary atrophy, diameter of retinal vessels at the disc border, and frequency of disc hemorrhages and localized retinal nerve fiber layer defects [40].

12.3
Pathophysiology

In 1958, Scheie and Fleischauer [83] described iris transillumination defects associated with PDS and attributed them to IPE atrophy. With no real evidence except a "somewhat waxy or pale" appearance of the ciliary body in a few patients, they extended the hypothesis of congenital atrophy to include this structure.

Fine, Yanoff and Scheie [25] found that IPE loss was accompanied by hyperplasia of the iris dilator muscle. Pigment epithelial cells appeared to be migrating anteriorly and differentiating into smooth-muscle-containing cells. Rodrigues et al. [80] on the other hand, reported a focally thickened dilator muscle with thinning in the areas of epithelial atrophy. They found an increased number of immature melanosomes in the IPE and suggested that a delay in melanogenesis occurred as part of a developmental defect. Kupfer et al. [46] considered the primary lesion in PDS to be an epithelial abnormality. The dilator fibers of the inner IPE appeared to be hypertrophic and hyperplastic, resembling the sphincter muscle, and were associated with degenerated neural elements. The relevance of dilator muscle hyperplasia and nerve fiber degeneration to the disease process remain unknown. The possibility of an adrenergic hypersensitivity in patients with PDS and PG might explain comments made in passing that epinephrine compounds, alone or in combination with other agents, seem to be more effective in patients with PG than in those with POAG [8, 84].

Campbell [13] proposed that posterior bowing of the iris brings it into contact with the anterior zonular bundles. The location and number of the transillumination defects correlated with the position and number of the underlying zonular bundles. He noted that hyperplasia of the iris dilator muscle was localized to areas of iridozonular contact and hypothesized that iridozonular friction during pupillary movement disrupts the IPE, releasing pigment into the posterior chamber. Scanning electron microscopic observations supported this hypothesis [16, 42],

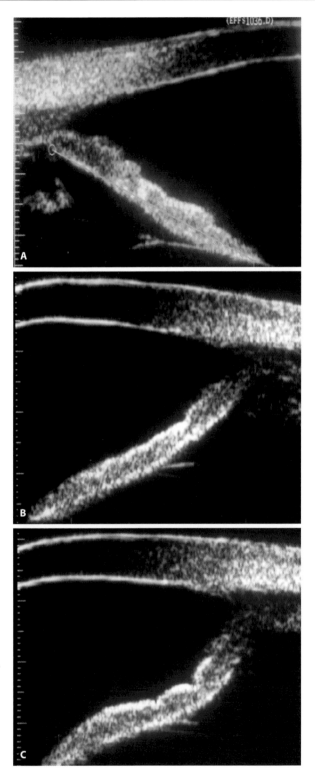

Fig. 12.4. Ultrasound biomicrograph of a normal eye (**A**), and an eye with pigment dispersion syndrome (**B**). The iris is large relative to the size of the anterior segment and the mid-peripheral concavity is prominent. There is extensive iridolenticular contact. **C** The same eye as in (**B**) during accommodation. Note the accentuation of the concavity

which is now accepted as the pathophysiologic mechanism of PDS.

Nevertheless, the question has again been raised as to whether posterior bowing of the iris and iridozonular contact is sufficient in itself to cause PDS [70]. Ultrasound biomicroscopy performed during accommodation reveals accentuation of the iris concavity, not only in patients with PDS but also in normals, particularly myopes. This accentuation also occurs in both normals and PDS patients after exercise [30]. It is possible that many people have iridozonular contact, but that a predisposing factor is required to produce disruption of the IPE. The IPE is continuous with those of the ciliary body and retina. Rare reports of retinal pigment epithelial dystrophies in association with PDS exist. More suggestively, Scuderi et al. [85] found psychophysical evidence of decreased retinal pigment epithelial function in eyes with PDS by electro-oculography, suggesting primary involvement of the retinal pigment epithelium in PDS. In another study, the mean ratios of the light-peak amplitude to dark-trough amplitude of patients with PDS and PG were significantly lower than the mean ratios of normal controls and patients with POAG, respectively [28].

Ultrasound biomicroscopy has enabled us to elucidate a number of facets of the pathophysiology of PDS. The size of the iris appears overly large relative to that of the anterior segment (Fig. 12.4). This may be the basic anatomic cause of the mid-peripheral iris concavity predisposing to iridozonular contact. Mathematical modeling, treating the aqueous humor as a Newtonian fluid and the iris as a linear elastic solid, suggests that passive iris deformation can produce the iris contours observed using UBM [33]. Sokol et al. [90] compared patients with PDS to age-, sex-, and refraction-matched controls and found a greater mean iris–trabecular meshwork distance in the PDS group. Thus, iridozonular contact appears to be facilitated by a congenitally more posterior iris insertion.

Electron microscopic examination of the trabecular meshwork shows cells lining the trabecular beams lifting off and disintegrating [67]. Trabecular cells are filled with pigment and show various stages of degeneration. The intertrabecular spaces contain free pigment granules as well as cell debris. These observations suggest that plugging of the trabecular spaces by pigment and cell debris together with fragmentation and collapse of trabecular sheets contribute to the decrease in the facility of outflow that occurs in PG [67, 87]. The mechanism of outflow obstruction may not be simple intertrabecular obstruction by pigment, but rather the result of a failure or breakdown of normal endothelial, phagocytic function. This is consistent with the report that trabecular aspiration in eyes with PG is much less effective than in eyes with exfoliative glaucoma [37].

12.4
Developmental Abnormalities Underlying PDS

Any hypothesis concerning the basic defect in PDS must account for the anatomic findings. Most difficult is explaining the relationship to lattice degeneration. A structural abnormality of the middle third of the eye causing an abnormally concave peripheral iris and the vitreous base/anterior retina to be drawn anteriorly could be consistent with previously proposed mechanisms. One hypothesis is that an abnormal persistence of connections between the zonular apparatus and the marginal bundle of Druault, a condensation of fibers during the formation of the secondary vitreous, which attaches strongly to the internal limiting membrane of the peripheral retina to form the vitreous base and also forms Weiger's ligament, might lead to tension on the peripheral retina [70]. A gene affecting the development of the middle third of the eye early in the third trimester appears as a reasonable explanation for these processes at the present time.

Loci for PDS have been reported at chromosome 7q35–36 [4] and 18q, suggesting genetic heterogeneity [5]. The gene for phenylthiocarbamide tasting is located in this region and was once associated with primary open-angle glaucoma [7]. A re-examination of this phenomenon showed no difference between patients with PDS, PG, and juvenile POAG [29]. The serotonin receptor 5A gene has been localized to 7q36.1 [82]. Ritch [70] hypothesized that a gene affecting either the serotonin or dopamine pathway is involved in the genesis of PDS.

A glaucoma associated with iris pigment dispersion and stromal atrophy with slit-like iris transillumination defects and secondary angle-closure has been identified in the DBA/2J (D2) mouse [39]. These defects result from mutations in related genes encoding melanosomal proteins [6]. Leakage of toxic intermediates of pigment production from melanosomes causes iris disease and subsequent PG, while eyes with decreased pigment production are protected [6].

AKXD-28/Ty mice, which also develop glaucoma, exhibit immune defects, including loss of ocular immune privilege [62]. Mice which have a homozygous deficiency of CYP1B1 have angle abnormalities resembling those of human congenital glaucoma, and the magnitude of the dysgenesis is increased by concomitant tyrosinase deficiency [50]. Administration of the tyrosinase product L-DOPA, alleviates the severity of the dysgenesis, potentially offering a novel avenue of treatment if human PDS is eventually shown to have a relationship to the tyrosinase pathway. Disruption of the iris pigment epithelium with release of melanin granules has also been reported in mice deficient in collagen XVI-II/endostatin deficient mice [56].

12.4.1
Blinking

Lid blinking may be important in determining iris configuration. When blinking is prevented in PDS patients, aqueous humor builds up in the posterior chamber and the iris assumes a planar and even a convex configuration [15, 52]. As the volume of the posterior chamber increases relative to that of the anterior chamber, the iris gradually flattens, iridolenticular contact diminishes, and iridozonular and iridociliary process distances increase. In the most pronounced cases, iridolenticular contact disappears, the iris sphincter lifting completely off the surface of the lens without the posterior chamber losing its expanded volume. Eyes with PDS take longer to reach a steady-state position because their initial iris concavity is greater than that of control eyes [52].

The mechanism by which blinking affects the anatomy of the anterior segment appears to be a mechanical one. Campbell [15] proposed that a blink initially deforms the cornea, transiently increasing IOP and pushing the iris posteriorly against the lens. When PDS patients are permitted to blink and then rescanned, the concave iris configuration returns in all eyes [52]. Chew et al. [20] demonstrated that during blinking of the nictitating membrane in the chick eye, the cornea indents in a wave from the periphery to the center and that anterior chamber depth similarly decreases. Extrapolating this finding to humans, we hypothesize that blinking acts as a mechanical pump to push a bolus of aqueous humor from the posterior chamber to the anterior chamber. A pressure wave is created, pushing the iris posteriorly toward the zonules. This wave begins at the iris periphery and moves centrally, pushing aqueous before it into the anterior chamber and emptying the posterior chamber.

Abnormally extensive iridolenticular contact in eyes with PDS prevents equilibration of aqueous between the anterior and posterior chambers, a situation which has been termed reverse pupillary block [43]. At the same time, the iris reassumes its concave configuration. The now increased volume of aqueous in the anterior chamber helps to maintain the mid-peripheral iris concavity, although whether or not there is a pressure gradient accentuating the concavity remains to be shown. As aqueous leaves the eye through the meshwork and enters via ciliary secretion, the anterior chamber volume decreases and the posterior chamber volume increases, until the next blink starts the cycle all over again. Interestingly, increasing myopia is also a predictor of increasing iridolenticular contact, independent of the presence of PDS [52]. This may explain why myopia enhances the phenotypic expression of the genetic abnormality underlying PDS. It also raises the question as to whether decreased trabecular function and reduction of the aqueous outflow coefficient might serve to accentuate the iris concavity.

12.4.2
Accommodation

Accommodation in normal, young individuals and PDS patients may also affect iris contour [52, 60, 95]. Accommodation in normal eyes causes an iris concavity indistinguishable from that in PDS. Contraction of the ciliary ring allows shallowing of the anterior chamber, anterior lens movement, and increased iridolenticular contact. Aqueous in the anterior chamber is forced into the angle recess and the peripheral iris becomes more concave. As accommodation is relaxed, the iris resumes its initial configuration.

Accommodation might enhance pigment liberation in two ways. In addition to posterior iris bowing during accommodation, the pupil constricts. Relaxation of accommodation accompanied by pupillary dilation might result in additional iridozonular friction. Ultrasound biomicroscopy during accommodation in eyes with PDS shows iridozonular contact at the lens margin, consistent with the usual position of iris transillumination defects [65].

Scanning following administration of pilocarpine shows resolution of the iris concavity and iridozonular contact in all eyes. Pilocarpine produces a convex rather than a planar configuration. Laser iridotomy relieves reverse pupillary block by allowing aqueous to flow from the anterior to the posterior chamber and produces a planar iris configuration. Iridotomy does appear to prevent the accentuation of the iris concavity which accompanies accommodation [65].

12.4.3
Exercise

Some PDS patients may develop IOP rises after shedding pigment with exercise or with pupillary dilation. The majority of patients do not appear to be affected. This is most commonly associated with jogging or bouncing, such as dancing or playing basketball. However, bicycle exercise increased the iris concavity by ultrasound biomicroscopy both in normals [30] and in eyes with PDS [38], an effect which was eliminated in the latter by laser iridotomy. The exercise-induced release of pigment and elevation of IOP can be blocked by pilocarpine [31]. Whereas pilocarpine completely inhibits exercise-induced pigment release and IOP elevation, iridotomy does so incompletely [32].

12.5
Clinical Correlations

12.5.1
Heredity

The above concept of the pathophysiology of PDS helps us to better understand a number of clinical aspects of the disorder. Structural abnormalities are characteristic of autosomal dominant disorders. Only occasional families with Krukenberg spindles were reported prior to the 1980s. Reports in the 1980s described familial PDS, but were inconclusive regarding the mode of inheritance. McDermott et al. [58] examined relatives of 21 probands, and found involvement in 36% of parents and 50% of siblings, indicative of autosomal dominant inheritance, but none in children under the age of 21 years. That Caucasians are almost exclusively affected is also consistent with a genetic origin.

12.5.2
Gender

Men and women are equally affected by PDS, women having predominated in some series and men in others. However, men develop glaucoma about three times as often as women and at a younger mean age. No population-based study has yet been performed. If myopia is the major determinant of phenotypic expression, then one would expect an equal incidence of men and women, since the prevalence of myopia in the United States is similar between men and women.

12.5.3
Race

Pigment dispersion syndrome occurs almost exclusively in Caucasians. African-American patients with PDS reported a significantly greater percentage of Caucasian ancestry and were more lightly complected than controls [78]. Rare cases have been reported in Asia. A form of pigment dispersion associated with retro-iridial lines of Vogt may occur in both blacks and whites [63, 79]. Pigment dispersion was described in a series of 20 black patients who were primarily older, hyperopic women, although lines of Vogt were not mentioned in this report [86].

12.5.4
Refractive Error

About 60%–80% of patients with PDS and PG are myopes and 20% are emmetropes (–1.00 to +1.00 diopters). In earlier series which reported about 10% of patients to be hyperopes, there appears to have been some confusion between PDS and exfoliation syndrome, particularly as the hyperopes in these series tended to be older and to be women. Eyes with PG are significantly more myopic than those with PDS and the higher the myopia, the earlier is the age of onset of glaucoma [9, 27].

12.5.5
Asymmetric Involvement

Since PDS is a bilateral disorder, asymmetric involvement requires explanation. A second disorder may make one eye worse. The most common cause in older patients appears to be the development of exfoliation syndrome in one eye in patients who had had PDS or PG glaucoma in earlier life [48]. Angle recession in one eye has also been reported [59, 71]. It is also possible for one eye to have a second disorder which reduces the severity of PDS, such as unilateral traumatic cataract extraction in youth prior to the onset of pigment dispersion or development of unilater-

al cataract during the pigment dispersion phase, which decreases iridozonular contact by causing pupillary block [73]. Trauma resulting in an iridectomy [88] and an iris coloboma [94] leading to protection against PDS have been reported. Horner's syndrome may achieve the same effect [44], while Adie's pupil has been associated with PDS in the same eye [64].

In other cases, mild to marked asymmetry may exist without any other evident process. Kaiser-Kupfer et al. [41] reported four normotensive patients with markedly asymmetric involvement and no obvious cause for asymmetry. Three had anterior chamber depths 0.2 mm greater in the affected eye. Liebmann et al. [51] examined four patients with markedly asymmetric PDS and no other ocular conditions to explain the asymmetry and found greater iridolenticular contact and a more posterior iris insertion in the more involved eye in all cases.

12.6
Natural History

12.6.1
Active Phase

The mean age of onset of PDS remains unknown, but is probably in the mid-20 s. Patients in their early teens have been reported. Although it seems logical that PDS might develop in the mid-teens, when myopia is commonly progressive, a screening of over 300 students at Stuyvesant High School, a school for above-average intelligent children in New York City, did not reveal a single case (unpublished results). Moreover, McDermott et al. [58] found no children of probands positive up to age 21. Further studies are warranted.

The phenotypic expression of PDS varies widely. More subtle manifestations may never be detected either because of a lack of suspicion on the part of the examiner, unawareness of the examiner of pathognomonic signs in patients with mild phenotypic involvement, failure to perform slit-lamp examination in patients presenting for refraction, and simply lack of an eye examination. Failure to perform gonioscopy may result in lack of diagnosis of patients with trabecular hyperpigmentation but without Krukenberg spindles, since transscleral transillumination is often the least likely test to be performed. It is not known whether the variability in phenotypic expression is hereditary, environmental, or a combination of both. For instance, the concavity due to iris position and size (genetic) could be affected by the cumulative amount of accommodation (environmental).

12.6.2
Regression Phase

Loss of accommodation with the onset of presbyopia and development of relative pupillary block secondary to increased lens thickness with age presumably lead to the cessation of pigment liberation in middle age. Older patients with PDS develop little or no accentuation of the iris concavity with accommodation [65]. The severity of involvement of both PDS and PG decreases in middle age when pigment liberation ceases. Transillumination defects may disappear [13, 23], most likely by migration of pigment epithelial cells adjacent to the defects. The IOP may return toward normal [23, 91, 93, 99]. Some patients treated with long-term miotic therapy have been able to reduce or discontinue treatment for glaucoma [14, 91]. Older patients presenting with glaucoma may have only very subtle manifestations, if any, of PDS, and may be misdiagnosed as primary open-angle glaucoma or normal-tension glaucoma [69]. Remission of PG has also been reported following glaucoma surgery [84] and following lens subluxation [72].

Trabecular pigmentation is initially dense and homogeneous for 360°. With age and clearance of pigment from the angle, it becomes lighter and more localized to the filtering portion of the meshwork, while it disappears from Schwalbe's line and the scleral spur. When the trabecular meshwork begins to recover, the normal pigment pattern reverses and the pigment band becomes darker superiorly than inferiorly. We have termed this the "pigment reversal sign" and, in older patients, it may be the only finding suggestive of previous PDS. Although it cannot be regarded as diagnostic, examination of the patient's offspring in such a case may be confirmatory. The pigment reversal sign may also be found in patients after long-term miotic therapy in patients with PDS/PG and also in patients with exfoliation syndrome, confirming that it occurs as a result of pigment clearing from the meshwork.

12.6.3
Conversion to Glaucoma

The frequency with which PDS converts to PG has probably been greatly overestimated. The three studies which have examined patients longitudinally suggest that up to 50% will eventually develop glaucoma [24, 61, 68]. However, the true rate of PDS in the general population may be an order of magnitude greater than has previously been suspected [76]. Wilensky et al. found only two of 43 patients with Krukenberg spindles developed visual field loss during a mean of 5.8 years of follow-up [98]. In a retrospective community-based study, 113 patients, of whom nine developed PG or elevated IOP requiring therapy, were newly diagnosed with PDS over 24 years [89]. The probability of converting to PG was 10% at 5 years and 15% at 15 years.

12.6.4
Differential Diagnosis

Other disorders can produce abnormal pigment dispersion. Exfoliation syndrome may produce dense trabecular pigmentation. A typical Krukenberg spindle does not develop; rather, a more evenly distributed flecking of pigment develops on the posterior surface of the corneal endothelium. The diagnosis is made by discerning the typical pattern of exfoliation material within the eye in association with pigment dispersion. Patients who have had PDS can develop exfoliation syndrome in later life [49, 77]. We are finding this combination increasingly common as patients with known PDS have been followed into middle age.

Secondary pigment dispersion has also been reported associated with iris pigment epithelial cysts [2], iris nevus [45], and melanocytoma of the ciliary body [10]. Peripheral iris and/or ciliary body cysts can occasionally cause dispersion of a moderate amount of pigment to the trabecular meshwork, but again there is no typical Krukenberg spindle. Iris, ciliary body, or even posterior segment melanomas (if the anterior hyaloid face is disrupted), can be associated with dispersed pigment [19]. The pigmented tumor cells, or pigment-laden macrophages, may cause considerable darkening of the anterior and posterior chambers. The typical signs of PDS/PG are absent: there is no Krukenberg spindle; there are no transillumination defects; and, the tumor is usually readily apparent. Inflammation involving the posterior surface of the iris can occasionally disperse a moderate amount of pigment often clumped in the inferior angle.

A secondary form of PDS capable of causing glaucoma has been described following implantation of a posterior chamber intraocular lens (PCIOL) [17, 21, 35, 81] and after penetrating keratoplasty with a PCIOL. In this situation, ongoing postoperative contact between the iris and the abnormally positioned IOL causes release of pigment. This entity has been termed pseudophakic posterior iris chafing syndrome [57]. Posterior chamber phakic refractive lenses have also been reported to induce PDS through contact between the lens and the iris [11, 34], as has piggyback lens implantation [36].

12.6.5
Treatment

Classically, PG has been treated identically with POAG. However, there are important differences based upon the mechanism of development of elevated IOP in PDS which warrant a very different approach to therapy. Prostaglandin analogues, which increase uveoscleral outflow, produce an excellent IOP response in patients with PDS and are now our first line choice of drug.

Miotics both constrict the pupil, eliminating iridozonular contact, and increase aqueous outflow, lowering IOP, thus allowing the pathophysiologic process to begin to reverse, and should be in principle the drug of choice with which to initiate therapy. Miotics may prevent progression of the disease and the development of glaucoma by both inhibiting iris pigment release and by enhancing clearance of the pigment through the trabecular meshwork. The peripheral retina should be examined carefully and appropriate steps taken if lattice is present.

Strong miotics are poorly tolerated because of accommodative spasm and induced myopia in young patients, causing difficulty functioning in work-related situations and activities such as sports and driving, particularly at night. Pilocarpine Ocuserts have proven to be the best delivery system for miotic therapy, and had excellent success with them. Ocuserts immobilize the pupil without causing extreme miosis, allowing normal functioning. Unfortunately, their manufacture has been discontinued.

Alpha-adrenergic antagonists, such as dapiprazole, constrict the pupil and may pull the peripheral iris away from the zonules to reduce pigment release. Unlike cholinergic agonists, which contract the iris sphincter and ciliary muscle, alpha$_1$-adrenergic antagonists produce miosis by relaxing the dilator muscle and do not affect the ciliary muscle. Although dapiprazole has been reported to be beneficial, we found it poorly tolerated due to burning and marked conjunctival hyperemia with chronic usage and it causes irregular and insufficient miosis.

Aqueous suppressants have theoretical disadvantages. They decrease IOP by reducing aqueous flow, which would diminish the rate of clearance of the pigment from the trabecular meshwork, and conceivably exacerbate the disease process. Furthermore, reduced aqueous flow into the posterior chamber may exacerbate reverse pupillary block, allowing for more rubbing of the posterior iris surface against the zonules to release more pigment. Nonselective beta-blockers are likely to suppress younger patients' exercise-induced tachycardia and interfere with exercise tolerance.

Laser peripheral iridotomy (LPI) has been advocated for treatment of PDS as a means of eliminating reverse pupillary block, just as it does in angle closure caused by relative pupillary block. In relative pupillary block, iridotomy results in opening of the angle and increased iridolenticular contact [18], while in reverse pupillary block, it produces narrowing of the angle and decreased iridolenticular contact [12]. The iris contour flattens after LPI, although perhaps not in all cases. A reduction of IOP has been reported to correlate with loss of the iris concavity [66].

The number of aqueous melanin granules in the anterior chamber has been correlated with IOP93 and is decreased after LPI [47]. In one study, 21 patients with PDS underwent unilateral LPI and a rise in IOP of more than 5 mmHg was reported in 11/21 untreated fellow eyes during a 2-year follow-up [26]. No other study of PDS has reported this high a proportion of rises in IOP in normotensive eyes with PDS in so short a time, nor have we seen such rises in our patients. In a review of 23 patients with PDS and elevated IOP with no or mild glaucomatous damage having undergone LPI, Wang et al. found no significant long-term IOP reduction in the lasered eyes compared to the medically treated fellow eyes [96]. Most of these eyes were treated with pilocarpine Ocuserts and/or latanoprost. Retrospective analysis showed no clear benefit of LPI in PDS. However, definitive conclusions were rendered difficult by selection bias, use or nonuse of miotics, and advent of latanoprost.

Who should undergo LPI? Ostensibly, by preventing further pigment liberation from the iris, the meshwork would have time to clear itself of pigment already deposited and reduce or eliminate further deposition. Therefore, patients should still be in the pigment liberation stage. If pigment is liberated into the anterior chamber with pupillary dilation, it is suggestive that the patient is still in this stage. Patients who have uncontrolled glaucoma and are facing surgery are also poor candidates for LPI, since perhaps years are required to achieve functional reconstitution of the trabecular meshwork [74].

As a rule of thumb, we have restricted iridotomy so far to patients under 45 years of age who have elevated IOP with no damage or early glaucomatous damage. Clinical trials are needed to determine whether Ocuserts or iridotomy can normalize IOP in eyes with glaucomatous damage, prevent glaucomatous damage in eyes with elevated IOP, and prevent elevated IOP in normotensive eyes. Since not all patients with PDS go on to develop elevated IOP, and since the iridotomy procedure itself results in significant pigment liberation, we do not advocate treating normotensive eyes at the present time.

The success rate of argon laser trabeculoplasty (ALT) in PG is greater in younger patients than in older ones and decreases with age [54, 75]. Pigment in younger patients is largely in the uveoscleral and corneoscleral meshworks, whereas in older patients, it if primarily localized to the juxtacanalicular meshwork and the back wall of Schlemm's canal [75]. A larger portion of patients fail within a shorter period of time compared to POAG patients [54, 75]. Initially successful trabeculoplasty may be followed by a sudden, late rise in IOP, similar to that seen in exfoliative glaucoma. Patients in the pigment liberation stage who undergo ALT should be maintained on miotics or undergo laser iridotomy after ALT to prevent further contact between the iris and zonules.

Summary for the Clinician

- Eyes with PDS differ from normal eyes in having an apparently larger iris, a mid-peripheral posterior iris concavity which increases with accommodation, a more posterior iris insertion, increased iridolenticular contact which is reversed by inhibition of blinking, possibly an inherent weakness of the iris pigment epithelium, and an increased incidence of lattice degeneration of the retina

- The classic clinical findings of PDS begin to reverse in middle age with the onset of presbyopia, and understanding of the mechanism underlying the iris pigment liberation allows planning treatment to not only lower IOP but to reverse the pathophysiology. In this instance, glaucoma is a preventable disease.

References

1. Alward WLM, Haynes WL (1991) Pupillometric and videographic evaluation of anisocoria in patients with the pigment dispersion syndrome. Invest Ophthalmol Vis Sci 32[Suppl]:1109
2. Alward WL, Ossoinig KC (1995) Pigment dispersion secondary to cysts of the iris pigment epithelium. Arch Ophthalmol 113:1574–1575
3. Alward WL, Munden PM, Verdick RE, Perell HR, Thompson HS (1990) Use of infrared videography to detect and record iris transillumination defects. Arch Ophthalmol 108:748–750
4. Andersen JS, Pralea AM, DelBono EA et al (1997) A gene responsible for the PDS maps to chromosome 7q35-q36. Arch Ophthalmol 115:384–388
5. Andersen JS, Delbono EA, Haines JL, Wiggs JL (1999) Identification and genetic analysis of pigmentary glaucoma loci on 7q36 and 18q. Invest Ophthalmol Vis Sci 40[Suppl]:S596
6. Anderson MG, Smith RS, Hawes NL et al (2002) Mutations in genes encoding melanosomal proteins cause pigmentary glaucoma in DBA/2J mice. Nature Genet 30:81–85
7. Becker B, Morton WR (1964) Phenylthiourea taste testing and glaucoma. Arch Ophthalmol 72:323–327
8. Becker B, Shin DH, Cooper DG, Kass MA (1977) The pigment dispersion syndrome. Am J Ophthalmol 83:161–166
9. Berger A, Ritch R, McDermott J et al (1987) Pigmentary dispersion, refraction and glaucoma. Invest Ophthalmol Vis Sci 28[Suppl]:134
10. Bhorade AM, Edward DP, Goldstein DA (1999) Ciliary body melanocytoma with anterior segment pigment dispersion and elevated intraocular pressure. J Glaucoma 8:129–133
11. Brandt JD, Mockovak ME, Chayet A (2001) Pigmentary dispersion syndrome induced by a posterior chamber phakic refractive lens. Am J Ophthalmol 131:260–263
12. Breingan PJ, Esaki K, Ishikawa H, Liebmann JM, Greenfield DS, Ritch R (1999) Iridolenticular contact decreases following laser iridotomy for pigment dispersion syndrome. Arch Ophthalmol 117:325–328
13. Campbell DG (1979) Pigmentary dispersion and glaucoma. A new theory. Arch Ophthalmol 97:1667–1672
14. Campbell DG (1983) Improvement of pigmentary glaucoma and healing of transillumination defects with miotic therapy. Invest Ophthalmol Vis Sci 23[Suppl]:173
15. Campbell DG (1993) Iridotomy, blinking and pigmentary glaucoma. Invest Ophthalmol Vis Sci 34[Suppl]:993
16. Campbell DG, Jeffery CP (1979) Pigmentary dispersion in the human eye. Scanning electron microscopy. In: O'Hare, SEM Inc, 329–334
17. Caplan MB, Brown RH, Love LL (1988) Pseudophakic pigmentary glaucoma. Am J Ophthalmol 105:320–321
18. Caronia RM, Liebmann JM, Stegman Z et al (1996) Iris-lens contact increases following laser iridotomy for pupillary block angle-closure. Am J Ophthalmol 122:53–57
19. Chaudhry IM, Moster MR, Augsburger JJ (1997) Iris ring melanoma masquerading as pigmentary glaucoma. Arch Ophthalmol 115:1480–1481
20. Chew SJ, Tello C, Wallman J, Ritch R (1994) Blinking indents the cornea and reduces anterior chamber volume as shown by ultrasound biomicroscopy. Invest Ophthalmol Vis Sci 35[Suppl]:1573
21. Cykiert RC (1986) Pigmentary glaucoma associated with posterior chamber intraocular lenses. Am J Ophthalmol 101:500–501
22. Davidson JA, Brubaker RF, Ilstrup DM (1983) Dimensions of the anterior chamber in pigment dispersion syndrome. Arch Ophthalmol 101:81–83
23. Epstein DL (1979) Pigment dispersion and pigmentary glaucoma. In: Chandler PA, Grant WM (eds) Glaucoma. Lea and Febiger, Philadelphia, p 122
24. Farrar SM, Shields MB, Miller KN, Stoup CM (1989) Risk factors for the development and severity of glaucoma in the pigment dispersion syndrome. Am J Ophthalmol 108:223–229
25. Fine BS, Yanoff M, Scheie HG (1974) Pigmentary "glaucoma". A histologic study. Trans Am Acad Ophthalmol Otolaryngol 78:OP314–325
26. Gandolfi SA, Vecchi M (1996) Effect of a YAG laser iridotomy on intraocular pressure in pigment dispersion syndrome. Ophthalmology 103:1693–1695
27. Gramer E, Thiele H, Ritch R (1998) Family history of glaucoma and risk factors in pigmentary glaucoma. A new clinical study. Klin Monatsbl Augenheilkd 212:454–464
28. Greenstein VC, Seiple W, Liebmann J, Ritch R (2001) Retinal pigment epithelial dysfunction in patients with pigment dispersion syndrome: implications for the theory of pathogenesis. Arch Ophthalmol 119:1291–1295
29. Gürses-Ozden R, Emarah A, Liebmann JM, Ritch R (2001) Phenylthiocarbamide taste testing in patients with pigmentary glaucoma. Arch Ophthalmol 119:309–310

30. Haargaard B, Jensen PK, Kessing SV, Nissen OI (2001) Exercise and iris concavity in healthy eyes. Acta Ophthalmol Scand 79:277–282

31. Haynes WL, Johnson AT, Alward WLM (1990) Inhibition of exercise-induced pigment dispersion in a patient with the pigment dispersion syndrome. Am J Ophthalmol 109:599–601

32. Haynes WL, Alward WL, Tello C, Liebmann JM, Ritch R (1995) Incomplete elimination of exercise-induced pigment dispersion by laser iridotomy in pigment dispersion syndrome. Ophthalmic Surg Lasers 26:484–486

33. Heys JJ, Barocas VH, Taravella MJ (2001) Modeling passive mechanical interaction between aqueous humor and iris. J Biomech Engin 123:540–547

34. Hoyos JE, Dementiev DD, Cigales M, Hoyos-Chacón J, Hoffer KJ (2002) Phakic refractive lens experience in Spain. J Cataract Refract Surg 28:1939–1946

35. Huber C (1984) The gray iris syndrome. An iatrogenic form of pigmentary glaucoma. Arch Ophthalmol 102:397–398

36. Häberle H, Wirbelauer C, Aurich H, Pham DT (2003) Piggyback lens implantation for anisometropia in pseudophakic eyes. Ophthalmologe 100:129–132

37. Jacobi PC, Dietlein TS, Krieglstein GK (2000) Effect of trabecular aspiration on intraocular pressure in pigment dispersion syndrome and pigmentary glaucoma. Ophthalmology 107:417–421

38. Jensen PK, Nissen O, Kessing SV (1995) Exercise and reversed pupillary block in pigmentary glaucoma. Am J Ophthalmol 120:110–112

39. John SW, Smith RS, Savinova OV, Hawes NL, Chang B, Turnbull D, Davisson M, Roderick TH, Heckenlively JR (1998) Essential iris atrophy, pigment dispersion, and glaucoma in DBA/2J mice. Invest Ophthalmol Vis Sci 39:951–962

40. Jonas JB, Dichtl A, Budde WM, Lang P (1998) Optic disc morphology in pigmentary glaucoma. Br J Ophthalmol 82:875–879

41. Kaiser-Kupfer MI, Kupfer C, McCain L (1983) Asymmetric pigment dispersion syndrome. Trans Am Ophthalmol Soc 81:310–324

42. Kampik A, Green WR, Quigley HA, Pierce LH (1981) Scanning and transmission electron microscopic studies of two cases of pigment dispersion syndrome. Am J Ophthalmol 91:573–587

43. Karickhoff JR (1992) Pigmentary dispersion syndrome and pigmentary glaucoma: a new mechanism concept, a new treatment, and a new technique. Ophthalmic Surg 23:269–277

44. Krebs DB, Colquhoun J, Ritch R, Liebmann JM (1989) Asymmetric pigment dispersion syndrome in a patient with unilateral Horner's syndrome. Am J Ophthalmol 108:737–738

45. Kremer I, Cohen S, Loya N, Sandbank U (1989) Massive pseudophakic pigment dispersion associated with an iris nevus. Ophthalmic Surg 20:182–185

46. Kupfer C, Kuwabara T, Kaiser-Kupfer M (1975) The histopathology of pigmentary dispersion syndrome with glaucoma. Am J Ophthalmol 80: 857–862

47. Küchle M, Nguyen NX, Mardin CY, Naumann GO (2001) Effect of neodymium:YAG laser iridotomy on number of aqueous melanin granules in primary pigment dispersion syndrome. Graefes Arch Clin Exp Ophthalmol 239:411–415

48. Layden WE, Shaffer RN (1974) Exfoliation syndrome. Am J Ophthalmol 78:835–841

49. Layden WE, Ritch R, King DG, Teekhasaenee C (1990) Combined exfoliation and pigment dispersion syndrome. Am J Ophthalmol 109:530–534

50. Libby RT, Smith RS, Savinova OV, Zabaleta A, Martin JE, Gonzalez FJ, John SW (2003) Modification of ocular defects in mouse developmental glaucoma models by tyrosinase. Science 299: 1578–1581

51. Liebmann JM, Langlieb A, Stegman Z et al (1995) Anterior chamber anatomy in asymmetric pigment dispersion syndrome. Invest Ophthalmol Vis Sci 36[Suppl]:S562

52. Liebmann JM, Tello C, Chew SJ, Cohen H, Ritch R (1995) Prevention of blinking alters iris configuration in pigment dispersion syndrome and in normal eyes. Ophthalmology 102:446–455

53. Lord FD, Pathanapitoon K, Mikelberg FS (2001) Keratometry and axial length in pigment dispersion syndrome: a descriptive case-control study. J Glaucoma 10:383–385

54. Lunde MW (1983) Argon laser trabeculoplasty in pigmentary dispersion syndrome with glaucoma. Am J Ophthalmol 96:721–725

55. Mardin CY, Küchle M, Nguyen NX, Martus P, Naumann GO (2000) Quantification of aqueous melanin granules, intraocular pressure and glaucomatous damage in primary pigment dispersion syndrome. Ophthalmology 107:435–440

56. Marneros AG, Olsen BR (2003) Age-dependent iris abnormalities in collagen XVIII/endostatin deficient mice with similarities to human pigment dispersion syndrome. Invest Ophthalmol Vis Sci 44:2367–2372

57. Masket S (1986) Pseudophakic posterior iris chafing syndrome. J Cataract Refract Surg 12:252–256

58. McDermott JA, Ritch R, Berger A, Wang RF (1987) Familial occurrence of pigmentary dispersion syndrome. Invest Ophthalmol Vis Sci 28[Suppl]: 136

59. McKinney JK, Alward WL (1997) Unilateral pigment dispersion and glaucoma caused by angle recession. Arch Ophthalmol 115:1478–1479

60. McWhae J, Crichton A (1994) International Society for Ophthalmic Ultrasound. Cortina, Italy
61. Migliazzo CV, Shaffer RN, Nykin R, Magee S (1986) Long-term analysis of pigmentary dispersion syndrome and pigmentary glaucoma. Ophthalmology 93:1528–1536
62. Mo JS, Anderson MG, Gregory M, Smith RS, Savinova OV, Serreze DV, Ksander BR, Streilein JW, John SW (2003) By altering ocular immune privilege, bone marrow-derived cells pathogenically contribute to DBA/2J pigmentary glaucoma. J Exp Med 197:1335–1344
63. Moroi SE, Lark KK, Sieving PA et al (2003) Retroiridial lines of Vogt and pigment dispersion. Am J Ophthalmol 136:1176–1178
64. Murthy S, Hawksworth N (2001) Asymmetric pigment dispersion in a patient with the unilateral Adie pupil. Am J Ophthalmol 132:410–411
65. Pavlin CJ, Macken P, Trope GE, Harasiewicz K, Foster FS (1996) Accommodation and iridotomy in the pigment dispersion syndrome. Ophthalmic Surg Lasers 27:113–120
66. Pillunat LE, Böhm A, Fuisting B, Kohlhaas M, Richard G (2000) Ultrasound biomicroscopy in pigmentary glaucoma. Ophthalmologe 97:268–271
67. Richardson TM, Hutchinson BT, Grant WM (1977) The outflow tract in pigmentary glaucoma: a light and electron microscopic study. Arch Ophthalmol 95:1015–1025
68. Richter CU, Richardson TM, Grant WM (1986) Pigmentary dispersion syndrome and pigmentary glaucoma. A prospective study of the natural history. Arch Ophthalmol 104:211–215
69. Ritch R (1982) Nonprogressive low-tension glaucoma with pigmentary dispersion. Am J Ophthalmol 94:190–196
70. Ritch R (1996) A unification hypothesis of pigment dispersion syndrome. Trans Am Ophthalmol Soc 94:381–405; discussion 405–409
71. Ritch R, Alward WL (1993) Asymmetric pigmentary glaucoma caused by unilateral angle recession. Am J Ophthalmol 116:765–766
72. Ritch R, Manusow D, Podos SM (1982) Remission of pigmentary glaucoma in a patient with subluxed lenses. Am J Ophthalmol 94:812–813
73. Ritch R, Chaiwat T, Harbin TS (1992) Asymmetric pigmentary glaucoma resulting from cataract formation. Am J Ophthalmol 114:484–488
74. Ritch R, Campbell DG, Camras C (1993) Initial treatment of pigmentary glaucoma. J Glaucoma 2:44–49
75. Ritch R, Liebmann J, Robin A, Pollack IP, Harrison R, Levene RZ, Hagadus J (1993) Argon laser trabeculoplasty in pigmentary glaucoma. Ophthalmology 100:909–913
76. Ritch R, Steinberger D, Liebmann JM (1993) Prevalence of pigment dispersion syndrome in a population undergoing glaucoma screening. Am J Ophthalmol 115:707–710
77. Ritch R, Mudumbai R, Liebmann JM (2000) Combined exfoliation and pigment dispersion: an overlap syndrome. Ophthalmology 107:1004–1008
78. Roberts DK, Ho LA, Beedle NL et al (2000) Heritage characteristics reported by a group of African-Americans who exhibit the pigment dispersion syndrome: a case-control study. Doc Ophthalmol 101:179–193. Erratum: Doc Ophthalmol 2001;102:81–82
79. Roberts DK, Lo PS, Winters JE, Castells DD, Alexander CC, Teitelbaum BA (2002) Prevalence of pigmented lens striae in a black population: a potential indicator of age-related pigment dispersal in the anterior segment. Optom Vis Sci 79:681–687
80. Rodrigues MM, Spaeth GL, Weinreb S, Sivalingam E (1976) Spectrum of trabecular pigmentation in open-angle glaucoma: a clinicopathologic study. Trans Am Acad Ophthalmol Otolaryngol 81:258–276
81. Samples JR, Van Buskirk EM (1985) Pigmentary glaucoma associated with posterior chamber intraocular lenses. Am J Ophthalmol 100:385–388
82. Schanen NC, Scherer SW, Tsui LC, Francke U (1996) Assignment of the 5-hydroxytryptamine (serotonin) receptor 5A gene (HTR5A) to human chromosome band 7q36.1. Cytogenet Cell Genet 72:187–188
83. Scheie HG, Fleischhauer HW (1958) Idiopathic atrophy of the epithelial layers of the iris and ciliary body; a clinical study. Ama Arch Opthalmol 59:216–228
84. Scheie HG, Cameron JD (1981) Pigment dispersion syndrome: a clinical study. Br J Ophthalmol 65:264–269
85. Scuderi GL, Ricci F, Nucci C, Galasso MJ, Cerulli L (1998) Electro-oculography in pigment dispersion syndrome. Ophthalmic Res 30:23–29
86. Semple HC, Ball SF (1990) Pigmentary glaucoma in the black population. Am J Ophthalmol 109:518–522
87. Shimizu T, Hara K, Futa R (1981) Fine structure of trabecular meshwork and iris in pigmentary glaucoma. Albrecht Von Graefes Arch Klin Exp Ophthalmol 215:171–180
88. Shuttleworth GN (1999) A traumatic "peripheral iridotomy" protects against pigment dispersion and glaucoma. Br J Ophthalmol 83:376
89. Siddiqui Y, Ten Hulzen RD, Cameron JD, Hodge DO, Johnson DH (2003) What is the risk of developing pigmentary glaucoma from pigment dispersion syndrome. Am J Ophthalmol 135:794–799

90. Sokol J, Stegman Z, Liebmann JM, Ritch R (1996) Location of the iris insertion in pigment dispersion syndrome. Ophthalmology 103:289–293

91. Speakman JS (1981) Pigmentary dispersion. Br J Ophthalmol 65:249–251

92. Strasser G, Hauff W (1985) Pigmentary dispersion syndrome. A biometric study. Acta Ophthalmol (Copenh) 63:721–722

93. Tarkkanen A, Kivelä T (1999) Unilateral capsular glaucoma after long-standing bilateral pigmentary glaucoma. Eye 13 (Pt 2):212–214

94. Tesser PM (2003) An iris coloboma preventing pigmentary glaucoma. Arch Ophthalmol 121: 1055–1056

95. Ueda J, Sawaguchi S, Watanabe J, Shirakashi M, Abe H (1997) Posterior iris bowing after accommodation – elucidation of the etiology of pigment dispersion syndrome. Nippon Ganka Gakkai Zasshi 101:187–191

96. Wang JC, Liebmann JM, Ritch R (2001) Long-term outcome of argon laser iridotomy in pigment dispersion syndrome. Invest Ophthalmol Vis Sci 42[Suppl]:S560

97. Weseley P, Liebmann J, Walsh JB, Ritch R (1992) Lattice degeneration of the retina and the pigment dispersion syndrome. Am J Ophthalmol 114:539–543

98. Wilensky JT, Buerk KM, Podos SM (1975) Krukenberg's spindles. Am J Ophthalmol 79:220–225

99. Yanoff M, Fine BS (1975) Ocular pathology: a text and atlas. Harper & Row, New York

Wound Modulation in Glaucoma Surgery

Holger Mietz

Core Messages

- Scarring of subconjunctival connective tissue is the main source of failure of trabeculectomy
- Preoperatively applied topical medications increase the wound healing response after trabeculectomy
- Potent topical corticosteroids after trabeculectomy strongly interfere with many of the wound healing cascades and are the basis for postoperative wound healing modulation
- 5-FU may be recommended as a series of postoperative injections. However, inconvenient side-effects have to be considered and discussed with the patient before surgery
- Mitomycin C is used mostly in refractory glaucomas (repeat-trabeculectomy), secondary glaucomas, and in normal pressure glaucoma. However, some surgeons use it also in primary trabeculectomies. Long-term side effects have to be considered
- MMC can be used postoperatively topically applied to the conjunctiva with a sponge at a 0.05-mg/ml concentration with few side effects
- Subconjunctival injections of TGF-β2 monoclonal antibodies are a new treatment regimen to specifically block excessive wound healing responses after trabeculectomy
- Suramin blocks various cellular wound healing processes and may be an alternative to presently used compounds like MMC or 5-FU

13.1
Introduction

13.1.1
Basics

At present, trabeculectomy is the most frequently performed procedure to surgically treat glaucoma. Alternative procedures such as visco-canalostomy and deep sclerectomy do not achieve the amount of reduction of intraocular pressure (IOP) that can be accomplished with trabeculectomy [25]. The AGIS study [1] has pointed out the importance of individual target pressures as opposed to a general cut-off line. The study has shown that eyes with advanced stages of glaucoma have target pressures that are well below usually accepted levels. This makes it important to reduce the IOP in selected cases markedly below values of 22 mmHg or 21 mmHg.

13.1.2
Wound Healing Following Trabeculectomy

Scarring at the episcleral and deep Tenon's level is the main cause of failure of trabeculectomy. Several factors influence and control the complicated mechanism of wound healing. Extracellular matrix components such as collagen and fibronectin, cell adhesion molecules such as selectins and integrins, and different growth factors are intimately involved with the fibroblasts (Fig. 13.1) [7].

Among other factors, the amount, duration and kind of pre-operatively topically applied medications have an impact on the conjunctival

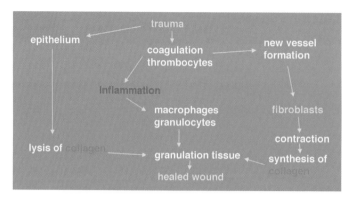

Fig. 13.1. Flow diagram showing a few important steps regarding conjunctival wound healing following surgical procedures involving the conjunctiva

fibroblasts and on the composition of the extracellular matrix. Conjunctival changes following topical antiglaucomatous therapy include a decrease in the number of epithelial goblet cells, an increase in subepithelial collagen deposition, and a higher number of macrophages, fibroblasts, lymphocytes, and mast cells in the substantia propria [8, 9, 46].

Ongoing studies address the issue of whether it is better to initially perform surgery as compared to medical treatment. Previous studies have suggested a better long-term success of trabeculectomies in eyes with no pre-operative long-term topical antiglaucomatous therapy.

13.1.3
Therapeutic Options

In an effort to influence the wound healing cascade at least with some rationale, potential substances should directly interfere with the subsequent single steps that lead to the deposition of new fibrous connective tissue, with fibrocytes being the main target cells.

Different substances have been tested and found effective to interfere with fibroblast proliferation using tissue cultures of human conjunctival fibroblasts. Such tissue samples are easy to obtain for laboratory studies during cataract surgery. Only some of the substances that were promising in tissue culture studies found their way to use in animal models and only a few of these have been reported to improve success rates in human studies [23, 37].

5-Fluorouracil (5-FU) and mitomycin have gained widespread acceptance among glaucoma surgeons [18, 33]. Many authors describe the use of mitomycin as the "gold standard" for trabeculectomies that have an increased risk for failure, and some even promote the use of mitomycin for every trabeculectomy performed.

In contrast to these two highly toxic drugs, attempts were recently made to use a different class of substances that are not antineoplastic. These substances use a new pathway in that they interfere with the action of growth factors on target cells [41]. During surgery, several growth factors are released from the blood, from the tissue, and from the aqueous humor. These growth factors play an important role in the activation of tissue fibroblasts to proliferate and produce ground substance and collagen fibrils [6, 16, 35, 45].

13.1.3.1
Steroids

It may be common sense, but the post-operative application of corticosteroids does have an important effect on the wound healing process. Corticosteroids reduce the deposition of fibrin, reduce leakage of capillaries, reduce the migration of leukocytes and makrophages, and reduce the activity of phagocytosis of these makrophages.

In addition to these effects, corticosteroids reduce the activity of fibroblasts to build and deposit new collagen fibers. The activity of phospholipase A2 is inhibited, which usually liberates arachidonic acid from the plasma membrane phospholipases. Through this mechanism, the synthesis of mediators that activate the lipooxygenase and cyclooxygenase pathways is down-regulated. Furthermore, the degranulation of granulocytes and mast cells is reduced, stabilizing the intracellular lysosomes and reducing chemotaxis.

These actions are important for the wound healing process itself, and this process runs its own time course as a biological phenomenon. Therefore, clinical impressions from the individual case should not influence the therapeutic regimen too much.

To obtain the optimum effect from the use of corticosteroids, only highly potent corticosteroids such as prednisolone and dexamethasone should be used. Corticosteroids with a more superficial action are less likely to have a strong enough effect on the conjunctiva, and non-steroidal anti-inflammatory substances (NSAID) may similarly not be effective enough.

The time period of intensified application of the corticosteroids should be at least 4–6 weeks after surgery and can be slowly tapered afterwards.

In a few instances, corticosteroids should be avoided or given with caution:

- In patients who are steroid-responders
- In eyes with a conjunctival wound healing problem following the use of antimetabolites

A systemic application of corticosteroids, regardless of the dosage, can not replace the effect of topical medication nor can it increase the efficacy. Therefore, systemic application is not necessary and should be avoided, reducing unnecessary side effects.

13.1.3.2
5-Fluorouracil

5-Fluorouracil was the first antimetabolite that found its way into routine use among glaucoma surgeons. 5-Fluorouracil is a fluorinated pyrimidine analogue that acts as a potent antimetabolite by competitively inhibiting thymidylate synthetase and cell division. Animal models demonstrated decreased fibroblast proliferation and scarring after filtration surgery.

13.1.3.3
Mitomycin

Mitomycin C is the most active fraction of the three different mitomycins A, B, and C, and exhibits both antibacterial and antineoplastic activity, the latter in a broad spectrum against transplanted and spontaneous tumors (Fig. 13.2). As an alkylating substance, MMC has three active groups, quinone, urethane, and aziridine. The binding to proteins seems to have a relation to the activity of mitomycin. In mammalian cells, DNA synthesis is inhibited, preformed DNA is degraded, and lysis of nuclei is induced. At markedly higher concentrations than necessary for these effects, RNA synthesis is affected. DNA synthesis inhibition by cross-linking of DNA requires the lowest concentrations of MMC and is the most important mechanism. DNA repair mechanisms do not tend to be influenced. Cells are most vulnerable in the G1 and S phases, although some effect is present at any time throughout the cell cycle (Fig. 13.3).

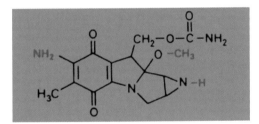

Fig. 13.2. Schematic drawing with the molecule structure of mitomycin C

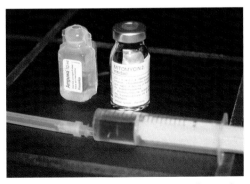

Fig. 13.3. Mitomycin is available as a sterile powder. After dissolving in BSS, the liquid gets a blue color and is light sensitive

13.1.3.4
Transforming Growth Factor-β

In humans, transforming growth factor-β (TGF-β) exists in the three different forms TGF-β1, TGF-β2, and TGF-β3. At least TGF-β1 and TGF-β2 have been shown to be an important component of conjunctival scarring, and it is not surprising that neutralization of its activity makes it a possible target for modulating the scarring response following glaucoma filtration surgery.

For the synthesis of antibodies against these TGF-βs, the technique of phage display is used. For identification, a human single chain Fv (scFv) fragment is isolated that neutralizes the hormone from a phage display repertoire. This is converted into a human IgG4 to determine its binding and neutralizing properties. The selected antibodies have a high affinity for TGF-β2 with only low cross-reactivity for TGF-β1 and TGF-β3. In bioassays, the antibodies strongly neutralize the anti-proliferative effect of TGF-β2 in special cell cultures. There is also strong inhibition of binding of TGF-β2 to cell surface receptors in radioreceptor assays.

In animal studies, it was found that repeated subconjunctival injections of 100 μl at a concentration of 1 mg/ml caused a slight chemosis, but no inflammation or change of the vascularity of that tissue, when examined both clinically and histopathologically.

13.1.3.5
Suramin

Suramin was originally synthesized and designed as an antiparasitic drug, and due to its inhibitory effect on reverse transcriptase, it has recently been used in clinical trials for AIDS, for metastatic disease, and for selected malignancies, including prostate, adrenal cortex, lymphoma, breast, and colon cancer. Because suramin is a heparin analog, it binds to heparin-binding proteins.

More important with relation to ocular wound healing, suramin blocks the effects of growth factors on tumor cells in vitro and interferes with the action of growth factors by competitive binding to growth factor receptors. Growth factors inhibited by suramin include

TGF-β1, TGF-β2, TGF-β3; PDGF A, PDGF B; EGF; bFGF; IGF-I; and IGF-II. Therefore, cytokines that play an important role in stimulating fibroblasts during wound healing are affected by suramin.

In other experiments, cell cultures from human ocular fibroblasts were used and the amount of collagen type I and type III produced under the influence of suramin was measured. The results established a dose response curve and demonstrated that suramin inhibits the production of collagen type I and type III while overall protein production is not affected. This suggests that suramin influences wound healing by blocking growth factor receptors and neutralizing antibodies and has the potential to effectively delay or inhibit the wound healing response.

13.1.3.6
Further Substances

Many more substances with antiproliferative potential have been identified in tissue studies, but at this time there are no drugs with a confirmed clinical efficacy or advantage as compared to the substances currently used.

13.2
Clinical Experience
with the Described Substances

13.2.1
Corticosteroids

13.2.1.1
Topical Post-operative Application
of Corticosteroids

There are a few studies that show the benefit of the use of topically applied corticosteroids following trabeculectomy in a clinical setting .

In a prospective fashion, standard trabeculectomies were performed [2]. Afterwards, patients received no steroids at all (group 1), topical 1 % prednisolone acetate every 3 h for 20 days (group 2), or in addition to group 2 80 mg oral prednisone, tapered over 16 days (group 3). The patients were followed for up to 10 years. At that time, the need for one or two topical antiglaucomatous medications was 73 % in group 1, 94 % in group 2, and 92 % in group 3. The need for three or more topical medications was 27 % in group 1, 6 % in group 2, and 8 % in group 3. At 5 years, the mean IOP was 19.3 mmHg in group 1, 13.2 mmHg in group 2, and 15.9 mmHg in group 3. The glaucoma status was worse in 24 % of the cases in group 1, 17 % in group 2, and 17 % in group 3.

These findings demonstrate, in a clinical setting, the importance of a post-operative application of corticosteroids. However, only one regimen of the topical corticosteroids was investigated, so that this study gives no clinically validated information of how much corticosteroids are actually needed.

▶ **Technique for Corticosteroids Following Trabeculectomy**
- Dexamethasone 0.1 % eye drops, prednisolone acetate 1 %, or similar should be given 5 times daily for the first 4 weeks
- The drops can then be tapered by one drop per week or slower, according to the clinical course

Summary for the Clinician
- The application of steroids following trabeculectomy is mandatory with only few exceptions:
  - In patients who are steroid-responders
  - In eyes with a conjunctival wound healing problem following the use of antimetabolites
- The application does not strictly follow the clinical course, but the biological process of wound healing. This means that the drops should not be reduced too early even when "everything looks fine"

13.2.1.2
Corticosteroids for Needling Procedures of Failing Blebs

Needling procedures can be performed as a slit-lamp procedure or under aseptic conditions in the operating room. First, the scar tissue is dissected with a sharp needle and the aim should be to restore filtration either by procedures that open the firm, prominent blebs themselves or by mobilization of the scleral flap. Thereafter, some of the corticosteroid can be injected in that area to produce some chemosis of the conjunctiva.

▶ **Technique for Post-operative Bleb Revision with Corticosteroids**
- Topical anesthesia with oxibuprocaine, proparacaine, tetracaine 0.5 %, or lidocaine 4 %
- A 28-gauge or 30-gauge needle attached to an insulin or tuberculin syringe
- The firm scar tissue is dissected with the needle, the scleral flap is elevated, if necessary to restore filtration
- Immediate injection of 0.5–1.0 ml of betamethasone 4 mg/ml or similar

Summary for the Clinician
- Well-accepted therapy to increase the success rate of failing blebs
- The technique may be combined with 5-fluorouracil injections over the following few days

13.2.2
5-Fluorouracil

13.2.2.1
Standard Trabeculectomy with Post-operative Injections of 5-Fluorouracil

For the use of 5-fluorouracil, a routine trabeculectomy is carried out first. The standard application of 5-fluorouracil includes repeated subconjunctival injections. These injections can be performed directly into the filtering bleb or directly opposite. The injections can be performed as often as twice per day for the first week and then once per day during the second post-operative week or less frequently. Usually, an amount ranging from 5 mg to 10 mg of 5-fluorouracil is injected each time. Frequent side effects include long-standing corneal erosions, and it has been reported that these injections are quite painful despite topical anesthesia. Typical dosages and results of this kind of application are listed in Table 13.1.

Table 13.1. Clinical data on trabeculectomies performed with post-operative subconjunctival injections of 5-fluorouracil

Study	Amount (mg)	Application (injections)	Success (%)	Follow-up (months)
5-FU study group [18]	105	21	51	36
Rockwood et al. [38]	105	21	65	36
Bansal and Gupta [3]	70	14	100	8–27
Jampel et al. [19]	33±10	10	100	8
Patitsas et al. [34]	60	14	71	34
Whiteside-Michel et al. [47]	28±9	14	100	11–50
Liebman et al. [24]	29±10	14	100	24

The use of 5-fluorouracil has been described both for eyes with complicated forms of glaucoma, as well as for primary procedures. A comment regarding this issue is found in Sect. 13.2.3.

▶ **Technique for Post-operative Injections of 5-Fluorouracil**
- Topical anesthesia of the conjunctiva using oxibuprocaine eye drops or similar
- Injection of 5–10 mg of 5-fluorouracil (5 mg is a good option)
- A total of up to 21 injections during the first 2 weeks after trabeculectomy

Summary for the Clinician
- Well-accepted therapy to increase the success rate. The patient should be aware of the sometimes painful injections before surgery

13.2.2.2
Standard Trabeculectomy with Intra-operative Application of 5-Fluorouracil

This option has been adopted from the routine application of mitomycin. Just like a trabeculectomy performed with the application of mitomycin, the intra-operative application of 5-fluorouracil is done just before dissection of the scleral flap. In the initial reports describing this technique, the scleral flap was dissected first and sponges, soaked with 5-fluorouracil, were then placed on the scleral bed and underneath the conjunctiva. Therefore, it appears that there are at least two different positions regarding sponge application in the literature. Concentrations of 5-fluorouracil range from 25 mg/ml to 50 mg/ml. In none of the publications is there a statement regarding the volume of the 5-fluorouracil solution used. While small pieces regarding sponge can usually hold 0.1 ml, it appears from printed figures of the surgical site that some surgeons used considerably larger volumes and more sponges. This makes it difficult to compare the data and give practical advice.

This technique of 5-fluorouracil application makes it possible to irrigate the surgical site and wash the solution away from the tissues. Typical dosages and results of this kind of application are listed in Table 13.2.

▶ **Technique for Intra-operative Application of 5-Fluorouracil**
- Standard trabeculectomy including dissection of the scleral flap. Then application of sponges soaked with 5-Fluorouracil
- Concentrations of 5-fluorouracil range from 25 mg/ml to 50 mg/ml
- Application time is uniformly 5 min
- Irrigation with BSS is recommended

Table 13.2. Clinical data on trabeculectomies performed with intra-operative application of 5-fluorouracil

Study	Amount (mg)	Application (injections)	Success (%)	Follow-up (months)
Smith et al. [43]	50 + 29 mg	1+6 injections	93	4–9
Dietze et al. [15]	50	1	95	3
Egbert et al. [17]	50	1	87	10

Summary for the Clinician

- Well-accepted therapy to increase the success rate
- The sponges may also be placed on top of the intact sclera
- The technique may be combined with post-operative injections of 5-fluorouracil

13.2.2.3
5-Fluorouracil for Failing Filtering Blebs

In order to recognize failing filtering blebs, it is necessary to monitor the patients frequently throughout the first few weeks following trabeculectomy. Failing blebs have been described as encapsulated blebs, characteristically highly elevated, localized, and firm with a patent sclerostomy. Encapsulated blebs develop typically at 2–8 weeks following surgery. However, in one large study, the mean time point of needling revision was 49 weeks with a range from 0.4 weeks to 216 weeks.

In different reports, needling procedures were performed as a slit-lamp procedure or under aseptic conditions in the operating room. It appears to be important to inject the 5-fluorouracil close to the scleral flap and to attempt to restore filtration by manipulating the needle over the scleral flap or underneath the flap. On average, 2.4 injections with a range of 1–7 injections appeared to be necessary to restore filtration. A typical amount of 5-fluorouracil used is 5 mg in 0.5 ml or 5 mg in 0.1 ml.

Other surgeons perform a dissection of the scar tissue with a needle first and inject 5-fluorouracil away from the bleb site on the next days.

▸ **Technique for Post-operative Injections of 5-Fluorouracil for Failing Blebs**
- Topical anesthesia with oxibuprocaine, proparacaine, tetracaine 0.5 % or lidocaine 4 %
- A 28-gauge or 30-gauge needle attached to an insulin or tuberculin syringe
- The firm scar tissue is dissected with the needle, the scleral flap is elevated, if necessary, to restore filtration
- Immediate or later injection of 5 mg 5-fluorouracil
- Injections may be repeated over the next days

Summary for the Clinician

- Well-accepted therapy to increase the success rate of failing blebs
- Frequent monitoring of the patient in the weeks following trabeculectomy is necessary

13.2.3
Mitomycin

A discussion or review of the current use of mitomycin to enhance the outcome of filtering surgery for glaucoma has to start with defining the situation one has to deal with and therefore, as a second step, setting the goal of the procedure.

Some authors advocate that a substance like mitomycin should be used for every trabeculectomy performed. This would mean that the authors do not fear the high incidence of possible side effects of the substance. In addition, this would mean that many primary trabeculectomies are done with mitomycin, since these are the trabeculectomies performed most frequently. This would also mean that especially low target pressures are attempted, since the use of mitomycin does not only lead to a reduced rate of episcleral scarring, but also to low and very low values of intraocular pressure over a long time. Low intraocular pressures are advocated for patients with only mildly elevated intraocular pressures but advanced glaucomatous damage of the optic nerve head for patients with low tension glaucoma, and for patients with a vascular component of their glaucomatous disease.

Therefore, it is important to distinguish between trabeculectomies performed with mitomycin as procedures for primary surgery and uncomplicated cases of glaucoma and repeat trabeculectomies and cases of complicated glaucoma.

13.2.3.1
Primary Procedures with Mitomycin

The issue of whether primary trabeculectomies should be performed with or without the use of an antimetabolite is still controversial and will probably remain such for a while. One should at least keep in mind that uncomplicated cases of glaucoma might have a good prognosis even without the use of antimetabolites (Fig. 13.4).

Summarized Information
from Important Publications:

In one study, [22] 33 eyes of mostly black patients were operated with a concentration of 0.5 mg/ml of mitomycin and a 3-min exposure. These eyes were compared to a historical control group of 30 eyes. At each time point of the follow-up period of up to 18 months, the mitomycin-operated eyes had a significantly lower intraocular pressure (e.g., 10.0 mmHg versus 17.2 mmHg). The complication of severe hypotony, here defined as an intraocular pressure of less than 6 mmHg, was 15 % in the mitomycin group and 0 % in the control group.

In a second publication [14], a total of 28 eyes were operated with 14 of these receiving mitomycin with a concentration of 0.2 mg/ml for 3 min. The mean follow-up was around 17 months. At the last visit, the intraocular pressure was below 16 mmHg in 12/14 mitomycin-treated eyes and in 4/14 control eyes. Complications such as choroidal effusion and shallow anterior chamber were more frequent in the mitomycin-treated eyes.

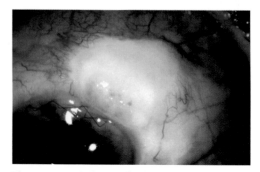

Fig. 13.4. Typical avascular filtering bleb following intra-operative application of mitomycin with a concentration of 0.2mg/ml

In one series [32], 25 eyes of 23 white patients underwent trabeculectomy with mitomycin with a concentration of 0.2 mg/ml for 5 min. Although there was no control group, the authors were pleased with the outcome, reduction of the mean intraocular pressure from 26.0 mmHg to 12.5 mmHg at a follow-up of 12 months. The only reported complication included a case of temporary hypotonous maculopathy.

In a different study, the effect of no mitomycin compared with a short-term and a longer-term exposure to mitomycin was described [20]. The concentration of mitomycin was 0.5 mg/ml, and a total of 124 eyes were included. In that report, the best control of the intraocular pressure combined with the lowest risk for severe complications was accomplished in the group with a short-term exposure to mitomycin, ranging from 30 to 60 s only.

Different concentrations of mitomycin with a standard application time of 5 min were applied in a study performed by Kitazawa et al. [21]. They treated 11 patients with a standard trabeculectomy with a concentration of mitomycin of 0.2 mg/ml in one eye and a concentration of 0.02 mg/ml in the fellow eye. No control group with no mitomycin was included. The eyes receiving the higher concentration of mitomycin were more successful with regard to control of the intraocular pressure, but had more complications such as hypotony maculopathy and cataract progression. The authors concluded that the best concentration for mitomycin might be in between the two concentrations tested.

The most recent study with the longest follow up was performed by Bindlish et al. [5]. These authors included a total of 123 eyes and had a follow-up period of 5 years. Concentrations of mitomycin ranged from 0.25 mg/ml to 0.5 mg/ml and exposure times from 0.5 to 5 min. Although the mean intraocular pressure was low with 9.9 mmHg, the rate of complications was relatively high and included hypotony maculopathy, bleb leaks, blebitis, endophthalmitis, and significant loss of central vision.

These authors concluded that the intraocular pressure control with the use of mitomycin is good, but the rate of complications is much higher than with no use of mitomycin. Regarding this study [44], it was mentioned that the mean intraocular pressure of trabeculectomies done without mitomycin is something around 15 mmHg, and that this level of the intraocular pressure is just the one which is sufficient in most cases.

▶ **Technique for Intra-operative Application of Mitomycin**
- Preparation of the surgical site where the scleral flap is to be dissected
- Mitomycin, freshly prepared solution of 0.1–0.5 mg/ml (0.2 mg/ml is a good option)
- Volume of 0.1 ml
- Sponge, size 5x5 mm
- After placing the sponge on the sclera, the mitomycin is applied to the sponge using a tuberculin or insulin syringe
- The mitomycin remains for 0.5– 5 min (2–3 min is a good option)
- The whole area is irrigated with at least 10 ml of BSS

Summary for the Clinician
- The use of mitomycin for primary trabeculectomy is still under discussion
- Maybe the topical post-operative application should be favored for these cases

13.2.3.2
Mitomycin for Complicated Forms of Glaucoma

The review of the literature regarding the use of mitomycin for specific forms of complicated glaucoma including repeat trabeculectomy is difficult, because many studies combine different forms of secondary glaucoma in their reports so that it becomes hard to get specific information for one group of these eyes or an-other.

A list of forms of secondary glaucoma is given in Table 13.3.

13.2.3.3
Young Patients

The problem with the definition of these cases of glaucoma starts with the definition. It can be assumed that all of the above-mentioned forms of glaucoma refer to patients up to about 20 years of age. For older patients, one would probably use the terms primary open-angle glaucoma or dysgenetic glaucoma. Some surgeons

Table 13.3. List of secondary forms of glaucoma and risk factors for failure of trabeculectomy

Inflammatory
Chronic angle closure
Pseudoexfoliation
Pigmentary
Neovascular
Traumatic
Black patients
Pseudophakia
Previous argon laser trabeculoplasty
Juvenile/infantile
Anterior segment dysgenesis
Iridocorneal endothelial syndrome

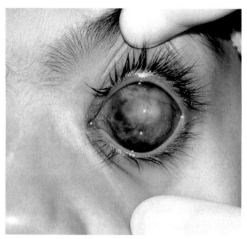

Fig. 13.5. Eye with a severe form of congenital glaucoma and enlargement of the cornea and vascularization. A challenging case for the glaucoma surgeon

tend to be very cautious when using mitomycin for children younger than 10 or 5 years of age, while others insist in using mitomycin especially in these patients because standard filtering procedures have a poor prognosis (Fig. 13.5).

Important Studies

In 1997, Mandal et al. [26] reported on 19 eyes of 13 patients with congenital glaucoma that underwent trabeculectomy with mitomycin with a concentration of 0.4 mg/ml for 3 min. Complete success was obtained in 18 of the 19 eyes after a mean follow-up period of 19 months. Beck et al. [4] in addition performed a retrospective study of 60 eyes in 49 patients. Trabeculectomy was performed with a concentration of 2.5 mg/ml or 0.5 mg/ml for 5 min. The probability of success was 67 % for 12 months and 59 % for 24 months. The most severe complication encountered was endophthalmitis, occurring in 8 % of the cases.

In another retrospective study published in 1999, Mandal et al. [27] evaluated 38 eyes in 29 patients. The concentration of mitomycin was 0.4 mg/ml, applied for 3 min. The success probability at 18 months was 65 %. No cases of endophthalmitis were reported. Most recently, Sidoti et al. [40] published a retrospective study of 29 eyes in 29 patients. The concentration of mitomycin was 0.5 mg/ml, and it was applied for

1.5–5 min. Success at 24 months was 59 %, and the rate of bleb-related infection was 17 %.

It appears that the overall outcome of the use of mitomycin for young patients is promising, but the long-term behavior of the thin and avascular blebs remains unclear. Infections were noted in three of the four cited studies, and this problem may give rise to severe disease.

13.2.3.4
Black Patients

In general, patients from African populations have a larger risk of post-operative scarring than white patients.

Important Studies

In 1993, Mermoud et al. [28] published a report on a prospective study evaluating 30 eyes of 26 black patients undergoing trabeculectomy with a concentration of 0.2 mg/ml of mitomycin applied for 5 min. These patients were compared to a historical group of eyes operated without mitomycin. Some 83 % of the mitomycin-operated eyes had an intraocular pressure of less than 21 mmHg at a mean follow-up time of 9.1 months as compared to only 37 % of eyes from the no-mitomycin group. Bleb fibrosis occurred at a rate of 7 % and 20 %, respectively. A late postoperative positive Seidel test was only seen in the mitomycin-treated eyes at a rate of 13 %.

In a study of 44 eyes receiving mitomycin in a concentration of 0.5 mg/ml for 3.5 min, the mean intraoperative pressure was 14.7 mmHg at a mean follow-up of 17.7 months [10]. The patients had advanced open-angle glaucoma. Similarly, Mwanza and Kabasele [31] performed a study with an intra-individual control group using mitomycin with a concentration of 0.4 mg/ml for 2.5 min. The success rate of mitomycin-treated eyes was 82 % compared to 63 % in the untreated controls.

Interestingly, in all three studies cited, no cases of hypotony maculopathy were reported, so that it can be assumed that these patients have a lower risk of developing this specific complication than non-black patients.

13.2.3.5
Uveitis

Uveitis is a challenging aspect for glaucoma surgeons, since the success of most surgical procedures appears to be limited in the long run.

In 1994, Prata et al. [36] published a retrospective, uncontrolled study of 24 eyes undergoing trabeculectomy with mitomycin with a concentration of 0.2 mg/ml, applied for 5 min. After a mean follow-up of around 10 months, a complete success was reached in 75 % of the eyes, but complications related to hypotony were quite high. In 1997, Wright et al. [48] published a similarly retrospective study of 24 eyes with a mean follow-up of around 15 months. Complete success was reported in 62 % of the cases. Recently, Ceballos et al. [11] published a report of a retrospective study of 44 eyes with uveitis that were operated with either mitomycin or 5-fluorouracil. The overall success rate was 62 % at 2 years. Interestingly, male gender was a significant risk factor for failure. Phakic patients developed significant cataracts in more than 50 %.

13.2.3.6
Repeat Trabeculectomy

Patients undergoing repeat trabeculectomy are probably those that profit the most from the use of mitomycin. Unfortunately, no studies exist that specifically address this problem. In most cases, these eyes are mixed with other forms of secondary glaucoma, so that no detailed information can be given for repeat trabeculectomies only. However, when looking at the abundant literature regarding this issue, it may be safe to conclude that a repeat trabeculectomy is the classic indication for the use of an antimetabolite. Typical dosages and results of this kind of application are listed in Table 13.4. Typical complications and side effects regarding the use of mitomycin in comparison to 5-fluorouracil are listed in Table 13.5 (Figs. 13.6–13.8).

▶ **Technique for Intra-operative Application of Mitomycin**
- Preparation of the surgical site where the scleral flap is to be dissected
- Mitomycin, freshly prepared solution of 0.1–0.5 mg/ml (0.2 mg/ml is a good option)
- Volume of 0.1 ml
- Sponge, size 5x5 mm
- After placing the sponge on the sclera, the mitomycin is applied to the sponge using a tuberculin or insulin syringe
- The sponge remains for 0.5 min - 5 min (2–3 min is a good option)
- The whole area is irrigated with at least 10 ml of BSS

Summary for the Clinician
- The use of mitomycin for repeat trabeculectomies and complicated forms of glaucoma is current practice in most glaucoma centers

Table 13.4. Clinical data on trabeculectomies performed with intra-operative application of mitomycin

Study	Mitomycin (mg/ml)	Time (min)	Success (%)	Follow-up (months)
Shields et al. [39]	0.25	2-5	59	2–12
Chen et al. [12]	0.1–0.4	5	76–100	12–60
Palmer [33]	0.2	5	84	6–42
Kitazawa et al. [21]	0.4	5	100	7–12
Skuta et al. [42]	0.5	5	95	6
Zacharia et al. [49]	0.4	3.5–7	100	2–12
Mermoud et al. [28]	0.2	5	93	3–18
Costa et al. [13]	0.4	1.5–2.5	95	6–7
Mietz andKrieglstein [29]	0.2–0.5	3–5	90	36

Table 13.5. Possible side effects following the use of 5-fluorouracil and mitomycin for trabeculectomy

Complication	5-Fluorouracil	Mitomycin
Painful injection	++	–
Conjunctival dehiscence	+	+
Corneal erosions	++	–
Corneal ulcer	(+)	–
Repeated applications	++	–
Blebitis or endophthalmitis	++	+
Post-operative hypotony	+	+
Hypotony maculopathy	+	+
Suprachoroidal hemorrhage	(+)	(+)
Intraocular toxic sideeffects	+	++
Conjunctival hemorrhages	++	+

–, Not frequent; +, typical complication; ++, frequently occurring; (+) typical, but rare complication

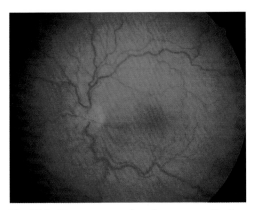

Fig. 13.6. Hypotony maculopathy as a complication of the intra-operative use of Mitomycin

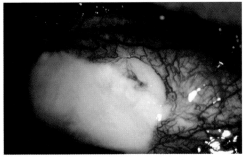

Fig. 13.8. A typical avascular filtering bleb. Note the conjunctival dehiscence superiorly. This may give rise to a blebitis

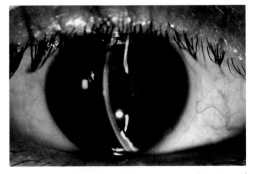

Fig. 13.7. Anterior synechiae as a complication of long-standing hypotony with a flat anterior chamber

13.2.3.7
Topical Application of Mitomycin

More recently, a topical application of Mitomycin was reported. With this technique, a standard trabeculectomy is performed first. For the first 3 days after surgery, a sponge with mitomycin is placed on the filtering bleb. This can be done under topical anesthesia as an office procedure and does not require aseptic conditions. The application is usually well tolerated by the patients. The main advantage is that a much lower concentration of mitomycin can be used. For the intra-operative application, a concentration of 0.2 mg/ml or higher is usually employed. For the post-operative application, a concentration of 0.05 mg/ml of mitomycin is used.

► **Technique for Post-operative Application of Mitomycin**
- Application on days 1, 2, and 3 after trabeculectomy
- Topical anesthesia using oxibuprocaine, proparacaine, tetracaine 0.5 %, or lidocaine 4 %
- Insertion of a lid-speculum.
- Sponge with 0.1 ml of 0.05 mg/ml m itomycin for 3 min
- Irrigation with 10 ml BSS

Summary for the Clinician
- The post-operative application of mitomycin is a new technique aimed to reduce intra-ocular toxicity
- It requires three applications after surgery and is therefore more time consuming

13.2.4
Transforming Growth Factor-β

With respect to this treatment modality, the results of two clinical phase II trials are available.

In a first trial, 24 patients underwent primary trabeculectomy. Sixteen patients of these received the specific antibody, while the remaining eight patients served as controls. The antibody was given as a sequence of four subconjunctival injections. Two injections were done on the day of surgery (pre- and post-operatively), one on the day after surgery and one a week after surgery.

After 1 year, the proportion of patients who had not required either intervention or resumption of topical medication was 11 of 16 (69 %) on the TGF-β antibody compared with 2 of 8 (25 %) on placebo. Mean IOP at 1 year was 3 mmHg lower in the TGF-β antibody group than in the placebo group. There were no significant differences in the incidence of complications between the two groups. Blebs after the TGF-β antibody were diffuse, noncystic and nonvascular. The

fall in IOP was greater in the TGF-β antibody group at 3 and 6 months ($p<0.05$) and approached significance at 12 months.

Follow-up results at 2 years showed that the TGF-β antibody patients achieved a significantly lower IOP than the control group. The mean values 2 years after surgery were 13.6 mmHg for the TGF-β antibody and 17.7 mmHg for the controls.

In a second trial, 56 patients underwent combined glaucoma and cataract surgery. Patients were randomized to receive either the TGF-β antibody (n=36) or matching placebo (n=20). The therapeutic regimen was similar to that in the first clinical trial. Follow-up results at 6 month revealed that the TGF-β antibody was safe and well tolerated with no serious drug-related adverse effects and no severe injection site reactions. There was no evidence of increased inflammation in the anterior chamber of the eye. IOP was successfully lowered by surgery in both patient groups. At 6 months after surgery, the achieved IOP was lower in patients receiving the TGF-β antibody (14.5 mmHg) compared with those receiving placebo (16.7 mmHg). In the early post-operative period, intervention with 5-FU injection was used in 28 % of TGF-β antibody eyes and in 10 % of placebo-treated eyes.

► **Technique for Application of TGF-β2 of TGF-β2 Antibodies:**
- The concentration of the TGF-β2 antibody is 1.0 mg/ml
- For each injection to the filtering bleb, the quantity injected is 100 µl
- The first injection is before surgery on the day of surgery
- The second injection is after surgery on the day of surgery
- The third injection is on the first day after surgery
- The fourth injection is at 1 week after surgery

Summary for the Clinician
- The use of the TGF-β antibody is only possible in ongoing clinical studies in participating study centers
- The synthetically engineered TGF-β antibody is not yet commercially available

13.2.5
Suramin

For this substance, only information from one clinical study is available [30].

Suramin was first applied during surgery at a concentration of 200 mg/ml and applied for 5 min. On days 1, 2, and 3 following surgery, the patients received a subconjunctival injection of 0.1 ml suramin solution (200 mg/ml) close to the filtering bleb. A historical group of eyes operated with mitomycin (0.2 mg/ml) served as a control.

The suramin- and mitomycin-treated eyes did not differ significantly for the mean IOP before surgery and at the final visit (32.7 vs. 29.5/19.7 vs. 19.3; both $p<0.0001$). Following surgery, the filtering blebs were slightly hyperemic in the suramin group, but this effect resolved over time without the need for increased topical therapy.

The most important complication encountered in both the early and late post-operative phase was hypotony. Hypotony as a transient phenomenon occurred frequently in all groups. Hypotony at some point within the first few days or weeks following trabeculectomy occurred twice in the suramin group, but not afterwards. Hypotony as a permanent complication developed in four mitomycin cases, causing hypotony maculopathy in one case. Using an ANOVA survival analysis, no difference was found between the suramin and mitomycin groups ($p<0.64$). The incidence of failures was not significantly different.

It appears, therefore, that suramin may be a potent substance, its efficacy comparable with that of mitomycin (Fig. 13.9).

► **Technique for Suramin Used**
  for Trabeculectomy
- Concentration of 200 mg/ml suramin dissolved in BSS
- One application during surgery using a sponge
- Subconjunctival injections directly to the filtering bleb on days 1, 2, and 3 (total of three injections)

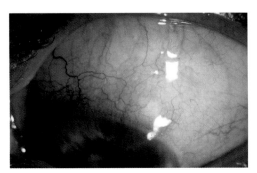

Fig. 13.9. Typical appearance of a filtering bleb at 2 years following trabeculectomy with Suramin. No avascularity is present

Summary for the Clinician

- At this time, only preliminary data are available. It is too early to recommend a specific therapeutic regimen

13.2.6
Additional Substances

Given the lack of data, the use of other substances that interfere with wound healing can not be recommended at this time.

13.3
Current Clinical Practice/Recommendations

Summarizing the previously given information, the following recommendations can be made:
- If primary trabeculectomies are performed, additionally used substances should have a low risk profile, if any are used to enhance the success.
- Repeat trabeculectomies or complicated cases should not be operated without the use of an antimetabolite.
- Both 5-fluorouracil and mitomycin are well accepted.
- New substances like TGF-β antibodies are on the horizon, but not yet well established.

13.4
Post-operative Intensified Care

The concept of intensified post-operative care is relatively new and includes the following issues:

- Regular visits following trabeculectomy
- High-dose topical corticosteroids for a longer period after surgery
- Detailed examination and description of the filtering bleb
- Early identification of risk factors for failing blebs
- Early intervention to interfere with the scarring process using injections with 5-fluorouracil or steroids

It was shown in clinical studies that the success rate of routine trabeculectomies could be significantly improved with this regimen of intensified care.

References

1. AGIS Investigators (2000) The advanced glaucoma intervention study (AGIS). 7. The relationship between control of intraocular pressure and visual field deterioration. Am J Ophthalmol 130: 429-440

2. Araujo SV, Spaeth GL, Roth SM, Starita RJ (1995) A ten-year follow-up on a prospective, randomized trial of postoperative corticosteroids after trabeculectomy. Ophthalmology 102: 1753-1759

3. Bansal RK, Gupta A (1992) 5-fluorouracil in trabeculectomy for patients under the age of 40 years. Ophthalmic Surg 23: 278-280

4. Beck AD, Wilson WR, Lynch MG, Lynn MJ, Noe R. (1998) Trabeculectomy with adjunctive mitomycin C in pediatric glaucoma. Am J Ophthalmol 126: 648-657

5. Bindlish R, Condon GP, Schlosser JD, D´Antonio J, Lauer KB, Lehrer R (2002) Efficacy and safety of mitomycin C in primary trabeculectomy: five-year follow-up. Ophthalmology 109: 1336-1341

6. Border WA, Noble NA (1994) Transforming growth factor b in tissue fibrosis. New Engl J Med 331: 1286-1292

7. Broadway D, Grierson I, Hitchings R (1993) The effect of topical anti-glaucomatous medications on the cell profile of the conjunctiva. Curr Opi Ophthalmol 4: 51-57

8. Broadway D, Grierson I, Hitchings R (1993) Adverse effects of topical antiglaucomatous medications on the conjunctiva. Br J Ophthalmol 77: 590-596

9. Broadway DC, Grierson I, O'Brien C, Hitchings RA (1994) Adverse effects of topical antiglaucoma medication. I. The conjunctival cell profile. Arch Ophthalmol 112: 1437-1445

10. Byrd SK, Egbert PR, Budenz D (1998) Risk of hypotony after primary trabeculectomy with antifibrotic agents in a black African population. J Glaucoma 1998; 7: 82-85

11. Ceballos EM, Beck AD, Lynn MJ (2002) Trabeculectomy with antiproliferative agents in uveitic glaucoma. J Glaucoma 11: 189-196

12. Chen CW, Huang HT, Bair JS, Lee CC (1990) Trabeculectomy with simultaneous topical application of mitomycin-C in refractory glaucoma. J Ocul Pharmacol 6: 175-182

13. Costa VP, Moster MR, Wilson RP, et al. (1993) Effects of topical mitomycin C on primary trabeculectomies and combined procedures. Br J Ophthalmol 77: 693-697

14. Costa VP, Comegno PEC, Vasconcelos JPC, Malta RFS, Jose NK (1996) Low-dose mitomycin C trabeculectomy in patients with advanced glaucoma. J Glaucoma 5: 193-199

15. Dietze PJ, Feldman RM, Gross RL (1992) Intraoperative application of 5-fluorouracil during trabeculectomy. Ophthalmic Surg 23: 662-665

16. Doxey DL, Ng MC, Dill RE, Iacopino AM (1995) Platelet-derived growth factor levels in wounds of diabetic rats. Life Sci 57: 1111-1123

17. Egbert PR, Williams AS, Singh K, Dadzie P, Egbert TB (1993) A prospective trial of intraoperative fluorouracil during trabeculectomy in a black population. Am J Ophthalmol 116: 612-616

18. The Fluorouracil Filtering Study Group (1996) Five-year follow-up of the fluorouracil filtering study. Am J Ophthalmol 121: 349-366

19. Jampel HD, Jabs DA, Quigley HA (1990) Trabeculectomy with 5-fluorouracil for adult inflammatory glaucoma. Am J Ophthalmol 109: 168-173

20. Kim YY, Sexton RM, Shin DH, Kim C, Ginde SA, Ren J, Lee D, Kupin TH (1998) Outcomes of primary phakic trabeculectomies without versus with 0.5- to 1- minute versus 3- to 5- minute mitomycin c. Am J Ophthalmol 126: 755-762

21. Kitazawa Y, Suemori-Matshushita H, Yamamoto T, Kawase K (1993) Low-dose and high-dose mitomycin trabeculectomy as an initial surgery in primary open-angle glaucoma. Ophthalmology 100: 1624-1628

22. Kupin TH, Juzych MS, Shin DH, Khatana AK, Olivier MDG (1995) Adjunctive mitomycin C in primary trabeculectomy in phakic eyes. Am J Ophthalmol 119: 30-39

23. Lee DA, Lee TC, Corres AE, Kitada S (1990) Effects of Mithramycin, Mitomycin, Daunorubicin, and Bleomycin on human subconjunctival fibroblast attachment and proliferation. Invest Ophthalmol Vis Sci 31: 2136-2144

24. Liebmann JM, Ritch R, Marmor M, Nunez J, Wolner B (1991) Initial 5-fluorouracil trabeculectomy in uncomplicated glaucoma. Ophthalmology 98: 1036-1041

25. Lüke C (2002) A prospective randomized trial of viscocanalostomy versus trabeculectomy in open-angle glaucoma: a 1-year follow-up study. J Glaucoma 11: 294-299

26. Mandal AK, Walton DS, John T, Jayagandan A (1997) Mitomycin C-augmented trabeculectomy in refractory congenital glaucoma. Ophthalmology 104: 996-1003

27. Mandal AK, Prasad K, Naduvilath TJ (1999) Surgical results and complications of mitomycinC-augmented trabeculectomy in refractory developmental glaucoma. Ophthalmic Surg Lasers 1999; 30: 473-480

28. Mermoud A, Salmon JF, Murray DN (1993) Trabeculectomy with mitomycin C for refractory glaucoma in blacks. Am J Ophthalmol 116: 72-78

29. Mietz H, Krieglstein GK (1998) Three-year follow-up of trabeculectomies performed with different concentrations of mitomycin-C. Ophthalmic Surg Lasers 29: 628-630.

30. Mietz H, Krieglstein GK (2001) Suramin to enhance glaucoma filtering procedures: a clinical comparison with mitomycin. Ophthalmic Surg Lasers 2001; 32: 358-369

31. Mwanza J-CK, Kabasele PM(2001) Trabeculectomy with and without mitomycin-C in a black African population. Eur J Ophthalmol 2001; 11: 261-263

32. Nuijts RMMA, Vernimmen RCJ, Webers C (1997) Mitomycin C primary trabecuelctomy in primary glaucoma of white patients. J Glaucoma 6: 293-297

33. Palmer SS (1991) Mitomycin as adjunct chemotherapy with trabeculectomy. Ophthalmology 98: 317-321

34. Patitsas CJ, Rockwood EJ, Meisler DM, Lowder CY (1992) Glaucoma filtering srugery with postoperative 5-fluorouracil in patients with intraocular inflammatory disease. Ophthalmology 99: 594-599

35. Pierce GF, Tarpley JE, Tseng J, et al m(1995) Detection of platelet-derived growth factor (PDGF)-AA in actively healing human wounds treated with recombinant PDGF-BB and absence of PDGF in chronic nonhealing wounds. J Clin Invest 96: 1336-1350

36. Prata JA, Neves RA, Minckler DS, Mermoud A, Heuer DK (1994) Trabeculectomy with mitomycin C in glaucoma associated with uveitis. Ophthalmic Surg 25: 616-620

37. Rabowski JH, Dukes AJ, Lee DA, Leong KW (1996) The use of bioerodible polymers and daunorubicin in glaucoma filtration surgery. Ophthalmology 103: 800-807

38. Rockwood EJ, Parrish RK II, Heuer DK, Skuta GL, Hodapp E, Palmberg PF, Gressel MG, Feuer W (1997) Glaucoma filtering surgery with 5-fluorouracil. Ophthalmology 94: 1071-1078.

39. Shields MB, Scroggs MW, Sloop CM, Sim-mons RB (1993) Clinical and histopathologic observations concerning hypotony after trabeculectomy with adjunctive mitomycin C. Am J Ophthalmol 116: 673-683

40. Sidoti PA, Belmonte SJ, Liebmann JM, Ritch R (2000) Trabeculectomy with mitomycin-C in the treatment of pediatric glaucomas. Ophthalmology 2000; 107: 422-429

41. Siriwardena D, Khaw PT, King AJ, Donalson ML, Overton BM, Migdal C, Cordeiro MF (2002) Human antitransforming growth factor beta (2) monoclonal antibody-a new modulator of wound healing in trabeculectomy: a randomized placebo controlled clinical study. Ophthalmology 109: 427-431

42. Skuta GL, Beeson CC, Higginbotham EJ, Lichter PR, Musch DC, Bergstrom TJ, Klein TB, Falck FY (1992) Intraoperative mitomycin versus postoperative 5-Fluorouracil in high-risk glaucoma filtering surgery. Ophthalmology 99: 438-444

43. Smith MF, Sherwood MB, Doyle JW, Khaw PT (1992) Results of intraoperative 5-fluorouracil supplementation on trabeculectomy for open-angle glaucoma. Am J Ophthalmol 114: 737-741

44. Spaeth GL, Terizidou C, Bhan A (2002) Discussion of above mentioned paper. Ophthalmology 109: 1341-1342

45. Sullivan KM, Lorenz HP, Meuli M, Lin RY, Adzick NS (1995) A model of scarless human fetal wound repair is deficient in transforming growth factor beta. J Ped Surg 30: 198-203

46. Thomas DW, O´Neill ID, Harding KG, Shepherd JP (1995)Cutaneous wound healing: a current perspective. J Oral Maxillofac Surg 53: 442-447

47. Whiteside-Michel J, Liebmann JM, Ritch R (1992) Initial 5-fluorouracil trabeculectomy in young patients. Ophthalmology 99: 7-13

48. Wright MM, McGehee RF, Pderson JE (1997) Intaoperative mitomycin-C for glaucoma associated with ocular inflammation. Ophthalmic Surg Lasers 1997; 28: 370-376

49. Zacharia PT, Deppermann SR, Schuman JS (1993) Ocular hypotony after trabeculectomy with mitomycin c. Am J Ophthalmol 116: 314-326

Core Messages

- Various outflow routes may be present in non-penetrating glaucoma surgery
- Deep sclerectomy and viscocanalostomy are the two most frequently used modifications of non-penetrating glaucoma surgery
- Non-penetrating surgery seems safer than trabeculectomy as far as immediate and long-term complications are concerned
- Trabeculectomy provides better IOP control

14.1
Introduction

Non-penetrating procedures have recently gained attention within the scientific community. An at times fierce debate concerning their role as a successor to the gold standard, trabeculectomy, has revolved around its relative effectiveness in short- to medium-term intraocular pressure control. Several controlled clinical trials, comparing both surgical procedures in terms of long-term IOP control, safety, and visual outcomes are underway and some short- to medium-term results are already available [4, 14]. However, we must remember that the goal of any glaucoma surgery is: (a) to reach the "guess"timated target IOP in the individual patient, (b) without threatening the patient's visual function, and (c) at a sustainable cost for the community. We will discuss what penetrating and non-penetrating surgery can offer.

14.1.1
Basics

14.1.1.1
Trabeculectomy

In this procedure (Fig. 14.1), aqueous flows from the anterior chamber onto the subconjunctival space through a sclerostomy, which involves a full-thickness penetration of the globe under a partial-thickness scleral flap. This flap is utilized to modulate aqueous flow in order to minimize the risk of post-surgical complications due to over-filtration and hypotony.

A peripheral iridectomy is mandatory to avoid entrapment of the iris root in the sclerostomy.

14.1.1.2
Non-penetrating Surgery

These procedures are designed to avoid full-thickness penetration of the anterior chamber. In theory, this would minimize the risk of over-filtration and hypotony. In principle, these procedures lower intraocular pressure by reducing resistance to aqueous outflow; however, the exact mechanism for the reduction of intraocular pressure following these procedures is not known but could be: (a) filtration onto the subconjunctival space with bleb formation (Fig. 14.2), (b) transscleral flow, (c) unrecognized micro-penetration into the anterior chamber, (d) opening of previously nonfunctional areas of Schlemm's canal, and (e) increased uveoscleral outflow may contribute to the overall decreased IOP in the operated eye. In a recent study per-

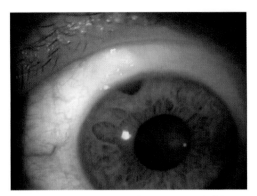

Fig. 14.1. An eye 1 year after an uneventful trabeculectomy. A localized filtering bleb and a patent iridectomy are clearly visible

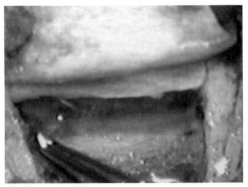

Fig. 14.3. Stripping of the inner wall of the Schlemm's canal together with inner meshwork. The stripping is followed by percolation of aqueous from the anterior chamber

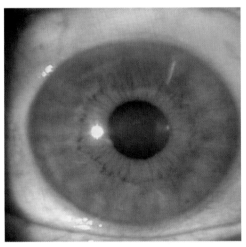

Fig. 14.2. An eye 1 year after an uneventful deep sclerectomy. A diffuse filtering bleb is seen. No iridectomy is visible since non-penetrating surgery does not require an iridectomy

14.1.1.2.1
Deep Sclerectomy

In this procedure, after preparing a limbus/fornix-based conjunctival flap, a superficial partial-thickness scleral flap is dissected into clear cornea. A second, deeper flap approximately 4 mm wide is then dissected forward to the Schlemm's canal; the canal is then de-roofed and stripped and the underlying trabecular meshwork is peeled off (Fig. 14.3). This is usually followed by a free percolation of aqueous through the trabeculodescemetic window previously created. The deep scleral flap is then excised, the superficial scleral flap is loosely approximated to create an open intrascleral space (the so-called intrascleral lake), and the conjunctival incision is closed. Re-absorbable devices, placed under the scleral flap, have been offered as a possible option to preserve the intra-scleral lake from long-term collapse. Some surgeons use 5-fluorouracil postoperatively or mitomycin-C under the flap to inhibit fibrosis.

14.1.1.2.2
Viscocanalostomy

This procedure does not require formation of a filtration bleb. In theory, its success is independent of conjunctival or episcleral fibrosis, which is a major cause of long-term failure of trabeculectomy. Although the initial part of the

formed by using ultrasound biomicroscopy in living human eyes, operated with a deep sclerectomy, filtering bleb formation, however frequent, was not the only surgically induced IOP-lowering mechanism. Increased uveoscleral and transscleral filtration have been observed and considered by the authors as equally important [13]. The possible mechanisms underlying the IOP-reducing effect of viscocanalostomy has been extensively reviewed elsewhere [8].

procedure resembles non-penetrating deep sclerectomy (NPDS), the viscocanalostomy differs in that Schlemm's canal is injected with high-molecular weight viscoelastic substance. In this procedure, upon preparation of a proper conjunctival flap, the superficial scleral flap is dissected to approximately one-third scleral thickness. A second, deeper flap is prepared to provide access to Schlemm's canal. A cannula with an outer diameter measuring approximately 150 µm is used to inject the viscoelastic into the Schlemm's canal. A Descemet's window is created by gently dissecting the deep flap anterior to Schlemm's canal and then excising the deep flap. The superficial scleral flap is tightly sutured, viscoelastic substance is injected into the "scleral lake," and the conjunctiva is closed.

14.2
Non-penetrating vs Penetrating Procedures: Clinical Evaluation

14.2.1
Efficacy

Efficacy is gauged by the degree to which the "*guess*timated" target IOP in the individual patient is achieved. Recent reports suggest that the progression of glaucomatous damage can be significantly reduced if the recorded IOP is consistently low. In particular, the AGIS study is providing evidence that, in clearly manifest glaucoma, the best outcome is reached when IOP never exceeds 18 mmHg. Incidentally, the "mean-IOP," measured in the study cohort fulfilling the above-mentioned criteria, proved to be 12.7 mmHg [22]. The glaucomas enrolled in the AGIS study are likely to be representative of the patient population usually requiring surgery. Therefore, any effective glaucoma surgery must be able to keep the IOP in the low-teens range.

Trabeculectomy can allow a good long-term IOP control. In particular, the CIGTS interim analysis showed that the mean "untreated" IOP in the surgical group proved to be 14 mmHg over a 5-year follow-up period [12]. Further controlled clinical trials are reporting an untreated

IOP of 16 mmHg or less in 45%–70% of eyes undergoing trabeculectomy supplemented with postoperative injections of 5-fluorouracil [1, 5, 24]. In fact, the success rate of conventional filtration surgery can vary according to possible intra- and postoperative supplement with antimetabolites (Mitomycin-C or 5-fluorouracil). Failure of trabeculectomies occur at a variable rate, the most frequent cause being the formation of a fibrovascular tissue at the epi-scleral level surrounding the flap. Thus, the use of antimetabolites has become increasingly popular among glaucoma surgeons. Any careful and realistic evaluation of the success rate of trabeculectomy, therefore, must take into account the need for supplementation with antimetabolites.

Non-penetrating surgery seems to be less effective. As reported in a recent review [21], the untreated mean IOP level, observed in non-penetrating procedures, is at best in the "high-teens." In particular, prospective randomized controlled trials (including postoperative injection of 5-fluorouracil) are reporting: (a) <15% of the study population show an untreated IOP of 16 mmHg or less 2 years after surgery upon an uneventful deep sclerectomy [5], while (b) a slightly higher success rate (approximately 30%) is achieved in a similarly controlled protocol by viscocanalostomy [1]. Concurrent intraoperative application of MMC has been suggested to offer slightly better IOP control [11]. However, the IOP outcome of deep sclerectomy can be greatly improved if the procedure is transformed into an "penetrating" one by means of an opening of the filtering membrane via a YAG-laser goniopuncture. Two long-term case series have been recently reported by the Mermoud's group in Lausanne. The first case series [19] shows results collected in 105 glaucomatous eyes on which deep sclerectomy with collagen implant (DSCI) was performed. The cohort was followed up to 5 years. At the end of follow-up, 65 eyes (61%) showed an untreated IOP of <21 mmHg. Of these 65, 29 had a YAG-laser goniopuncture performed during follow-up due to an uncontrolled IOP. Therefore, the percentage of the study population which achieved an *IOP of <21 mmHg* as a result of an actual "non-penetrating" procedure, drops to

34%. However, it is worth pointing out that 45.7% of the overall population (including both the goniopunctured and the non-goniopunctured eyes) completed the study with an untreated IOP of <16 mmHg. The authors do not provide information enabling us to identify among this subgroup those eyes on which non-penetrating surgery was converted by laser treatment into penetrating surgery. Nevertheless, a 5-year 45.7% success rate, with <16 mmHg as a cutoff, is a figure comparable to what was reported for trabeculectomy.

The second case series [6] offers results of deep sclerectomy with collagen implant (DSCI) performed on myopic eyes (refractive error between –6.0 and –23.0 D, mean –11.8±5.8 D). A total of 21 eyes were followed for up to 4 years. At the end of the follow-up, seven eyes (33%) reached an IOP of <16 mmHg without medication. In all, 15 eyes (71%) underwent YAG-laser goniopuncture. Therefore, the vast majority of the non-penetrating procedures were transformed into "penetrating" procedures during follow-up.

Summary for the Clinician

- Early prospective randomized control trials are unanimous in showing that standard trabeculectomy (supplemented with antimetabolites) produces lower and better sustained IOP control than non-penetrating surgery (either deep sclerectomy supplemented with 5-fluorouracil or viscocanalostomy)
- While IOP control diminishes over time in non-penetrating surgery, this seems to be better maintained in trabeculectomy and is in agreement with previously published data
- Transformation of the NPDS into a penetrating procedure, by means of a laser goniopuncture, leads to better IOP control with time

14.2.2
Safety

Safety is measured by the extent to which vision is spared. Generically speaking, the ultimate goal of glaucoma therapy is to maintain the quality of vision of the affected patient. Glaucoma filtration surgery can be followed by sight-threatening complications. Postoperative management of the trabeculectomy patient can sometimes be more difficult than the procedure itself. The adoption of releasable sutures and the availability of viscoelastics have made flat anterior chamber and delayed postoperative suprachoroidal hemorrage less common [7]. However, the extensive use of potent antimetabolites led to a dramatic increase of chronic hypotony, late bleb leaks scleral melting (Fig. 14.4) and late endophthalmitis [15, 20]. Furthermore, a commonly voiced concern about trabeculectomy surgery is the risk of late postoperative cataract development. The Collaborative Normal Tension Glaucoma Study showed that cataract developed in 26% of the treatment group (of which 16% occurred in operated eyes) compared with 11% of the non-treated group [3]. A 78% increased risk of developing a cataract was reported by the investigators of the AGIS, the risk being not surprisingly higher in case of postoperative complications [23]. The development of a clinically relevant cataract is not irrelevant to the ultimate success rate of a filtration procedure. In fact, a planned cataract extraction in a previously filtered eye may be paralleled by malfunction of the filtration bleb [7].

As far as an uneventful NPDS is concerned, the avoidance of ocular entry obviates the need for an iridectomy and theoretically limits early postoperative hypotony. This in turn minimizes the attendant sequelae of hyphaema, choroidal effusions, shallow anterior chambers, and cataract [4, 14]. However, as pointed out correctly by Tan and Hitchings [21] "…concern has repeatedly been expressed about the steep learning curve associated with this type of surgery." In fact, one report found that inadvertent perforation of the trabecular meshwork occurred in approximately one third of initial cases [2]. Should an inadvertent perforation occur during

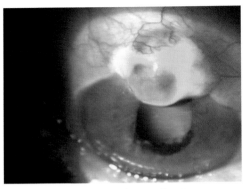

Fig. 14.4. An eye 7 years after a trabeculectomy supplemented with intraoperative application of 0.4 mg/ml Mitomycin, 3 min. A localized melting of the sclera over the sclerostomy site has occurred, leading to a prolapse of the iris-ciliary body. A thin layer of conjunctiva-scarred tissue is visible over the prolapsed uveal tissue

surgery, the unavoidable conversion to a penetrating filtering procedure will result in suboptimal flap construction, leading to overdrainage. Following such conversion, the incidence of postoperative hypotony is reported to be 90 %, while hyphaema is 68 % [17]. As far as cataract formation is concerned, proper monitoring of lens transparency, via a slit-lamp evaluation according to the LOCS II grading system, confirmed the postulated low incidence of newly onset nuclear cataracts [5]. However, no data are as yet available to evaluate the impact of deep sclerectomy (compared with trabeculectomy) in eyes with already significant lens opacity. In a case series, Karlen et al. showed a 7 % progression rate of pre-existing cataract in a 36-month follow-up in eyes operated with a NPDS [9]. In another case series, the same group reports a 21 % progression rate in 5 years of a pre-existing cataract upon NPDS [19]. Finally, it is worth recalling that non-penetrating procedures have been associated with some "new" late complications such as: (a) detachment of the Descemet membrane [10], and (b) iris incarceration on YAG-laser goniopuncture [16]. Both complications seem manageable, but they might require further surgery in the affected eye.

Summary for the Clinician

- Complications of trabeculectomy (supplemented with antimetabolites) are still not negligible, can be managed successfully in most cases but: (a) may occur late in the course of the disease, and (b) can have a detrimental impact on the patients' visual function
- Non-penetrating surgery seems safer both in the short and the long term
- However, the surgeons must be aware of some types of complications with which a planned trabeculectomy can be associated

14.2.3
Affordability

There is a growing requirement for the health benefits of new interventions to be verified in randomized control trials in order that their costs may be justified. Non-penetrating surgery: (a) is more time-consuming than the conventional trabeculectomy, (b) the learning curve is longer, (c) may require the intraoperative application of devices to keep the intrascleral lake patent [18], (d) surgeons must consider the need for postoperative YAG-laser goniopuncture, and (e) application of antimetabolites may nevertheless be required. Conversely, uneventful non-penetrating surgery: (a) can be routinely performed on an outpatient basis, (b) is likely to be followed by less requirement for cataract surgery, (c) is likely to be associated with a lower incidence of surgery-related blindness in high-risk glaucomatous eyes.

Summary for the Clinician

- In summary, the cost-efficacy profile of NPDS requires the completion of appropriate long-term clinical trials to be accurately traced

14.3
Conclusions

The ultimate outcome of any glaucoma treatment has so far been "to spare vision by decreasing the IOP." Trabeculectomy, in spite of alone being an effective means to achieve low target IOPs, ends in a high rate of lens opacification. A cataract extraction in a previously filtered eye often leads to an eventual failure of the filtration bleb and can be affected by a higher rate of complications. Again, a penetrating procedure is affected by a high rate of vision-threatening complications in selected phenotypes, high myopia included. Deep sclerectomy, if followed by a timely YAG-laser goniopuncture, can achieve a success rate comparable to a planned trabeculectomy. This is by no means unexpected, since NPDS becomes a penetrating procedure thereafter. However, once NPDS becomes penetrating, the efficacy improves but the traditional trabeculectomy-like complication rate does not seem to increase. Conversely, viscocanalostomy seems to offer a slightly better efficacy profile than pure non-penetrating procedures. No data are so far available to verify whether a YAG-laser goniopuncture can ameliorate the long-term success rate of viscocanalostomy. According to the available controlled clinical evidence, non-penetrating viscocanalostomy does not seem to offer the required efficacy profile in the majority of those glaucomatous eyes who are candidates for surgery. However, most of the available randomized trials have been performed on Caucasians affected by primary open angle glaucoma. These eyes are the best candidates for a planned filtering surgery. We do not know how non-penetrating surgery compares with trabeculectomy in eyes with a poor prognosis (i.e., uveitic glaucoma, black race, etc.). Prospective clinical trials, performed on patients who are at high risk for failure after a planned trabeculectomy, are then needed to establish an ultimate role for pure non-penetrating (and "non-filtering") surgeries in the overall management of glaucoma.

References

1. Carassa R, Bettin P (2003) Viscocanalostomy vs trabeculectomy. A two-year clinical trial. Ophthalmology 110:882–887
2. Chiou AG, Mermoud A, Jewelewicz DA (1998) Post-operative inflammation following deep sclerectomy with collagen implant versus standard trabeculectomy. Graefes Arch Clin Exp Ophthalmol 236:593–596
3. Collaborative Normal-Tension Glaucoma Study Group (1998) Comparison of glaucomatous progression between untreated patients with normal-tension glaucoma and patients with therapeutically reduced intraocular pressures. Am J Ophthalmol 126:487–497
4. El Sayyad F, Helal M, El-Kholify H, Khalil M, El-Maghraby A (2000) Nonpenetrating deep sclerectomy versus trabeculectomy in bilateral primary open-angle glaucoma. Ophthalmology 107: 1671–1674
5. Gandolfi SA and Cimino L (2000) Deep sclerectomy without absorbable implants and with unsutured scleral flap: prospective, randomised 2-year clinical trial vs. trabeculectomy with releasable sutures. Inv Ophthalmol Vis Sci (ARVO Suppl), S83
6. Hamel M, Shaarawy T, Mermoud A (2001) Deep sclerectomy with collagen implant in patients with glaucoma and high myopia. J Cataract Refract Surg 27:1410–1417
7. Haynes WL, Alward WM (1999) Control of intraocular pressure after trabeculectomy. Surv Ophthalmol 43:345–355
8. Johnson DH, Johnson M (2002) Glaucoma surgery and aqueous outflow: how does nonpenetrating glaucoma surgery work. Arch Ophthalmol 120:67–70
9. Karlen ME, Sanchez E, Schnyder CC, Sickenberg M, Mermoud A (1999) Deep sclerectomy with collagen implant: medium term results. Br J Ophthalmol 83:6–11
10. Kim CY, Hong YJ, Seong GJ, Koh HJ, Kim SS (2002) Iris synechia after laser goniopuncture in a patient having deep sclerectomy with a collagen implant. J Cataract Refract Surg 28:900–902
11. Kozobolis VP, Christodoulakis EV, Tzanakis N, Zacharopoulos I, Pallikaris IG (2002) Primary deep sclerectomy versus primary deep sclerectomy with the use of mitomycin C in primary open-angle glaucoma. J Glaucoma 11:287–293
12. Lichter PR, Musch DC, Gillespie BW, Guire KE, Janz NK, Wren PA, Mills RP (2001) Interim clinical outcomes in the Collaborative Initial Glaucoma Treatment Study comparing initial treatment randomized to medications or surgery. Ophthalmology 108:1943–1953

13. Marchini G, Marraffa M, Brunelli C, Morbio R, Bonomi L (2001) Ultrasound biomicroscopy and intraocular-pressure-lowering mechanisms of deep sclerectomy with reticulated hyaluronic acid implant. J Cataract Refract Surg 27:507–517

14. Mermoud A, Schnyder CC, Sickenberg M, Chiou AG, Hédiguer SE, Faggioni R (1999) Comparison of deep sclerectomy with collagen implant and trabeculectomy in open-angle glaucoma. J Cataract Refract Surg 25:323–331

15. Nuyts RM, Greve EL, Geijssen HC, Langerhorst CT (1994) Treatment of hypotonous maculopathy after trabeculectomy with mitomycin C. Am J Ophthalmol 118:322–331

16. Ravinet E, Tritten JJ, Roy S, Gianoli F, Wolfensberger T, Schnyder C, Mermoud A (2002) Descemet membrane detachment after nonpenetrating filtering surgery. J Glaucoma 11:244–252

17. Sanchez E, Schnyder CC, Mermoud A (1997) Comparative results of deep sclerectomy transformed to trabeculectomy and classical trabeculectomy. Klin Monatsbl Augenheilkd 210:261–264

18. Sanchez E, Schnyder CC, Sickenberg M, et al. (1997) Deep sclerectomy: results with and without collagen implant. Int Ophthalmol 20:157–162

19. Shaarawy T, Karlen M, Schnyder C, Achache F, Sanchez E, Mermoud A (2001) Five-year results of deep sclerectomy with collagen implant. J Cataract Refract Surg 27:1770–1778

20. Stamper RL, McMenemy MG, Lieberman MF (1992) Hypotonous maculopathy after trabeculectomy with subconjunctival 5-fluorouracil. Am J Ophthalmol 114:544–553

21. Tan JC, Hitchings RA (2001) Non-penetrating glaucoma surgery: the state of play. Br J Ophthalmol 85:234–237

22. The AGIS Investigators (2000) The advanced glaucoma intervention study, 6: effect of cataract on visual field and visual acuity. Arch Ophthalmol 118:1639–1652

23. The AGIS Investigators (2001) The Advanced Glaucoma Intervention Study, 8: risk of cataract formation after trabeculectomy. Arch Ophthalmol 119:1771–1780

24. The Fluorouracil Filtering Surgery Study Group (1996) Five-year follow-up of the Fluorouracil Filtering Surgery Study. Am J Ophthalmol 121:349–366

Subject Index

Printing: Mercedes-Druck, Berlin
Binding: Stein+Lehmann, Berlin